Respiratory Disease

Principles of Patient Care

Respiratory Disease

Principles of Patient Care

Robert L. Wilkins, MA, RRT
Associate Professor
Program Director,
Associate in Science Degree Program
Department of Respiratory Therapy
School of Allied Health Professions
Loma Linda University
Loma Linda, California

James R. Dexter, MD, FACP, FCCP
Associate Clinical Professor
School of Medicine
Loma Linda University
Loma Linda, California
and
Medical Director
Department of Respiratory Care
Redlands Community Hospital
Redlands, California

 F. A. DAVIS COMPANY • Philadelphia

F. A. Davis Company
1915 Arch Street
Philadelphia, PA 19103

Printed in the United States of America

Last digit indicates print number: 10 9 8 7 6 5 4 3 2 1

Allied Health Editor: Lynn Borders Caldwell
Production Editor: Gail Shapiro
Designer: Donald B. Freggens, Jr.
Cover Design by: Donald B. Freggens, Jr.

As new scientific information becomes available through basic and clinical research, recommended treatments and drug therapies undergo changes. The author(s) and publisher have done everything possible to make this book accurate, up to date, and in accord with accepted standards at the time of publication. The authors, editors, and publisher are not responsible for errors or omissions or for consequences from application of the book, and make no warranty, expressed or implied, in regard to the contents of the book. Any practice described in this book should be applied by the reader in accordance with professional standards of care used in regard to the unique circumstances that may apply in each situation. The reader is advised always to check product information (package inserts) for changes and new information regarding dose and contraindications before administering any drug. Caution is especially urged when using new or infrequently ordered drugs.

Library of Congress Cataloging-in-Publication Data

Respiratory disease : principles of patient care / [edited by] Robert
  L. Wilkins, James R. Dexter.
       p. cm.
    Includes bibliographical references.
    ISBN 0-8036-9326-5 :
    1. Respiratory organs — Diseases.   I. Wilkins, Robert L.
  II. Dexter, James R., 1948–
       [DNLM: 1. Respiration Disorders — physiopathology — case studies.
  2. Respiration Disorders — physiopathology — problems.   3. Respiration
  Disorders — therapy — case studies.   4. Respiration Disorders —
  therapy — problems.   WF 18 R434]
  RC731.R466   1993
  616.2 — dc20
  DNLM/DLC
  for Library of Congress   92-48263
                                                                        CIP

This book is dedicated to our wives,
Kris and Kathy,
and our children,
Tyler, Nicholas, Kimberly,
and Scott.

Foreword

The treatment of respiratory disease requires a breadth and depth of knowledge that challenges even the most dedicated respiratory therapist. Analyses of respiratory disturbances require an understanding of the etiology, pathophysiology, and clinical signs of the disease, thus leading to a plan for treatment, establishment of therapeutic goals, and a schedule for ongoing assessment. Today, microprocessor controlled ventilators, because they have so many possible modes of operation, demand an even greater understanding of the underlying causes of respiratory failure.

Many respiratory care books focus on equipment, respiratory therapy or pathophysiology, but unlike *Respiratory Disease: Principles of Patient Care,* few organize this information by specific medical and surgical problems. Wilkins and Dexter have assembled a text written specifically for respiratory therapists that addresses the most crucial aspects of twenty-two commonly encountered respiratory diseases.

Once you review this text, I'm sure you'll agree that a great deal of thought went into what to include, or perhaps more importantly, what *not* to include. The writing style is clear without being boring; the material in each chapter is comprehensive with just the right depth of coverage; and the medical terminology is appropriate for health professionals with treatment and assessment responsibilities.

Educators will better prepare their students if this book is assigned as required reading since it will help them understand a lecture on the pathophysiology of a particular respiratory disease and prompt thought about assessment and a therapeutic plan. Having this understanding will help new therapists begin their practice at a high level. The text should be used during the student's second clinical rotation and before studying advanced critical care topics. Individual chapters should be assigned prior to lectures on each disease entity with lectures focusing on the pathophysiology and etiology of the disease as found in the book. Discussion of each chapter's case study(ies) will enhance class time and reinforce the concepts presented in each chapter, especially since questions accompanying each case will trigger a discussion of the treatment plan and the assessment of therapeutic goals.

In addition to being of great value to students, this book is also a good reference for the beginning therapist. Its format summarizes pertinent information and makes it easy to locate quickly.

Candidates for the National Board for Respiratory Care registry written and clinical simulation examinations will find this to be an excellent review text. It covers important information about each disease and offers case studies so that readers can verify their knowledge of clinical application.

Loma Linda University has a reputation for having an excellent respiratory therapy program, and the Medical Center Respiratory Care Department has been a role model for others. Students enrolled at Loma Linda University have been fortunate to benefit from this great resource. Now, with this text, Loma Linda educators have made it possible for *all* students to benefit from their experience in treating respiratory disease.

I plan to make this a required text for a course I teach called "Respiratory Care for Medical and Surgical Patients."

Thomas A. Barnes, EdD, RRT
Associate Professor of Cardiopulmonary Sciences
Northeastern University
Boston, Massachusetts

Preface

This text is written to help the reader understand the assessment and treatment of patients with respiratory disease. In the clinical setting, caregivers need insight to ask the right questions, to look for the important physical findings and laboratory data, and to be able to integrate this information into an accurate assessment that leads to appropriate therapy. This text provides the reader with that insight into respiratory care that conventional textbooks do not describe. This is done through the use of case studies that illustrate key concepts.

The goals of this text are to describe (1) the pathophysiology related to the signs and symptoms of pulmonary disorders; (2) the appropriate information to gather in the assessment of the various pulmonary diseases; and (3) the appropriate treatment of each disorder. Twenty-three chapters review specific adult, pediatric, and neonatal respiratory diseases. Each chapter begins with an overview of background information related to the topic. This is followed by presentation of one or more illustrative case studies. Pertinent questions and answers are strategically presented at appropriate places throughout each case study to reinforce key points. It is not necessary to read the chapters in the order in which they are presented, although it may be helpful first to read Chapter 1 on acute respiratory failure.

The text is written for respiratory care, nursing, and medical students, as well as for clinicians who want to improve their pulmonary management skills. Because we have emphasized assessment (information gathering) and treatment (decision making) of respiratory care patients, the text should be especially useful to the student preparing for clinical simulation examinations offered by the National Board of Respiratory Care.

Background courses in pulmonary anatomy and physiology, diagnostic techniques, cardiopulmonary pharmacology, and medical terminology are essential if the reader is to understand the case reports presented in this text.

We have provided a glossary of the terms and abbreviations at the end of the text. In addition, tables that list normal values for clinical laboratory tests, pulmonary function tests, arterial blood gases, and hemodynamic monitoring data are provided in the appendix to help the reader interpret data and answer questions presented in the case studies.

RLW and JRD

Acknowledgments

We would like to acknowledge the reviewers of this text, who carefully reviewed the manuscript and provided many useful suggestions for improvement:

Thomas A. Barnes, EdD, RRT
Associate Professor of Cardiopulmonary Sciences
College of Pharmacy and Allied Health Professions
Northeastern University
Boston, Massachusetts

Dean Hess, MEd, RRT
Assistant Director
Department of Research
York Hospital
York, Pennsylvania

Allen Marangoni, MMSc, RRT
Program Director
Department of Respiratory Therapy
Wheeling Jesuit College
Wheeling, West Virginia

Anna W. Parkman, MBA, RRT
Associate Professor and Program Director
Department of Respiratory Therapy
University of Charleston
Charleston, West Virginia

Yvonne Jo Robbins, MEd, RRT
Program Director
Department of Respiratory Therapy
Bryn Mawr Hospital/West Chester University
Bryn Mawr, Pennsylvania

Although they did not review the entire manuscript, the following two people helped us shape the book in its early stages:

John H. Riggs, BA, RRT
Manager of Specialty Services
Western Wake Medical Center
Cary, North Carolina

Lee J. Robinson, MEd, RRT
Department of Respiratory Therapy
Springfield Tech Community College
Springfield, Massachusetts

We thank Rick Murray, MD, and Douglas Deming, MD, for their review of the neonatal chapters. We also thank medical illustrator Nathan Lindsey for the art work in this text.

Contributors

Gregory A.B. Cheek, MD, MSPH
Clinical Instructor
Department of Internal Medicine
Pulmonary/Critical Care Fellow
Loma Linda University
Loma Linda, California

George H. Hicks, MS, RRT
Instructor of Respiratory Care and Anatomy and
Physiology
Allied Health Division
Mt. Hood Community College
Gresham, Oregon

Patrice A. Johnson, BS, RRT
Instructor
Department of Respiratory Therapy
School of Allied Health Professions
Loma Linda University
Loma Linda, California

Cynthia Malinowski, MA, RRT
Assistant Professor
Department of Respiratory Therapy
School of Allied Health Professions
Loma Linda University
Loma Linda, California

Thomas P. Malinowski, BS, RRT
Assistant Director
Respiratory Care Services
Loma Linda University Medical Center
Loma Linda, California

Kenneth D. McCarty, MS, RRT
Assistant Professor
Director of Clinical Education
Department of Respiratory Therapy
School of Allied Health Professions
Loma Linda University
Loma Linda, California

Victoria C. Sciacqua, BS, RRT
Clinical Instructor
Department of Respiratory Therapy
School of Allied Health Professions
Loma Linda University
Loma Linda, California

N. Lennard Specht, MD
Assistant Professor of Medicine
School of Medicine
Medical Director,
Department of Respiratory Therapy
School of Allied Health Professions
Loma Linda University
Loma Linda, California

David M. Stanton, MS, CPFT, RCP, RRT
Assistant Professor
Department of Respiratory Therapy
School of Allied Health Professions
Loma Linda University
Loma Linda, California

Hoai Tran, RCP, CRTT
Staff Therapist
Loma Linda Community Hospital
Loma Linda, California

Contents

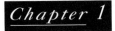

Robert L. Wilkins, MA, RRT
James R. Dexter, MD, FCCP

INTRODUCTION to RESPIRATORY FAILURE 1

INTRODUCTION 1
ETIOLOGY 2
PATHOPHYSIOLOGY 4
CLINICAL FEATURES 5
TREATMENT 6
CASE STUDY 9
REFERENCES 13

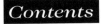

Robert L. Wilkins, MA, RRT
James R. Dexter, MD, FCCP

ASTHMA 15

INTRODUCTION 15
ETIOLOGY 15
PATHOPHYSIOLOGY 16
CLINICAL FEATURES 16
TREATMENT 18
CASE STUDY 20
REFERENCES 26

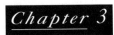

Robert L. Wilkins, MA, RRT
James R. Dexter, MD, FCCP

CHRONIC BRONCHITIS 29

INTRODUCTION 29
ETIOLOGY 29
PATHOLOGY AND PATHOPHYSIOLOGY 30
CLINICAL FEATURES 31
TREATMENT 32
CASE STUDY 33
REFERENCES 42

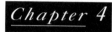

Chapter 4

Kenneth D. McCarty, MS, RRT

EMPHYSEMA 45

INTRODUCTION 45
ETIOLOGY 45
PATHOPHYSIOLOGY 46
CLINICAL FEATURES 46
TREATMENT 47
CASE STUDY 49
REFERENCES 57

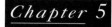

Chapter 5

N. Lennard Specht, MD

CYSTIC FIBROSIS 59

INTRODUCTION 59
ETIOLOGY 59
PATHOLOGY AND PATHOPHYSIOLOGY 60
CLINICAL FEATURES 61
TREATMENT 65
PROGNOSIS 67
CASE STUDY 67
REFERENCES 74

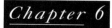

Chapter 6

Robert L. Wilkins, MA, RRT
James R. Dexter, MD, FCCP

**HEMODYNAMIC MONITORING and
SHOCK** 77

INTRODUCTION 77
WHAT IS CARDIAC OUTPUT? 78
WHAT DETERMINES CARDIAC OUTPUT? 78
ETIOLOGY 82
PATHOPHYSIOLOGY 82
CLINICAL FEATURES 83
TREATMENT 85
CASE STUDY 86
REFERENCES 91

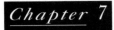

Chapter 7

Kenneth D. McCarty, MS, RRT

PULMONARY THROMBOEMBOLIC DISEASE 93

INTRODUCTION 93
ETIOLOGY AND PATHOLOGY 93
PATHOPHYSIOLOGY 93
CLINICAL FEATURES 94
TREATMENT 97
CASE STUDY 98
REFERENCES 105

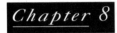

Chapter 8

George H. Hicks, MS, RRT

HEART FAILURE 107

INTRODUCTION 107
ETIOLOGY 107
PATHOPHYSIOLOGY 109
CLINICAL FEATURES 113
TREATMENT 115
CASE STUDY 118
REFERENCES 126

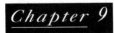

Chapter 9

George H. Hicks, MS, RRT

SMOKE INHALATION and BURNS 129

INTRODUCTION 129
ETIOLOGY 130
PATHOPHYSIOLOGY 131
CLINICAL FEATURES 135
TREATMENT 137
CASE STUDY 139
REFERENCES 148

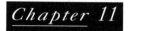

David M. Stanton, MS, RRT

NEAR DROWNING 151

INTRODUCTION 151
PATHOLOGY AND PATHOPHYSIOLOGY 152
CLINICAL FEATURES 154
INITIAL ASSESSMENT AND PROGNOSIS 155
TREATMENT 157
CASE STUDY NO. 1 159
CASE STUDY NO. 2 162
REFERENCES 170

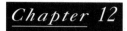

Kenneth D. McCarty, MS, RRT

ADULT RESPIRATORY DISTRESS SYNDROME 173

INTRODUCTION 173
ETIOLOGY 173
PATHOLOGY 174
PATHOPHYSIOLOGY 174
CLINICAL FEATURES 175
TREATMENT 176
CASE STUDY 179
REFERENCES 187

Chapter 12

George H. Hicks, MS, RRT

CHEST TRAUMA 191

INTRODUCTION 191
ETIOLOGY 192
INJURY PATHOPHYSIOLOGY 193
CLINICAL FEATURES 199
TREATMENT 200
CASE STUDY 202
REFERENCES 213

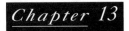
Chapter 13

Thomas P. Malinowski, BS, RRT

POSTOPERATIVE ATELECTASIS 217

INTRODUCTION 217
ETIOLOGY 217
PATHOPHYSIOLOGY 219
CLINICAL FEATURES 219
TREATMENT 220
CASE STUDY 221
REFERENCES 227

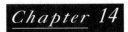
Chapter 14

N. Lennard Specht, MD

INTERSTITIAL LUNG DISEASE 229

INTRODUCTION 229
ETIOLOGY 229
PATHOLOGY AND PATHOPHYSIOLOGY 232
CLINICAL FEATURES 232
TREATMENT 237
PROGNOSIS 238
CASE STUDY 238
REFERENCES 247

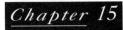
Chapter 15

N. Lennard Specht, MD
Robert L. Wilkins, MA, RRT

NEUROMUSCULAR DISORDERS 249

INTRODUCTION 249
RESPIRATORY CENTERS 249
CHEMORECEPTORS 250
NERVE TRANSMISSION 250
NEUROMUSCULAR JUNCTION 250
RESPIRATORY MUSCLES 250
PATHOLOGY AND PATHOPHYSIOLOGY 252
CLINICAL FEATURES 254
TREATMENT 256
CASE STUDY NO. 1 257
CASE STUDY NO. 2 262
REFERENCES 267

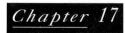

Chapter 16

Robert L. Wilkins, MA, RRT
James R. Dexter, MD, FCCP

BACTERIAL PNEUMONIA 269

INTRODUCTION 269
ETIOLOGY 269
PATHOLOGY AND PATHOPHYSIOLOGY 270
CLINICAL FEATURES 271
TREATMENT 274
CASE STUDY 275
REFERENCES 282

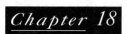

Chapter 17

Gregory A.B. Cheek, MD, MSPH

LUNG CANCER 285

INTRODUCTION 285
ETIOLOGY 285
PATHOLOGY 286
CLINICAL FEATURES 287
METASTATIC DISEASE 288
DIAGNOSIS 289
STAGING 293
TREATMENT AND PROGNOSIS 295
CASE STUDY 297
REFERENCES 306

Chapter 18

Robert L. Wilkins, MA, RRT
James R. Dexter, MD, FCCP

SLEEP APNEA 309

INTRODUCTION 309
SLEEP AND BREATHING 310
ETIOLOGY 312
PATHOPHYSIOLOGY 313
CLINICAL FEATURES 313
TREATMENT 315
CASE STUDY 316
REFERENCES 322

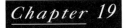

Robert L. Wilkins, MA, RRT
James R. Dexter, MD, FCCP

CROUP and EPIGLOTTITIS

CROUP and EPIGLOTTITIS 325

INTRODUCTION 325
CROUP 325
EPIGLOTTITIS 327
CASE STUDY NO. 1 329
CASE STUDY NO. 2 333
REFERENCES 337

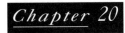

Victoria C. Sciacqua, BS, RRT

RESPIRATORY SYNCYTIAL VIRUS

RESPIRATORY SYNCYTIAL VIRUS 339

INTRODUCTION 339
ETIOLOGY 339
PATHOLOGY AND PATHOPHYSIOLOGY 340
CLINICAL FEATURES 340
TREATMENT 342
CASE STUDY 344
REFERENCES 350

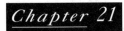

Patrice A. Johnson, BS, RRT
Cynthia Malinowski, MA, RRT

RESPIRATORY DISTRESS SYNDROME in the NEWBORN

**RESPIRATORY DISTRESS SYNDROME in
the NEWBORN** 353

INTRODUCTION 353
ETIOLOGY 353
PATHOPHYSIOLOGY 354
MATERNAL HISTORY 355
CLINICAL FEATURES 355
TREATMENT 355
CASE STUDY 356
REFERENCES 362

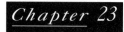

Chapter 22

Cynthia Malinowski, MA, RRT

BRONCHOPULMONARY DYSPLASIA 365

INTRODUCTION 365
ETIOLOGY 365
PATHOPHYSIOLOGY 366
CLINICAL FEATURES 367
TREATMENT 368
OUTCOME 369
CASE STUDY 369
REFERENCES 376

Chapter 23

Cynthia Malinowski, MA, RRT

PERSISTENT PULMONARY
HYPERTENSION of the NEWBORN 379

INTRODUCTION 379
ETIOLOGY 379
PATHOPHYSIOLOGY 380
CLINICAL FEATURES 381
DIAGNOSIS 381
TREATMENT 383
CASE STUDY 383
REFERENCES 391

GLOSSARY 393

APPENDIX 401

NORMAL LABORATORY VALUES   Hoai N. Tran, RCP, CRTT   401

INDEX 405

In addition to giving you a working knowledge of the most commonly encountered respiratory diseases, this text has been specifically designed to help improve your clinical reasoning skills. Each chapter begins with background information about a certain disease, then a detailed case study is presented. The case study will help bring the information to life and give you the opportunity to test your knowledge.

To use this text most effectively, we recommend that you approach each chapter in the following manner:

- Study the background information at the beginning of each chapter. This information about etiology, pathophysiology, clinical features, and treatment will be very helpful to you as you review the related case study.

- If, during the study of any chapter, you see a term or abbreviation with which you are unfamiliar, take a moment to look it up in the glossary provided at the back of the book.

- Key questions appear throughout each case study; the questions are there to make you think about important issues related to the case. After reading each question, take a moment to write your answer either in the space provided in the text or on a separate sheet of paper. If you need to review normal values to interpret data presented in the cases, refer to the tables of normal values for clinical laboratory tests, pulmonary function tests, arterial blood gases, and hemodynamic monitoring values in the Appendix.

- Compare your answer with the one we provide.

We hope you enjoy reading each chapter with its accompanying case study and find the information helpful to your understanding and treatment of respiratory diseases.

Robert L. Wilkins
James R. Dexter

Chapter 1

Robert L. Wilkins, MA, RRT
James R. Dexter, MD, FCCP

INTRODUCTION to RESPIRATORY FAILURE

INTRODUCTION

The production of energy in the body, which is necessary to maintain life, requires a constant supply of oxygen and nutrients to the tissues. Breathing provides a steady intake of oxygen to the lungs, where the oxygen diffuses through the alveolar capillary membrane into the blood (external respiration). The circulatory system distributes the oxygenated blood to the various vascular beds, where oxygen is given to the tissues (internal respiration). In addition to providing oxygenation of the blood, the lungs also serve to rid the body of carbon dioxide (CO_2), a waste product of metabolism. CO_2, which is brought to the lungs by the venous blood, diffuses into the alveoli and is subsequently exhaled into the atmosphere. This chapter is an introduction to the various medical problems that can lead to inadequate gas exchange. Subsequent chapters provide specific examples of diseases that affect the heart and lungs in adults, children, and neonates.

Respiratory failure is failure of the lungs to provide adequate oxygenation or ventilation for the blood.[1,2] **Oxygenation failure** more specifically refers to a partial pressure of oxygen in the arterial blood (Pao_2) of less than 60 mm Hg, in spite of an increase in the concentration or fraction of oxygen in the inspired gas (Fio_2) to 0.50 or higher. **Ventilatory failure** is inadequate ventilation between the lungs and atmosphere, resulting in an inappropriate elevation of the partial pressure of CO_2 in the arterial blood ($Paco_2$) to a level greater than 45 mm Hg.

Respiratory failure may also be used more generally to describe failure of either external or internal respiration. For example, if the circulatory system fails to move the blood at a sufficient rate to meet metabolic demands, the transport of oxygen is inadequate and the tissues may suffer from hypoxia (see Chapters 6 and 8). Although this example more accurately describes circulatory failure, it does represent a breakdown in the system needed for respiration.

The amount of oxygen consumed and CO_2 produced each minute is dictated by the metabolic rate of the patient. Exercise and fever are examples of factors that increase the metabolic rate and place more demands on the cardiopulmonary system. When the cardiopulmonary reserve is limited by disease, fever may represent an added stress that precipitates respiratory failure and tissue hypoxia.

This chapter provides an overview of the concepts important for managing respiratory failure and applies the concepts to a specific case of drug overdose.

1

Drug overdose can often cause neuromuscular deficiency leading to ventilatory failure. This chapter provides specific information about drug overdose in addition to information about respiratory failure.

ETIOLOGY

Oxygenation Failure

Hypoxemia is present when the arterial Po_2 is below the predicted normal for the patient. Hypoxemia is classified as mild (Pao_2 equals 60 to 79 mm Hg), moderate (Pao_2 equals 40 to 59 mm Hg), or severe (Pao_2 less than 40 mm Hg).[3] These classifications are based on predicted normal values for a patient under age 60 breathing room air. For older patients, the practitioner should subtract from the limits of mild and moderate hypoxemia 1 mm Hg for each year of the patient's age over 60 years. A Pao_2 less than 40 mm Hg represents severe hypoxemia at any age.

Hypoxemia has potentially serious consequences, as it may lead to inadequate tissue oxygenation (hypoxia). When hypoxemia is present, tissue oxygenation may be preserved by an increase in cardiac output. Patients with severe hypoxemia or marginal cardiac function may not be able to compensate adequately for the hypoxemia and may develop tissue hypoxia.

The most common cause of hypoxemia is ventilation to perfusion ($\dot{V}/\dot{Q}$) mismatching. $\dot{V}/\dot{Q}$ mismatching occurs when some regions of the lung are poorly ventilated but remain perfused by pulmonary blood (low $\dot{V}/\dot{Q}$) (Fig. 1–1). Although regional vasoconstriction typically occurs in the pulmonary capillaries of the affected region, blood flow is not entirely stopped. As a result, some blood leaves the lungs without receiving adequate oxygenation and lowers the Po_2 of arterial blood. $\dot{V}/\dot{Q}$ mismatching also occurs when perfusion of a portion of the lung is reduced or absent despite adequate ventilation of the affected region (high $\dot{V}/\dot{Q}$).

Shunt, another cause of hypoxemia, refers to blood moving from the right side of the heart to the left side without coming into contact with ventilated alveoli. One cause of shunt is congenital heart defects (anatomic shunt) that allows the venous blood to bypass the pulmonary circulation through abnormal channels (e.g., ventricular septal defect). The most common cause of shunt, however, is pulmonary disease that results in collapsed or unventilated alveoli (physiologic shunt).[4] In this situation, blood flow through the affected lung regions does not participate in gas exchange and may result in severe hypoxemia (Pao_2 less than 40 mm Hg) that does not respond well to oxygen therapy (see Fig. 1–1).

Hypoxemia can occur when an individual inhales a gas mixture that does not

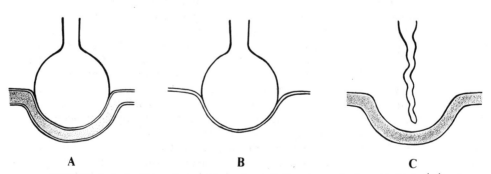

FIGURE 1–1 A, Normal matching of ventilation to perfusion; B, high $\dot{V}/\dot{Q}$ where ventilation is in excess of perfusion; and C, low $\dot{V}/\dot{Q}$ where perfusion is in excess of ventilation (shunt).

contain an adequate partial pressure of oxygen. Breathing gas that lacks adequate oxygen results in an alveolar P_{O_2} below normal and arterial hypoxemia. This situation can occur at high altitude, during fires in an enclosed structure, and with equipment failure while the patient is attached to a ventilator circuit.

Hypoventilation increases the alveolar P_{CO_2} (P_{ACO_2}) and decreases alveolar P_{O_2} (P_{AO_2}). If the patient is breathing room air, hypoventilation may result in hypoxemia. Hypoxemia is less likely if the hypoventilating patient is breathing an elevated F_{IO_2}. Causes of hypoventilation are described subsequently.

Ventilatory Failure

The ability to inhale requires a healthy neurologic system that stimulates the respiratory muscles. Contraction of the diaphragm decreases the intrathoracic pressure and causes gas to flow into the lungs. Minimal effort is required if the chest cage is intact, the airways are patent, and the lungs are compliant. The ability to exhale requires patent airways and lung parenchyma that has sufficient elastic recoil to hold the bronchioles open until exhalation is complete.

Causes of ventilatory failure include depression of the respiratory center by drugs, diseases of the brain, spinal cord abnormalities, muscular diseases (see Chapter 15), thoracic cage abnormalities (see Chapter 12), and upper and lower airway obstruction (Table 1–1). Upper airway obstruction may occur with acute infection (see Chapter 19) and during sleep when muscle tone is reduced (see Chapter 18).

Table 1–1 Causes of Ventilatory and Respiratory Failure

Ventilatory Failure
Dysfunction of the central nervous system
    Drug overdose
    Head trauma
    Infection
    Hemorrhage
    Sleep-related apnea
Neuromuscular dysfunction
    Myasthenia gravis
    Guillain-Barré syndrome
    Poliomyelitis
    Amyotrophic lateral sclerosis
    Spinal cord trauma
    Long-term use of aminoglycosides
Musculoskeletal dysfunction
    Chest trauma (flail chest)
    Kyphoscoliosis
    Malnutrition
Pulmonary dysfunction
    Emphysema
    Chronic bronchitis
    Asthma
    Cystic fibrosis

Respiratory Failure
    Pneumonia
    ARDS
    Congestive heart failure
    Obstructive lung diseases (e.g., asthma, bronchitis)
    Pulmonary embolism
    Restrictive lung disease (e.g., pulmonary fibrosis, kyphoscoliosis)

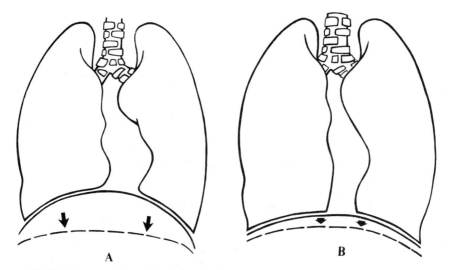

FIGURE 1–2 A, Normal position of the diaphragm at end exhalation and end inhalation *(dotted line)*. B, Abnormal position of the diaphragm demonstrating the mechanical disadvantage associated with pulmonary hyperinflation.

A number of factors may contribute to weakness of the inspiratory muscles and may tip the balance in favor of acute ventilatory failure. Malnutrition and electrolyte disturbances can weaken the ventilatory muscles, and pulmonary hyperinflation (e.g., emphysema) can make the diaphragm less efficient. Lung hyperinflation causes the diaphragm to assume an abnormally low position that results in a mechanical disadvantage (Fig. 1–2). These problems are common in patients with acute and chronic obstructive lung disease (e.g., asthma, chronic bronchitis, and emphysema; see Chapters 2 through 4).

PATHOPHYSIOLOGY

Oxygenation Failure

The severity of the hypoxemia and the patient's preexisting condition will determine the response to hypoxemia. A previously healthy patient will be unaffected by mild hypoxemia. A patient with severe cardiopulmonary disease, however, is likely to be in grave danger.

Patients usually respond to hypoxemia by increasing the rate of breathing (tachypnea). Tachypnea increases minute ventilation, decreases P_{ACO_2}, and to some extent increases P_{AO_2}. Since anatomic dead space (parts of the lung ventilated but not perfused) is fixed, the work of breathing increases. If the patient's respiratory system is not healthy (e.g., airways are obstructed), tachypnea may represent a serious increase in the work of breathing.

Alveolar hypoxia stimulates the pulmonary capillaries to constrict in the affected regions.[5] The pulmonary vasoconstriction will be widespread if the disease causing hypoxemia is prevalent throughout the lungs. Pulmonary vascular resistance (PVR) will be markedly increased when widespread pulmonary vasoconstriction is present. This increases right heart workload and, if it continues for many months, may result in right heart failure. Right heart failure is characterized by increased pressure and dilatation of the right heart (as the heart pumps against the constricted capillaries). The combination of lung disease and right heart failure is known as **cor pulmonale.**

Cardiac rate and strength of contraction increase in an effort to compensate for hypoxemia. If coronary artery disease is present, the increased cardiac workload may lead to ischemia and irreversible damage (infarction).

The brain may be affected by hypoxemia if the hypoxemia is severe or if the heart cannot increase cardiac output sufficiently to maintain adequate oxygen transport. In such cases the sensorium and cognitive function of the patient will diminish. If the brain continues to be hypoxic, the patient will lose consciousness and lapse into a coma.

Ventilatory Failure

An acute increase in Pa_{CO_2} decreases arterial blood pH. The combination of an elevated Pa_{CO_2} and acidosis may have a profound effect on the body, especially when the ventilatory failure is severe. Severe acute respiratory acidosis results in a diminished cognitive function because of depression of the central nervous system.[6] The cerebral and peripheral blood vessels dilate in response to hypercapnia.[6]

CLINICAL FEATURES

Oxygenation Failure

Inspection of the patient with severe hypoxemia typically reveals one who appears to be in acute respiratory distress. Use of the accessory muscles to breathe is common and indicates an increase in the work of breathing. The patient is likely to have central cyanosis unless anemia is present and obscures the cyanosis. Central cyanosis is a bluish discoloration of the tongue and mucous membranes caused by desaturation of hemoglobin. The presence of anemia will reduce the clinician's ability to detect cyanosis because insufficient hemoglobin is present for the discoloration to show. Vital signs are typically abnormal and demonstrate tachycardia, tachypnea, and hypertension. Severe hypoxemia may leave the patient confused, agitated, and slow to respond (because the brain is suffering from lack of adequate oxygenation).

If the hypoxemia is chronic, right heart failure due to a persistent increase in pulmonary vascular resistance (cor pulmonale) may develop and cause jugular venous distension. Chronic hypoxemia also leads to other signs of right heart failure including enlarged liver (hepatomegaly), pedal edema, loud pulmonic valve closure,[7] and digital clubbing.

Laboratory abnormalities associated with hypoxemia include low P_{O_2}, S_{O_2}, and O_2 content on arterial blood gas (ABG) analysis. If the hypoxemia is chronic, bone marrow is stimulated to produce red blood cells, which results in polycythemia and elevated hemoglobin and hematocrit values. When the hemoglobin increase is significant, the oxygen content of the arterial blood may be normal or near normal, even in the presence of hypoxemia.

The chest radiograph is usually abnormal in oxygenation failure. Typical abnormalities include infiltrates consistent with pulmonary edema, adult respiratory distress syndrome, atelectasis, or pneumonia (see Chapters 8, 11, 13, and 16, respectively). When the primary cause of the hypoxemia is outside the lung (e.g., shunting from a congenital heart defect), the chest radiograph is often normal unless a complicating respiratory problem is present.

Ventilatory Failure

There are few clinical findings specifically suggestive of an elevated Pa_{CO_2}. Clinical findings that suggest ventilatory failure include headache, diminished alertness, warm flushed skin, and bounding peripheral pulses. These findings are very nonspecific as they occur in a variety of conditions other than ventilatory failure. Because hypoxemia is often present in the patient with ventilatory failure, the clinical signs of inadequate oxygenation are often simultaneously present.

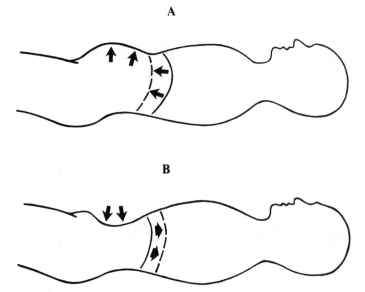

FIGURE 1–3 A, Normal movement of the diaphragm and abdominal contents with breathing. B, Abnormal, inward movement of the abdomen with each inspiratory effort as seen with diaphragm fatigue. This is known as abdominal paradox.

Hypothermia and loss of consciousness are common when the ventilatory failure is the result of drug overdose from sedatives. Sedatives and tricyclic antidepressants often cause the pupils to become fixed and dilated. Tricyclic antidepressants frequently increase heart rate and blood pressure. Breath sounds are often clear with drug overdose unless aspiration has occurred. Aspiration is more likely when sedatives and alcohol are abused (owing to a diminished gag reflex) and may result in crackles in the right lower lobe.

The clinical signs of diaphragm fatigue provide an early warning of respiratory failure in the patient in respiratory distress. It strongly suggests that the patient needs immediate ventilatory assistance (see Treatment, farther on). Fatigue of the diaphragm initially results in tachypnea, followed by periods of **respiratory alternans** or **abdominal paradox.**[8–10] Respiratory alternans is alternating for short periods between breathing with the accessory muscles and breathing with the diaphragm. Abdominal paradox is recognized by inward movement of the abdomen with each inspiratory effort (Fig. 1–3). This is due to the flaccid status of the diaphragm, causing it to be drawn upward when the accessory muscles create a negative intrathoracic pressure.

Blood gas measurements are very helpful in assessing the patient with ventilatory failure. The severity of ventilatory failure is indicated by the amount of Pa_{CO_2} increase. Measurement of arterial pH identifies the degree of respiratory acidosis present and suggests the urgency of treatment. The patient needs immediate care when the pH drops below 7.2 (see Treatment).

TREATMENT

Oxygenation Failure

The initial treatment of hypoxemia requires elevation of the concentration of oxygen in the inspired gas (FI_{O_2}). Oxygen supplementation rapidly corrects hypoxemia associated with V̇/Q̇ mismatching or hypoventilation. Oxygen therapy in this situation can be given by nasal cannula, simple mask, or entrainment mask. The entrainment mask delivers a specific FIO_2, regardless of the patient's breathing pattern; however, the FIO_2 of the nasal cannula and simple mask will vary in accordance with the patient's rate and volume of breathing.

Hypoxemia due to either anatomic or physiologic shunting usually does not respond to increases in FIO_2. This is because blood traversing the shunt does not come into contact with ventilated alveoli. Treatment of anatomic shunt requires closure of the defect, if that is possible. Treatment of physiologic shunt requires reopening of alveoli. Shunt caused by collapse of alveoli often responds to positive pressure ventilation, which may decrease the patient's work of breathing and may open collapsed alveoli to allow better gas exchange.

Positive pressure is generally used to treat hypoxemia when the patient's Pao_2 is less than 60 mm Hg despite increasing the FIO_2 to 0.50 or higher (Table 1–2). The application of continuous positive airway pressure (CPAP) by mask is an acceptable temporary measure as long as ventilation is adequate and the patient's problem is likely to resolve quickly (e.g., postoperative atelectasis). Intubation and mechanical ventilation are needed if mask CPAP does not correct the hypoxemia or reduce the patient's work of breathing, or when the problem is not likely to resolve quickly, as with patients having adult respiratory distress syndrome (ARDS). The application of positive end-expiratory pressure (PEEP) in conjunction with mechanical ventilation is usually needed to treat patients with severe hypoxemia due to shunting. PEEP and CPAP allow adequate oxygenation at a lower FIO_2, reducing the risk for oxygen toxicity. The use of PEEP and its potential complications are described in more detail in Chapter 11.

Conventional modes of mechanical ventilation are adequate for most patients. These include assist-control or intermittent mandatory ventilation (IMV). A ventilator set to assist-control delivers a preset tidal volume at a specified rate. The ventilator will also deliver a full mechanical breath each time the patient initiates an inspiratory effort. A ventilator set to IMV delivers preset tidal volumes at a present rate but does not provide mechanical breaths when the patient takes spontaneous breaths in between the mechanical breaths. As a result, the patient may receive numerous mechanical and spontaneous breaths each minute. Although IMV was popularized initially as a mode for weaning patients from mechanical ventilation, it is now also popular as a form of ventilator support.

Mechanical ventilation is almost always initiated with inspiratory times much shorter than expiratory times. A long expiratory time allows adequate time for exhalation and reduces the chance of inadvertent air trapping. Prolonged inspiratory times with short expiratory times (inverse inspiratory to expiratory [I:E] ratio) may improve oxygenation in some patients with low lung compliance and poor gas exchange. Inverse-ratio ventilation (IRV) was first applied in neonates but is now also used in adult patients with refractory hypoxemia.[4]

Ventilatory Failure

An acute elevation in arterial Pco_2 indicates that the patient cannot maintain adequate alveolar ventilation and may need ventilatory assistance. The $Paco_2$ does

---

Table 1–2 Clinical Guidelines for Initiation of Mechanical Ventilation (Adult Patients)

Respiratory rate	>35/min
Vital capacity	<15 cc/kg
Minute ventilation	>10 L/min
Maximum inspiratory pressure	<−20 cm H_2O
$Paco_2$	>50 mm Hg
Pao_2	<60 mm Hg on O_2

not have to be higher than the normal range to indicate the need for mechanical ventilation. For example, if the $Paco_2$ had been 30 mm Hg, and now, because of muscle fatigue had risen to 40 mm Hg, the patient would benefit from immediate intubation and mechanical ventilation. This example illustrates how documenting $Paco_2$ trends helps determine the need for mechanical ventilation.

Once the patient is intubated, the tidal volume selected should be in the range of 10 to 15 cc/kg of ideal body weight (e.g., obese patients do not need enormous tidal volumes). Tidal volumes smaller than this tend to result in collapse of peripheral lung units (atelectasis; see Chapter 13). Tidal volumes larger than 10 to 15 cc/kg tend to overinflate the lungs and may result in barotrauma (pneumothorax or pneumomediastinum). The respiratory rate needed by the patient depends on his or her metabolic rate, but adults typically require 8 to 15 breaths/minute. Ventilation is adjusted in most patients to keep the $Paco_2$ between 35 and 45 mm Hg. One exception is the patient with cerebral edema in whom a lower $Paco_2$ may lower intracranial pressure. Another exception is the patient with a chronically elevated $Paco_2$ in whom the goal of mechanical ventilation is to return the pH to normal range and the Pco_2 to the patient's baseline. If patients with chronic hypoventilation and CO_2 retention are ventilated with enough vigor to achieve a normal Pco_2, respiratory alkalosis becomes a problem in the short term and weaning a problem in the long term.

Clinicians should determine the cause of the ventilatory failure while initiating symptomatic treatment. In the case of drug overdose, attempts should be made to identify the involved drug, the amount of drug ingested, the length of time since ingestion, and whether or not trauma occurred. General goals in management of drug overdose are to prevent toxin absorption (stomach lavage or inducement of vomiting and use of charcoal), to enhance drug excretion (dialysis), and to prevent accumulation of toxic metabolic products (e.g., acetylcysteine is the antidote for acetaminophen overdose).

Weaning the patient from mechanical ventilation can begin as soon as the cause of the respiratory failure has been corrected and the patient's medical problems have stabilized. Weaning parameters help determine when weaning is likely to be successful (Table 1–3). Clinicians should use numerous parameters to make the decision about when to begin weaning, as any one parameter can be misleading. The combination of a spontaneous tidal volume of greater than 325 cc and a spontaneous respiratory rate of less than 38/minute appears to be a good predictor of weaning success in adults.[11]

Methods for weaning include IMV, pressure support, and T piece. Each method has advantages and disadvantages, but any of the methods should effectively wean most patients when they are ready.[12] Each method depends on decreasing the patient's ventilatory support under controlled circumstances while closely monitoring the patient. Extubation can occur when the patient's gag reflex is intact and the endotracheal tube is no longer needed.

Table 1–3 Weaning Criteria

Cause of respiratory or ventilatory failure is remedied
Patient condition is stable and improving
Vital capacity is >10–15 cc/kg
Resting minute volume is <10 L/min
Maximum inspiratory pressure is >−20 cm H_2O
Adequate oxygenation on an FIO_2 <0.50
Spontaneous respiratory rate <35/min
Spontaneous tidal volume >325 cc

IMV weaning is done by decreasing the number of mechanical breaths/minute every few hours until the patient either no longer needs mechanical support or demonstrates poor tolerance of the weaning (e.g., 20 percent changes in pulse rate and blood pressure). The primary disadvantage of IMV is the potential increase in the work of breathing imposed on the patient during spontaneous breaths.[13] This increased workload is primarily due to excessive resistance at the demand valve. Newer ventilators are attempting to correct this problem.

Pressure support helps overcome the workload imposed by the resistance of the artificial airway and ventilator circuitry by providing a set amount of positive airway pressure during inspiration.[14,15] Weaning with pressure support requires the practitioner to lower the preset pressure support gradually while monitoring the patient. Once the patient can tolerate a low-pressure support level (e.g., less than 5 cm H_2O), mechanical assistance can be discontinued.

T-piece weaning is done by discontinuing mechanical ventilation for short periods of time and placing the patient on "blow-by" at the appropriate F_{IO_2}. The duration of time the patient is breathing spontaneously is gradually increased until the patient shows signs of stress or no longer requires mechanical ventilation.

Case Study

HISTORY

Ms. N is a 47-year-old white woman who was found unconscious on the floor of her apartment by a relative. Empty bottles of Valium, amitriptyline (an antidepressant), and beer cans were nearby. The relative dialed 911 and the patient was transported to a local emergency room. During transportation the patient had an adequate pulse but required ventilatory assistance with a bag-valve-mask on oxygen. An emergency arterial blood gas measurement was obtained and a drug screen ordered.

Questions

1. What complications are likely to occur in this patient?
2. What information should the attending physician attempt to identify from the relative or paramedics?
3. Is this patient most likely to be experiencing ventilatory or oxygenation failure?
4. Should the patient be intubated? If so, why?
5. What treatment should be provided?

Answers

1. Common complications include respiratory depression, hypothermia or hyperthermia, and vomiting and aspiration.
2. The physician should attempt to identify how much medication the patient swallowed and how much time has passed since ingestion. Some of the pertinent information could be obtained from the prescription labels on the bottles.
3. The patient is most likely to experience ventilatory failure due to depression of the central nervous system. Oxygenation failure would be expected only if gastric acid aspiration has occurred.
4. Yes, the patient should be intubated to ensure adequate ventilation and to protect the airway from aspiration.
5. The most urgent treatment needed after establishing an airway and ensuring adequate ventilation is to prevent further absorption of the overdose medication. This is accomplished with the use of charcoal to absorb and

bind with the toxins. If the patient is awake and alert, vomiting is induced with ipecac syrup; however, if the patient is lethargic or if mental status is rapidly deteriorating, stomach lavage is preferable. Placement of an endotracheal tube for protection of the lungs is important before performing stomach lavage.

PHYSICAL EXAMINATION

General *An unconscious, slightly obese woman who has an 8.0-mm endotracheal tube in place orally and is being ventilated with a hand resuscitator. A Ewald tube is in her left nostril. The gastric lavage fluid contains a large number of pill fragments. A strong smell of alcohol is emanating from the patient. She is approximately 5 feet, 8 inches tall and weighs 70 kg.*

Vital Signs *Pulse 124/minute; respiratory rate 12 to 16/minute with bag-valve; temperature 35.3°C; and blood pressure 120/75 mm Hg*

HEENT *No signs of trauma; pupils dilated, and response to light sluggish*

Heart *Normal heart sounds with no murmurs*

Lungs *Breath sounds clear except in right lower lobe, where inspiratory crackles heard*

Abdomen *Soft, obese, with no organomegaly or tenderness; bowel sounds hypoactive but present*

Extremities *Warm to palpation with no edema, clubbing, or cyanosis*

Initial ABG findings while the patient is being ventilated with an FIO_2 of 1.0 via a bag-valve-mask before intubation reveal pH 7.28, Pco_2 54 mm Hg, Po_2 135 mm Hg, So_2 99 percent, Hco_3^- 26 mEq/liter.

Questions

6. What accounts for the hypothermia?
7. What accounts for the dilated and sluggishly reactive pupils?
8. What could account for the crackles heard in the right lower lobe?
9. How do you interpret the ABG findings?
10. What is the significance of the pill fragments found in the contents of the stomach? Why is the charcoal given?

Answers

6. Hypothermia is common in patients with drug overdose due to sedatives. Amitriptyline overdose especially disrupts temperature regulation.
7. Dilated and slowly reactive pupils are common in patients who overdose on sedatives and tricyclic antidepressants.
8. Crackles in the right lower lobe are most likely due to aspiration of stomach contents. Sedatives and alcohol decrease mental acuity and depress the pharyngeal muscle function, both of which contribute to a disturbed gag reflex and increase the chance of aspiration.

9. The ABG measurements reveal an acute respiratory acidosis with adequate oxygenation. Respiratory acidosis is common in patients who overdose on sedatives, as they depress the central nervous system and diminish the drive to breathe. Ventilation with a bag-valve-mask is often less effective than ventilation with a bag-valve and a properly placed endotracheal tube because of face mask leaks and gastric inflation.

10. The presence of pill fragments in the stomach indicates that at least some of the pills were ingested somewhat recently. Gastric lavage and the use of charcoal will probably prevent absorption of a large amount of the medication in the stomach.

The patient was transferred from the emergency room to the intensive care unit (ICU), where she was given continuous mechanical ventilation with a volume ventilator and cardiac monitoring was continued.

Questions

11. What laboratory tests do you suggest at this time?
12. What ventilator settings do you recommend? Specifically suggest the mode of ventilation and tidal volume, rate, FIO_2, and PEEP levels.

Answers

11. A repeat of the ABG measurements after initiation of mechanical ventilation would help ensure adequate ventilation. A chest radiograph would be helpful to investigate the crackles in the right lower lobe.

12. The patient should be ventilated using the assist-control or IMV mode. The tidal volume should be in the range of 600 to 900 ml because Ms. N's ideal body weight is approximately 60 kg. The mechanical rate should be about 10 to 12/minute. The presence of inspiratory crackles indicates that the patient may have some abnormal lung pathology that could lead to $\dot{V}/\dot{Q}$ mismatching or shunting. This suggests that an elevated FIO_2 will be needed to maintain adequate oxygenation. An FIO_2 in the range of 0.40 to 0.60 is a reasonable place to start because the patient has more than adequate oxygenation on an FIO_2 of 1.0. PEEP levels greater than 5 cm H_2O should not be necessary unless the patient requires an FIO_2 of greater than 0.60 on mechanical ventilation.

The ventilator was set to deliver a tidal volume of 800 ml at a rate of 12/minute with an FIO_2 of 0.45 in the assist-control mode. Twenty minutes after initiation of mechanical ventilation an arterial blood sample was drawn and revealed pH 7.51, PcO_2 32 mm Hg, PO_2 88 mm Hg, HcO_3^- 25 mEq/liter. The chest radiograph demonstrated patchy infiltrates in the right lower lobe consistent with aspiration pneumonia (Fig. 1–4). The electrocardiogram (ECG) monitor revealed a sinus rate of 115 to 130/minute. Breath sounds were clear in all areas except the right lower lobe.

A drug screening demonstrated that the patient had also taken acetaminophen. The patient's blood alcohol level was 0.155, and the presence of amitriptyline was confirmed through analysis of a urine sample.

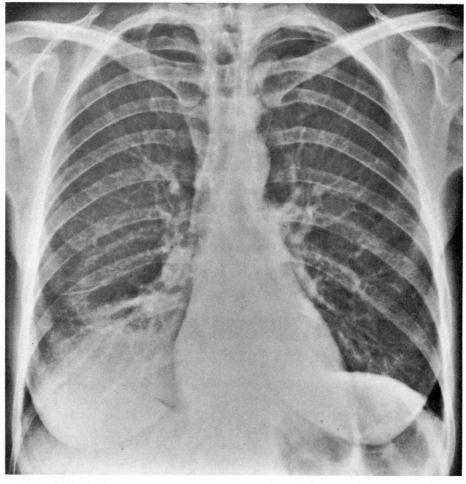

FIGURE 1–4 Chest radiograph demonstrating infiltrates in the right lower lobe.

Questions

13. Interpret the ABG analysis results.
14. What changes in the ventilator settings do you suggest, based on the ABG results?
15. What is the treatment for acetaminophen overdose?

Answers

13. The ABG analysis reveals an acute respiratory alkalosis with adequate oxygenation on an F_{IO_2} of 0.45. The respiratory alkalosis is the result of the mechanical ventilation with an excessive minute ventilation.
14. The ventilator should be adjusted to deliver a lower minute volume. A reduction in the tidal volume or rate would reduce alveolar ventilation and allow the arterial P_{CO_2} to increase to a more normal range.
15. The antidote for acetaminophen overdose is N-acetyl-L-cysteine (acetylcysteine, or Mucomyst). The need for treatment with the antidote is determined by the use of a nomogram that calls for comparing the amount of time passed since ingestion and the acetaminophen plasma blood level. If the acetaminophen plasma level is on or above the minimum treatment level, the patient should be given an oral loading dose

of acetylcysteine (140 mg/kg) followed by 17 maintenance doses of 70 mg/kg each at 4-hour intervals. The acetylcysteine should be diluted with water, juice, or soda. Acetylcysteine is also given when acetaminophen plasma level is not available and the history of ingestion is greater than 7.5 g or 140 mg/kg.[15]

The rate of the mechanical ventilator was reduced to 8/minute at the same tidal volume. Acetylcysteine was given to the patient to treat the overdose from acetaminophen. Over the next 24 hours the patient regained consciousness and was able to respond to commands and communicate by writing. T-piece weaning was started and the patient carefully observed. After 4 hours her vital signs were normal and her arterial blood gas analysis revealed pH 7.43, P_{CO_2} 36 mm Hg, P_{O_2} 79 mm Hg on an F_{IO_2} of 0.40. Based on these findings the patient was extubated and placed on oxygen by mask with aerosol at an F_{IO_2} of 0.45. Over the next 24 hours her pneumonia and general condition improved and she was transferred to the psychiatric ward on day 3. The remainder of her hospital stay was uneventful.

REFERENCES

1. Bryan CL: Classification of respiratory failure. In Kirby, RR and Taylor, RW (eds): Respiratory Failure. Year Book Medical, Chicago, 1986, pp 17–21.

2. George, RB: Pathophysiology of acute respiratory failure. In Bone, RC, George, RB, and Hudson, LD (eds): Acute Respiratory Failure. Churchill Livingstone, New York, 1987, pp 1–10.

3. Shapiro, BA, Harrison, RA, Cane, RD, and Templin, R: Clinical Application of Blood Gases, ed 4. Year Book Medical, Chicago, 1989, p 93.

4. Marini, JJ and Wheeler, AP: Critical Care Medicine—The Essentials. Williams & Wilkins, Baltimore, 1989, p 176.

5. Murray, JF: The Normal Lung. WB Saunders, Philadelphia, 1986, p 159.

6. Guyton, AC: Textbook of Medical Physiology, ed 6. WB Saunders, Philadelphia, 1981, p 459.

7. Butler, J: Cardiac evaluation. In Murray, JF and Nadel, JA (eds): Textbook of Respiratory Medicine. WB Saunders, Philadelphia, 1988.

8. Barrett, TA: Nutrition and respiratory failure. In Bone, RC, George, RB, and Hudson, LD (eds): Acute Respiratory Failure. Churchill Livingstone, New York, 1987, pp 265–304.

9. Cohen, CA: Clinical manifestations of inspiratory muscle fatigue. Am J Med 73:308, 1982.

10. Mier-Jedrzejowicz, A, et al: Assessment of diaphragm weakness. Am Rev Respir Dis 137:877, 1988.

11. Yang, KL and Tobin, MJ: A prospective study of indexes predicting the outcome of trials of weaning from mechanical ventilation. N Engl J Med 324:1445, 1991.

12. Balk, RA and Bone, RC: Mechanical ventilation. In Bone, RC, George, RB, and Hudson, LD (eds): Acute Respiratory Failure. Churchill Livingstone, New York, 1987, pp 213–239.

13. Fiastro, JF, Habib, MP, and Quan, SF: Pressure support compensation for inspiratory work due to endotracheal tubes and demand continuous positive airway pressure. Chest 93:499, 1988.

14. Beydon, L, Chasse, M, and Harf, A: Inspiratory work of breathing during spontaneous ventilation using demand valves and continuous flow systems. Am Rev Respir Dis 138:300, 1988.

15. Hall, AH and Rumack, BH: Diagnosis and treatment of poisoning. In Shoemaker, WC, et al (eds): Textbook of Critical Care. WB Saunders, Philadelphia, 1989, p 1174.

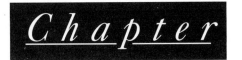

Chapter 2

Robert L. Wilkins, MA, RRT
James R. Dexter, MD, FCCP

ASTHMA

INTRODUCTION

Asthma is an obstructive pulmonary disease characterized by diffuse bronchospasm that, in many cases, occurs in response to various stimuli. A key feature of asthma is that the airway obstruction is reversible. In fact, between episodes the patient often is without symptoms and may experience normal pulmonary function. When the patient has an asthmatic attack that does not respond to conventional treatment, the condition is called **status asthmaticus.**

Although much overlap occurs, it is helpful to classify asthma into two categories: extrinsic and intrinsic. Extrinsic asthma is characterized by bronchospasm that occurs in an atopic patient (someone who has an allergic reaction in response to exposure to allergens) when exposed to environmental irritants. Intrinsic asthma is present when the patient suffers asthma attacks without evidence of atopy. Extrinsic asthma occurs most commonly in childhood, whereas intrinsic asthma often starts in adult life.

Occupational asthma is the term used for bronchospasm that develops in response to a provoking agent in the workplace. Typically the individual with this type of asthma becomes asymptomatic during times spent away from work such as on weekends and vacations.

Stable asthma is present when a period of 4 weeks has passed in which an asthma-prone patient has not had increased symptoms or a need for an increase in medication. Conversely, unstable asthma is present when the patient has experienced increased symptoms sometime during the past 4 weeks.[1]

ETIOLOGY

In some cases of extrinsic asthma, a specific provoking situation can be linked to the patient's asthma attacks; thus, terms such as exercise-induced asthma or pollen asthma are frequently used. Most patients with extrinsic asthma can have attacks provoked by many different allergens such as house dust mites, animal dander, and certain foods or food additives such as sulfites. In addition to allergens, asthma attacks may be provoked by pharmacologic agents such as β-adrenergic receptor antagonists and aspirin, air pollutants such as sulfur dioxide, oxidants, exercise, cigarette smoke, and airway infections.

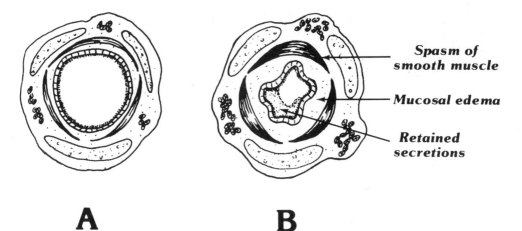

*Spasm of
smooth muscle*

Mucosal edema

*Retained
secretions*

A   B

FIGURE 2–1 Cross-sectional view of a normal airway (A) and from a patient with asthma (B). A combination of airway secretions, edema, and bronchospasm contribute to a reduction in the airway diameter.

PATHOPHYSIOLOGY

In addition to experiencing bronchospasm, airways of the patient with asthma may be obstructed by mucosal edema and excessive secretions (Fig. 2–1). Frequently patients with asthma have thick, tenacious mucus in the lung that causes plugging in the distal airways. The lack of uniform ventilation throughout the lung causes ventilation-perfusion ratio ($\dot{V}/\dot{Q}$) mismatching, which results in hypoxemia.

Initially the airway obstruction primarily hinders exhalation, resulting in air trapping and progressive hyperinflation of the lungs. With air trapping the residual volume increases at the expense of the vital capacity. The combination of increased airway resistance and lung hyperinflation significantly elevates the work of breathing in patients with asthma.

CLINICAL FEATURES

Medical History

Typically the patient suffering from an acute asthma attack complains of chest tightness, difficulty breathing, wheezing, and/or cough. The onset of these symptoms may be rapid or more gradual. When the symptoms occur rapidly they may disappear rapidly as well, with appropriate treatment. Although some idea of the seriousness of an asthma attack can be determined from the patient's history, the degree of dyspnea is not a reliable predictor of severity.

While dyspnea and wheezing suggest asthma, other disorders such as congestive heart failure, bronchitis, pulmonary embolism, and upper airway obstruction can cause similar findings. In most cases the patient's age, medical history, physical findings, and radiographic and laboratory test results will confirm the diagnosis.

Physical Examination

The physical examination can provide important objective information that will assist in confirming the diagnosis and in identifying the severity of the obstruction. Inadequate assessment of the patient's status can be a fatal mistake that may result in insufficient treatment and monitoring.[1-3] Common findings associated with asthma include tachypnea, use of accessory muscles for breathing, a prolonged exhalation, increased anteroposterior (AP) diameter of the chest, expiratory wheezing, and intercostal retractions. Severe asthma is suggested by pronounced use of accessory muscles, paradoxic pulse, tachypnea, and wheezing on inhalation and exhalation (Fig. 2–2).[4–7]

Use of accessory muscles to breathe is due to the pulmonary hyperinflation that causes the diaphragm to assume a flat position less capable of effective ventilation.[7] A prolonged expiratory phase occurs as the intrapulmonary airways become obstructed and slow the movement of gas out of the lungs. Increased AP diameter occurs when air-trapping and pulmonary hyperinflation are present. Wheezing is produced as rapid airflow occurs through narrowed airways, causing the airway walls to vibrate.[8] Retractions are an intermittent depression of the skin around the rib cage occurring with each inspiratory effort. Retractions result when a significant drop in intrapleural pressure causes the skin overlying the chest wall to sink inward. This suggests that the patient's work of breathing is markedly increased. The significant drop in intrapleural pressure is also responsible for the drop in pulse pressure during inspirations (paradoxic pulse).[9,10]

It is not uncommon to see patients lean forward and brace their hands or elbows on a nearby table during an acute asthma attack. This position may provide a better mechanical advantage for the accessory muscles to assist breathing.

> ## Laboratory Evaluation

The chest radiograph is most helpful in identifying the presence of complications such as pneumonia, atelectasis, or pneumothorax. In the absence of complications the chest radiograph typically demonstrates hyperinflation of the lung fields with asthma.

Complete pulmonary function studies are not typically done when the patient is suffering an acute asthma attack. Simple bedside spirometry, however, is appropriate and very useful in determining the severity of obstruction and the response to therapy. Measurement of peak flow and forced expiratory volume in 1 second (FEV_1) is commonly used and easy to obtain unless the patient has severe dyspnea.

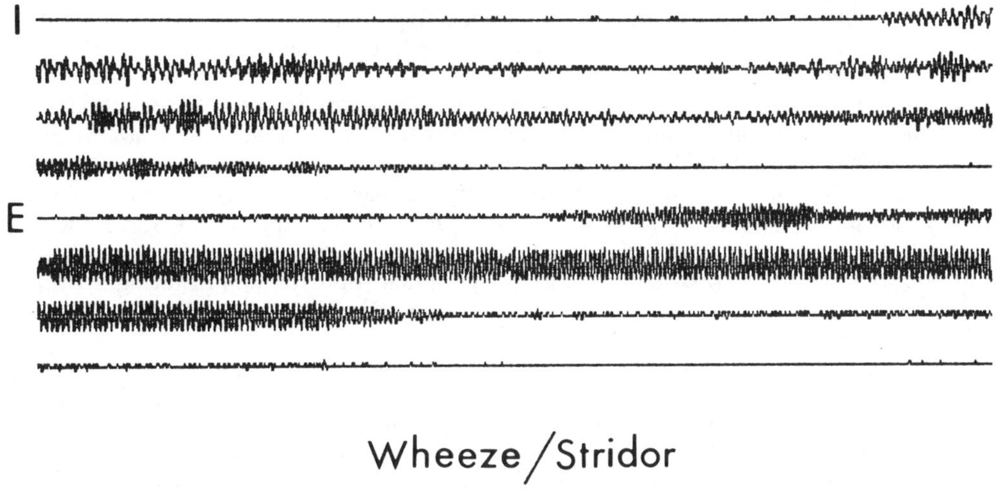

Wheeze/Stridor

FIGURE 2–2 Waveform analysis demonstrating an inspiratory and expiratory high-pitched wheeze. Time is represented on the horizontal axis and intensity (loudness) on the vertical axis. The pitch is indicated by the number of deflections per time period. Each horizontal line represents 0.34 second. Reprint from Respir Care 35: 969, 1990 with permission.

A peak flow of less than 100 liters/minute or an FEV_1 less than 1.0 liter suggests severe obstruction.[7]

Bronchial provocation testing is useful in identifying the degree of airway reactivity in patients with symptoms typical for asthma but with normal pulmonary function study results. Methacholine is most often used for bronchial provocation testing because it increases parasympathetic tone in the smooth muscles of the airways, resulting in bronchospasm. Patients with asthma will have more than a 20 percent decrease in FEV_1 in response to methacholine, whereas healthy persons have little or no response.

Arterial blood gases (ABGs) are extremely useful for assessing the severity of the asthma attack especially when the bronchospasm is severe enough to prevent the patient from performing a forced expiratory maneuver. The degree of hypoxemia and hypercapnia present is a reliable guide to the severity of the airway obstruction.[7] Typically the $Paco_2$ is decreased with the onset of an asthma attack.[3,4] A normal or increased $Paco_2$ indicates that a more severe degree of obstruction is present or the patient has started to fatigue. Additional signs of fatigue include tachypnea, diaphoresis, abdominal paradox, disturbed consciousness, and decreasing peak flow.[7] Abdominal paradox is seen as an inward movement of the abdominal wall during inspiration and is associated with fatigue of the diaphragm (see Chapter 1).

One important goal of assessment in acute asthma is related to the efficiency of evaluation. Most asthmatic patients need immediate care and the experienced clinician will perform an efficient yet effective assessment without delaying the onset of treatment. Avoiding unnecessary evaluation tools is an essential part of any assessment, especially when the patient is acutely ill.

TREATMENT

Initially treatment should be directed toward achieving adequate oxygenation, providing bronchodilation, and decreasing airway inflammation. The majority of patients suffering from an acute asthma attack will develop hypoxemia resulting from $\dot{V}/\dot{Q}$ mismatching. In some cases the hypoxemia will be severe enough to represent a serious threat to the patient's life but can almost always be corrected with appropriate oxygen therapy.

Numerous pharmacologic agents are available to promote bronchodilatation and reduce airway inflammation, such as β-adrenergics, xanthines, parasympatholytics, and steroids. In the majority of mild cases, the bronchospasm can be reversed by use of an aerosolized β_2-adrenergic. Inhaled β-agonist bronchodilators offer the following advantages over oral bronchodilators: more rapid onset, lower dosage requirements, a lower incidence of systemic side effects, and better protection of the airways against provoking agents.[1,11] A popular route for administering the bronchodilator is the metered-dose inhaler (MDI). The MDI is popular because it is simple for the patient to use.

Aerosolized bronchodilator treatments with a small-volume nebulizer (SVN) are useful for patients unable to use the MDI. The SVN treatments are most often given every 4 to 6 hours, but during severe bronchospasm may be provided more often with careful monitoring. Continuous nebulization therapy for the administration of a bronchodilator may prove useful when the patient with asthma does not respond to conventional therapy and is on the verge of respiratory failure.[12,13] Oral or intravenous theophylline is indicated for patients who fail to respond to aerosolized β-agonist treatments or when the asthma attack is severe.

During an acute, severe asthma attack, if the patient fails to respond adequately to inhaled β-agonists and intravenous theophylline, intravenous corticosteroids can be added to the treatment plan. The anti-inflammatory effects of corticosteroids may take several hours to cause beneficial results and therefore should be started as soon as indicated. In addition, inhaled Atrovent or atropine may be added when conventional bronchodilators are not effective.[7]

Clinicians should avoid giving asthmatic patients certain medications during an acute asthma attack. Sedatives may induce ventilatory failure and should be used only if the patient is intubated and being mechanically ventilated. Inhaled corticosteroids, Mucomyst, cromolyn sodium, and dense aerosols may increase bronchospasm because these agents tend to irritate the airways.[7]

Other goals of management include the treatment of airway infections, mucolysis, and adequate hydration. Hydration improves the patient's pulmonary condition by aiding in the expectoration of secretions.

Favorable prognostic signs include improvement in the vital signs, Pa_{O_2}, Pa_{CO_2}, breath sounds, sensorium, and breathing pattern. Because any one of these parameters alone can be misleading, it is always best to assess numerous values to obtain a more accurate clinical picture of the patient's response to therapy.

If the patient becomes fatigued in spite of treatment, mechanical ventilation is necessary. The decision to intubate and mechanically ventilate the patient can be difficult, especially when the clinical findings are not convincing (Table 2–1). Use of the physical findings, ABGs, and peak flow parameters described earlier and in the case study that follows will provide the most reliable data for evaluating the need for mechanical ventilation.

Table 2–1 Decision Making in Asthma

Admit Patient? Yes, if:	How to Recognize
The attack is severe	Use of accessory muscles at rest Paradoxic pulse present Inspiratory and expiratory wheezing present Peak flow is <100 L/min FEV_1 <1.0 L Significant hyperinflation noted on chest radiograph
The patient does not respond to initial therapy	Vital signs not improving Continued use of accessory muscles Pa_{O_2} responds minimally to O_2 therapy
Intubate and Initiate CMV? Yes, if:	**How to Recognize?**
The patient fatigues	Pa_{CO_2} rising Sensorium deteriorates Abdominal paradox present Peak flow decreasing
Respiratory failure present	Hypoxemia is present despite high F_{IO_2} Severe respiratory acidemia (pH <7.25) occurs Central cyanosis
Cardiopulmonary arrest occurs	Pulse and respiratory effort absent Pallor Patient becomes unconscious

The ultimate goal in the management of asthma is to prevent or at least minimize future attacks by decreasing the level of airway responsiveness. Consequently, once the episode is over and the patient has recovered, the severity of the underlying asthma should be assessed. This is accomplished through a careful history, pulmonary function testing, and, in selected cases, investigations of provoking agents. The latter is especially helpful in evaluating patients with suspected occupational asthma. Patient education regarding the avoidance of provoking agents, the use of medications, and medication side effects is especially helpful in allowing the patient to lead an active, independent lifestyle. The use of cromolyn sodium helps stabilize the mast cells to prevent the release of mediators such as histamine that can cause bronchospasm.[14] Training the patient to use a peak flow meter to monitor the degree of airway obstruction can help the patient know when to increase the medication or seek medical attention.

Case Study

HISTORY

Ms. B is a 19-year-old bareback bronco rider seen in the emergency room because of shortness of breath. The dyspnea began during a particularly hard ride that culminated in the patient landing on the rodeo floor and inhaling a modest amount of dust. She stated that the tightness in her chest and shortness of breath were so severe that she had to leave the rodeo eventually and seek medical help. She was now very uncomfortable, even at rest. During the past week she had had a cough productive of greenish-yellow sputum, mild fever, malaise, and fatigue but had not felt seriously ill until the dyspnea developed at the rodeo earlier in the day. She denied previous lung problems except for mild "whistling" in her chest, occurring off and on during the past several years. She denied the use of any prescription medications or any previous episodes of dyspnea, chest pain, leg pain, hemoptysis, sinusitis, or allergies. Her family history was negative for lung disease.

Questions

1. What is the key symptom to explore in greater detail?
2. What is the differential diagnosis of this patient's problem, and what is the most likely diagnosis?
3. To what details should the physical examination be specifically directed?
4. Why is the patient having trouble now rather than 2 months ago?

Answers

1. Dyspnea; the patient should be questioned to evaluate the severity of the dyspnea because this determines the speed at which further evaluation and treatment should be pursued.
2. Asthma, acute bronchitis, congestive heart failure, flu syndrome, pneumothorax, pulmonary embolus, and psychogenic dyspnea are possible causes of the patient's symptoms. Asthma exacerbated by acute bronchitis is the most likely diagnosis.
3. The physical examination should be directed toward identifying signs that confirm or rule out the aforementioned diagnoses and toward identifying the severity of the airway obstruction (see farther on).
4. The patient is having trouble now because she has had a triple airway insult consisting of respiratory tract infection, allergen (dust) inhalation, and recent severe exertion.

PHYSICAL EXAMINATION

General   Patient is alert but restless and in moderate respiratory distress, mildly diaphoretic, sitting up on the edge of the bed and leaning forward with her arms braced on her knees. Her cough is frequent and productive of small amounts of greenish sputum.

Vital Signs   Temperature 37.5°C; respiratory rate 38/minute; blood pressure 170/95 mm Hg; pulse 140/minute; paradoxic pulse 25 mm Hg

HEENT   Sinuses not tender to palpation; alae nasii flare with inspiration

Neck   Trachea midline, mobile to palpation, with no stridor; carotid pulsations ++ and symmetric bilaterally, without bruit; no lymphadenopathy, thyroidomegaly, or jugular venous distension present; sternomastoid muscles tense during inspiration

Chest   Increased AP diameter with decreased expansion during breathing; resonance to percussion moderately increased bilaterally; mild abdominal paradox with respiratory efforts

Lungs   Rapid respiratory rate with prolonged expiratory phase and polyphonic wheezing heard over the entire chest during inhalation and exhalation (see Fig. 2–2)

Heart   Regular rhythm with rate of 140/minute; no murmurs, gallops, or rubs; the point of maximum impulse (PMI) in normal position

Abdomen   Soft, nontender, bowel sounds present, no masses or organomegaly

Extremities   No clubbing, cyanosis, or edema; pulses ++ and symmetric in all areas

Questions

5. What is causing the patient's wheezing?
6. What is causing the paradoxic pulse, and what is the significance of this finding?
7. What is the cause and significance of the accessory muscle usage?
8. What is the cause and significance of the paradoxic breathing pattern?
9. Why do patients in respiratory distress lean forward and brace themselves on their hands or elbows?
10. What pathophysiology accounts for the patient's increased AP diameter?
11. Does the physical examination provide evidence that hypoxemia is present, and if so, what are the signs?

Answers

5. Wheezing is caused by a decreased airway diameter that results from bronchospasm, airway edema, and secretions. Rapid airflow through the partial obstruction causes the airway walls to "flutter" much like the reed in a musical instrument.[8] It is important to note that relatively rapid airflow is needed to cause the flutter, and wheezing stops when the patient fatigues to the point that airflow is no longer rapid enough to vibrate the airway wall.

6. Paradoxic pulse (variation of the systolic pressure greater than 10 mm Hg caused by breathing efforts) can be caused by wide swings in intrathoracic pressure or by cardiac tamponade.[9,10] In this case the airway obstruction is requiring vigorous respiratory muscle effort, which causes large changes in intrathoracic pressure. Although this finding has been shown to occur in more severe cases of asthma,[15,16] its absence does not preclude severe airway obstruction.[7]

7. Accessory muscle usage occurs when the lung hyperinflation associated with asthma causes the diaphragm to become flattened and therefore less effective. Retraction of the sternomastoid muscle is a reliable sign of severe airway obstruction.[7]

8. The paradoxic breathing pattern is a sign of diaphragm fatigue.[17,18] It is recognized by inward movement of the abdomen during inspiration. Normally, diaphragm contraction pushes the abdominal contents downward and the anterior abdominal wall out during inspiration. Fatigue of the diaphragm allows it to be "sucked" upward into the chest when the accessory muscles create a negative intrathoracic pressure during inspiration.

9. Patients in respiratory distress who have developed diaphragmatic fatigue lean forward and brace themselves on their arms or elbows to stabilize the shoulder girdle and provide a better mechanical advantage for the accessory respiratory muscles.

10. The increased AP diameter is caused by air trapping, which occurs when partial airway obstruction is present in the medium to small bronchi.

11. Although cyanosis is not present, there are other clues that the patient is probably hypoxemic. The tachycardia, tachypnea, diaphoresis, restlessness, and wheezing suggest that oxygenation is not optimal.

LABORATORY EVALUATION

Chest Radiograph	*Shows moderate hyperexpansion with no evidence of infiltrates (Fig. 2–3).*
ABGs	*pH 7.38, $Paco_2$ 43 mm Hg, Pao_2 49 mm Hg on room air*
Spirometry	*FEV_1 1.5 liter (27 percent of predicted)* *Peak flow = 140 liter/minute* *Forced vital capacity (FVC) = 2.1 liters (40 percent of predicted)*
Hematology	*Results pending*

Questions

12. How would you interpret the ABG and spirometry results?
13. What treatment should be planned?
14. What are the possible medication side effects?
15. Should you leave the patient to go take care of other patients while you are waiting for other test results?
16. Should the patient be admitted?
17. How would you evaluate the patient's response to therapy?
18. What therapies should be avoided for this patient?

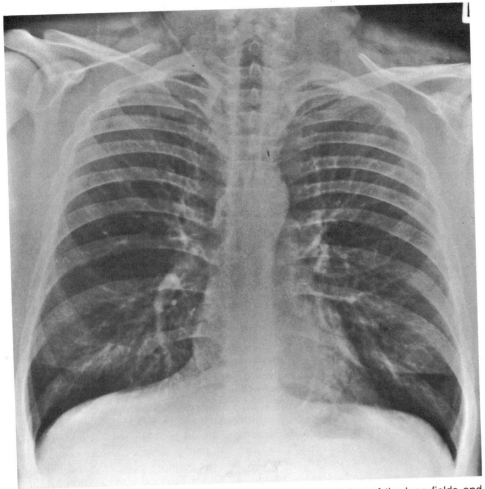

FIGURE 2–3 Chest radiograph demonstrating hyperinflation of the lung fields and no evidence of infiltrates.

19. If the patient fails to improve with conventional bronchodilators and corticosteroids, what other medication should be added to the treatment regimen?
20. When should mechanical ventilation be considered?

Answers

12. The ABG results suggest that the patient is tiring because the Pa_{CO_2} is now in the upper limits of normal. In most patients with asthma, the Pa_{CO_2} is reduced below normal until the patient becomes fatigued. The Pa_{O_2} of 49 mm Hg indicates moderate hypoxemia on room air. These ABG results would strongly suggest the need for mechanical ventilation if the patient had been receiving maximum treatment before the arterial sample was obtained.

    The spirometry results are consistent with an obstructive lung disease such as asthma. The peak flow of 140 liters/minute and FEV_1 of 1.5 liters indicate moderate obstruction. The significant reduction in the

FVC indicates air trapping, which is most likely in this case (but could indicate restrictive lung disease).

13. Treatment should include oxygen, aerosolized and intravenous bronchodilators, antibiotics, and hydration. Oxygen should be started at 4 to 6 liters/minute via nasal cannula or with 40 percent by entrainment mask and should be adjusted to keep the Sao_2 greater than 90 percent (or the Pao_2 in the 60 to 80 mm Hg range). Both β-adrenergic and xanthine types of bronchodilator should be administered. This is typically accomplished by administering aerosolized albuterol or other $β_2$-specific bronchodilator by a MDI or SVN and intravenous aminophylline. Aminophylline is given to achieve a blood level of 10 to 20 mg/liter. These may be supplemented by a subcutaneous injection of a β-agonist when a rapid peak effect is desired. High-dose parenteral corticosteroids should be started if the patient fails to respond adequately to β-adrenergic and xanthine bronchodilators. Intravenous fluids are given to establish optimum thinning of airway secretions. Antibiotics may be needed to treat the upper respiratory tract infection if evidence of bacterial infection exists (e.g., purulent sputum with numerous pus cells).

14. The bronchodilator can cause tachycardia, tremor, nausea, and dysrhythmias. Oxygen therapy is not likely to cause any side effects, as most asthmatic patients are not CO_2 retainers and do not depend on their hypoxic drive.

15. This patient should not be left unattended for any reason. The patient needs close monitoring and evaluation because respiratory failure could occur at any moment.

16. Unless the patient improves dramatically with treatment in the emergency room, she should be admitted to the intensive care unit (ICU). If she improves significantly in the emergency room she could be admitted to the pulmonary ward for treatment and observation (see Table 1–1).

17. The patient's response to therapy should be evaluated using the same techniques used for the initial assessment. It is important to monitor the sensorium as this will help evaluate the patient's condition and her ability to cooperate with treatment.[7] Other physical examination findings such as the degree of accessory muscle usage and the vital signs can also be very useful. Results of simple spirometry tests such as the FEV_1 or peak flow, or both, can provide objective data regarding the course of recovery. ABGs should be analyzed when the physical examination findings suggest a change in the patient's status.

18. In this patient, sedatives,[19] inhaled corticosteroids, cromolyn sodium, acetylcysteine, and dense aerosols should be avoided.[7] In the presence of airway obstruction, cromolyn sodium could be added to the treatment plan once bronchodilator therapy has stabilized lung function.[11,14] If this patient had had a history of hypertension, she may have been given an β-adrenergic antagonist that increases bronchospasm (e.g., Inderal). If this had been the case, she could have been given a trial of calcium channel blockers to treat the hypertension. Calcium channel blockers do not increase airway resistance.

19. Inhaled Atrovent or atropine could be added to her treatment plan if the more conventional bronchodilators are not effective. The effects of atropine are additive to those of the theophylline and the adrenergic agonists.[1,20]

20. Mechanical ventilation should be considered if the patient's mental status deteriorates significantly, especially if this is associated with a rising $Paco_2$ (see Table 1–1) despite bronchodilator and oxygen therapy. Once

mechanical ventilation is started, sedation can be used to make the patient more comfortable. Because the patient is alert and treatment has not been initiated, mechanical ventilation is not yet mandatory.

In the emergency room the patient was given oxygen via nasal cannula at 4 liters/minute. This resulted in the saturation improvement from 87 percent to 97 percent as obtained by pulse oximetry. An intravenous line was established to deliver aminophylline, steroids, fluids, and antibiotics. A loading dose of aminophylline 300 mg was given over 10 minutes. (This loading dose is based on the recommendation that 6 mg/kg of ideal body weight be given when the patient has not been taking oral theophylline.) Additionally, SVN treatment with 0.5 mL of albuterol diluted in 3 mL of saline was provided.

While this treatment resulted in improvement in the patient's dyspnea, the peak flow improved only slightly (150 liters/minute) and the patient continued to depend heavily on her accessory muscles to breathe. Based on the minimal improvement 1 hour after the initiation of bronchodilator therapy, it was decided to admit the patient for further care and close observation.

The patient was admitted to the respiratory ICU where the oxygen therapy, steroids, fluids, and aminophylline therapy were continued. The nebulized albuterol treatment was repeated. Ninety minutes after admission to the ICU ABG results revealed:

pH 7.43
$Paco_2$ 36 mm Hg
Pao_2 84 mm Hg
HCO_3^- 25 mEq/liter

Peak flow measurement at this point was 145 liters/minute. The clinical examination revealed polyphonic wheezing throughout exhalation, normal sensorium, respiratory rate of 32/minute, and pulse rate of 126/minute. Because it was determined that the patient responded only minimally to aerosolized bronchodilator and aminophylline, the attending physician started intravenous methylprednisolone with a bolus of 30 mg to be repeated every 4 to 6 hours. The Gram's stain revealed numerous pus cells and gram-positive organisms.

Questions

21. Should the use of methylprednisolone result in rapid improvement in the patient's airway obstruction?
22. What are the potential side effects of steroids?
23. Is this patient a candidate for continuous nebulization of bronchodilator?
24. Are any favorable prognostic signs present at this point?

Answers

21. The use of intravenous corticosteroids is not expected to result in rapid improvement in airway obstruction.[7] In most cases 4 to 6 hours is needed before significant improvement in peak flow or FEV_1 can be expected.
22. The potential systemic side effects of high-dose oral corticosteroids taken for prolonged periods of time are significant. Depletion of bone calcium, impairment of immunologic response, increased fat cell production and deposition in the subcutaneous tissues of the neck and trunk, and hypertension are commonly associated with long-term use of systemic steroids. With the use of aerosolized corticosteroids, candidiasis (oral thrush) and dysphonia can occur.[1] Because the patient in this

case is expected to need only a short course of intravenous steroids, these side effects are not of concern at this point.

23. This patient could be a candidate for continuous nebulization therapy for the administration of an aerosolized bronchodilator. This therapy has been shown to be safe and effective for the treatment of acute asthma in children[12,13] and adults. Continuous nebulization of a bronchodilator has been suggested as a treatment alternative to intermittent therapy because the continuous administration could allow more optimal delivery of nebulized medication. Prolonged inhalation should promote better distribution of the aerosolized drug and a more consistent topical administration of the bronchodilator to the bronchial smooth muscle. To avoid toxic side effects, a more diluted solution of the medication should be used; the dose typically given in a 15-minute treatment is thus given over 1 hour. In addition, bronchodilators with a more specific β_2 response such as terbutaline and salbutamol are recommended to avoid cardiac side effects (e.g., tachycardia, palpitations).

Continuous nebulization therapy appears to be indicated in asthmatic patients with impending respiratory failure not responding optimally to conventional therapy. More studies need to be conducted to identify the role of this therapy in severe cases of asthma and the exact criteria for its use.

24. The improvement in arterial P_{O_2} and P_{CO_2} is a favorable prognostic sign.[7]

Over the next 24 hours the patient steadily improved. The patient's peak flow improved to 220 liters/minute the next day and her vital signs returned to nearly normal. The wheezing improved so that it was heard only during the latter half of exhalation, and the use of accessory muscles was minimal at this point. The patient was transferred to the general floor for maintenance therapy and evaluation of prophylactic therapy.

The remainder of the patient's hospital stay was uneventful and she was discharged 3 days later with a follow-up outpatient appointment in 2 weeks. The patient was discharged on a regimen of oral antibiotics and an MDI bronchodilator (albuterol). She was counseled on the avoidance of dust inhalation, how to recognize and what to do in response to respiratory infections, and how to use the MDI bronchodilator. She was advised to use the MDI before anticipated heavy exercise.

REFERENCES

1. Woolcock, AJ: Asthma. In Murray, JF and Nadel, JA (eds): Textbook of Respiratory Medicine. WB Saunders, Philadelphia, 1988, pp 1030–1068.

2. Rebuck, AS and Read, J: Assessment and management of severe asthma. Am J Med 51:788, 1971.

3. Kelsen, SG, et al: Emergency room assessment and treatment of patients with acute asthma: Adequacy of the conventional approach. Am J Med 64:622, 1978.

4. Shim, CS and Williams, MH Jr: Relationship of wheezing to the severity of obstruction in asthma. Arch Intern Med 143:890, 1983.

5. McFadden, ER Jr, Kiser, R, and DeGroot, WJ: Acute bronchial asthma: Relations between clinical and physiologic manifestations. N Engl J Med 288:221, 1973.

6. George, RB: Monitoring of patients during asthma attacks. In Lavietes, M and Reichman, LB (eds): Diagnostic aspects and management of asthma. Purdue Frederick, Norwalk, CT, 1981.

7. George, RB: Management of the acute asthma attack. In Bone, RC, George, RB, and

Hudson, LD (eds): Acute Respiratory Failure. New York, Churchill Livingstone, 1987, pp 143–154.

8.   Forgacs, P: The functional basis of pulmonary sounds. Chest 73:399, 1978.

9.   Henkind, SJ, Benis, AM, and Teichholz, LE: The paradox of pulsus paradoxus. Am Heart J 114:198, 1987.

10.   Rebuck, AS and Pengelly, LD: Development of pulsus paradoxus in the presence of airway obstruction. N Engl J Med 288:66, 1973.

11.   Canny, GJ and Levison, H: Aerosols—therapeutic use and delivery in childhood asthma. Ann Allergy 60:11, 1988.

12.   Moler, FW, Hurwitz, E, and Custer, JR: Improvement in clinical asthma score and PaCO2 in children with severe asthma treated with continuously nebulized terbutaline. J Allergy Clin Immunol 81:1101, 1988.

13.   Portnow, J and Aggarwal, J: Continuous terbutaline nebulization for the treatment of severe exacerbation of asthma in children. Ann Allergy 60:368, 1988.

14.   Blumenthal, MN, et al: A multicenter evaluation of the clinical benefits of cromolyn sodium aerosol by metered-dose inhaler in the treatment of asthma. J Allergy Clin Immunol 81:681, 1988.

15.   Shim, C and Williams, MH, Jr: Pulsus paradoxus in asthma. Lancet 1:530, 1978.

16.   Knowles, GK and Clark, TJH: Pulsus paradoxus as a valuable sign indicating severity of asthma. Lancet 2:1356, 1973.

17.   Mier-Jedrezejawicz, A, et al: Assessment of diaphragm weakness. Am Rev Respir Dis 137:877, 1988.

18.   Cohen, CA, et al: Clinical manifestations of inspiratory muscle fatigue. Am J Med 73:308, 1982.

19.   Neder, GA, et al: Death in status asthmaticus: Role of sedation. Dis Chest 44:263, 1963.

20.   Brady, RE and Easton, JG: The value of atropine in the documentation of reversible airways obstruction. Ann Allergy 42:211, 1979.

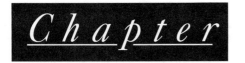

Chapter 3

Robert L. Wilkins, MA, RRT
James R. Dexter, MD, FCCP

CHRONIC BRONCHITIS

INTRODUCTION

Chronic bronchitis is a pulmonary disease in which the patient has a chronically productive cough due to inflamed bronchi. Because the term "chronic" is open to different interpretations, most experts have agreed on specific criteria with regard to time the productive cough has been present (at least three consecutive months of the year for two successive years) to make the diagnosis. In a patient with a chronic productive cough, other potential causes of this problem such as tuberculosis, lung cancer, and congestive heart failure must be excluded before the diagnosis of chronic bronchitis can be made.

This chapter on chronic bronchitis and the following one on emphysema present two components of a commonly encountered problem today known as chronic obstructive pulmonary disease (COPD). COPD occurs worldwide and is a major cause of death and disability in adults. Although it is true that the majority of patients with COPD have a combination of emphysema and chronic bronchitis, for teaching purposes we present these two components separately. A third condition that some experts include under the heading of COPD is asthma (Fig. 3–1). Chapter 2 provides background information and a case presentation on asthma.

ETIOLOGY

The most important factor contributing to the onset of chronic bronchitis is cigarette smoking.[1] Compared with nonsmokers, cigarette smokers have a more rapid decline in lung function[2-4] and a higher incidence of respiratory infections, chronic bronchitis, and emphysema. The differences between smokers and nonsmokers in terms of lung function increase as the quantity of cigarette consumption increases.[1] Pipe and cigar smokers have morbidity and mortality rates for COPD higher than nonsmokers but not as high as cigarette smokers.[1]

Because nonsmokers rarely develop chronic bronchitis, it appears that factors other than smoking are much less important causes of chronic bronchitis.[1] Other factors may, however, be important in the overall decline of the chronic bronchitis patient's clinical condition. Infection (viral or bacterial), air pollution, occupational exposure to irritants, and the like, may play a key role in the exacerbation of the patient with chronic bronchitis.

FIGURE 3-1 Schema of chronic obstructive pulmonary disease. A nonproportional Venn diagram shows subsets of patients with chronic bronchitis, emphysema, and asthma in three overlapping circles. Subset of patients lying within the rectangle have airway obstruction. Patients with asthma, subset 9, are defined as having completely reversible airway obstruction and lie entirely within the rectangle; their diagnosis is unequivocal. Patients in subsets 6 and 7 have reversible airway obstruction with chronic productive cough or emphysema, respectively. Patients in subset 8 have features of all three disorders. It may be difficult to be certain whether patients in subsets 6 and 8 indeed have asthma or whether they have developed bronchial hyperactivity as a complication of chronic bronchitis or emphysema; the history helps. Patients in subset 3 have chronic productive cough with airway obstruction but no emphysema; it is not known how large this subset is because epidemiologic studies are not available using computed tomographic (CT) scan, the most sensitive in vivo imaging technique for diagnosing or excluding emphysema. It is much easier to identify patients with emphysema in the chest radiograph who do not have chronic bronchitis (subset 4). Most patients who require medical care for their disease fall into subsets 5 and 8. Patients in subsets 1 and 2 do not have airway obstruction, as determined by the FEV_1, but have clinical or radiographic features of chronic bronchitis or emphysema, respectively. Because chronic obstructive pulmonary disease (COPD), when defined as a process, does not have airway obstruction as a defining characteristic, and because pure asthma is not included in the term COPD, patient subsets 1 through 8 are included within the area outlined by the shaded band that denotes COPD. (From Snider, GL: Chronic bronchitis and emphysema. In Murray, JF and Nadel, JA: Textbook of Respiratory Medicine. WB Saunders, Philadelphia, p 1071, 1988, with permission.)

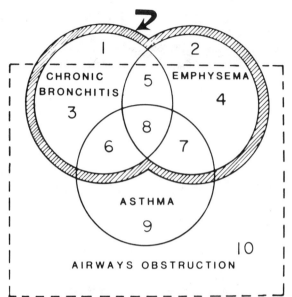

PATHOLOGY AND PATHOPHYSIOLOGY

Chronic cigarette smoking causes the airways to undergo a variety of pathologic changes. The bronchial mucous glands enlarge (hypertrophy) and the goblet cells increase in number,[1,5] resulting in an abnormal increase in mucus production. The increased mucus is hardly noticeable early in the disease, but as exposure to cigarette smoke continues the airways produce ever-increasing amounts of mucus. The bronchial walls often become inflamed and lose cilia either as a result of exposure to smoke or as a complication of airway infection. The combination of excessive mucus production and reduced ciliary function leads to mucus plugging of the smaller airways. Many patients with chronic bronchitis also develop emphysematous changes in the lung (see Chapter 4).

The patient with chronic bronchitis may have only a minimal increase in airway resistance. With more complicated disease the flow through the larger bronchi is abnormally low owing to the inflammation and excessive mucus. Mucus plugging and airway obstruction cause ventilation-perfusion ratio ($\dot{V}/\dot{Q}$) mismatching. This leads to significant changes in gas exchange such as hypoxemia.

In response to the hypoxemia, the pulmonary vasculature constricts (hypoxic vasoconstriction). Acidosis adds to the contraction of smooth muscles in the pulmonary blood vessels.[6] This added resistance to blood flow through the pulmonary circulatory system puts an abnormally high workload on the right side of the heart. The added workload causes the right ventricle gradually to dilate. If the problem continues for many months or years, the right ventricle will not be able to continue effectively pumping blood through the pulmonary circulation. This results in right heart failure caused by chronic lung disease and is known as **cor pulmonale.**[7]

CLINICAL FEATURES

Medical History

Patients with chronic bronchitis essentially always acknowledge chronic cough and sputum production. In many patients the onset of these symptoms is very gradual and, as a result, the patient may not consider these symptoms serious or be able to identify the date of onset. Typically the patient seeks medical attention when either a superimposed acute problem such as infection is present or when the chronic problem is severe enough to cause concern. Dyspnea is often present during acute episodes of exacerbation but may not be a primary symptom when the patient is stable.

Mucus is typically white or mucoid, or both, in patients with stable chronic bronchitis. With the onset of infection, the mucus changes to yellow-green and appears thick and purulent. The change in color of mucus may also occur with allergic reactions and when stagnation of secretions within the airways is a problem. As a result, microscopic examination of the sputum sample will help determine the cause of the change in mucus character.

Hemoptysis (coughing up blood from the lung) may occur in patients with chronic bronchitis.[1] Airway inflammation, coughing, and infection can contribute to the rupture of superficial blood vessels in the bronchi. This may result in blood-streaked sputum.

The patient's smoking history is frequently positive when chronic bronchitis is present. The interviewer should report the smoking history with regard to the age when the patient started smoking, how many packs of cigarettes are typically smoked each day, any attempts to stop smoking, and duration of periods in which the patient refrained from smoking. It is also important to report the use of other forms of tobacco such as pipes and cigars.

The family history is often positive for COPD, as the tendency to acquire this disease appears to be genetically transferable.[8] The occupational history should be obtained to identify any significant exposure to dusts or fumes in the workplace.

Physical Examination

In patients with mild, stable chronic bronchitis, no significant findings are discovered during the physical examination. With more severe disease or during acute exacerbations, numerous findings are typically revealed. Fever may indicate that an infection is present. Chest examination may reveal use of accessory muscles with a prolonged expiratory phase. Heavy use of accessory muscles indicates a more severe case of airway obstruction. Coarse crackles and expiratory wheezes and rhonchi are often present during auscultation. The coarse crackles indicate excessive airway secretions and the expiratory wheezes or rhonchi suggest airway obstruction. A loud pulmonic valve closer is typically heard when pulmonary hypertension is present. The examiner may refer to this abnormal heart sound as a "loud

P$_2$," suggesting that the pulmonic component of the second heart sound is abnormally loud. Jugular venous distension may be present, suggesting cor pulmonale. Pedal edema and hepatomegaly (enlarged liver) are often present when cor pulmonale complicates the case. The right ventricular hypertrophy associated with cor pulmonale may result in a heave (systolic pulsation) at the left sternal border.

Cyanosis of the tongue and mucous membranes is often present in patients with complicated cases of chronic bronchitis, and suggests significant hypoxemia. With severe hypoxemia and hypercapnia the patient typically develops disturbances in consciousness.

Laboratory Evaluation

The complete blood count (CBC) generally reveals an elevated red blood cell count if chronic hypoxemia is present. The white blood cell count may increase if an infectious process such as pneumonia is occurring. Otherwise the CBC is not significantly abnormal in most patients with chronic bronchitis.

The arterial blood gases (ABGs) are very useful to assess the oxygenation and acid-base status. Typically, with mild chronic bronchitis ABGs are normal. With acute exacerbations complicating more advanced disease, hypoxemia is often severe and respiratory acidosis is commonly seen. If the respiratory acidosis has been present chronically, compensatory elevation of serum bicarbonate occurs and the pH is within normal limits.

The chest radiograph does not demonstrate obvious abnormalities in stable or mild cases of chronic bronchitis. In more severe cases, as during an exacerbation, the chest radiograph may demonstrate hyperinflation and increased lung markings. The increased lung markings refer to the radiologist's ability to identify airway walls within the chest that have enlarged as a result of bronchial wall thickening. The chest radiograph may demonstrate an enlarged right heart when cor pulmonale is present. The chest radiograph must be inspected for evidence of complications such as pneumonia in any patient with acute exacerbation of chronic bronchitis.

Pulmonary function studies are useful in quantifying the severity of the disease and in identifying the response to therapy. In mild chronic bronchitis the routine pulmonary function study results are typically normal. With more significant disease measurements of expiratory flow and vital capacity decrease and residual volume increases. If bronchospasm is also present the expiratory flow rates may improve with bronchodilator therapy. The total lung capacity and diffusion capacity are usually normal in patients with chronic bronchitis. Complete pulmonary function studies should be done only when the patient is clinically stable. An electrocardiogram (ECG) may demonstrate right-axis deviation if cor pulmonale is present. The right-axis deviation is seen as a negative (downward) deflection of the QRS complex in lead I.

TREATMENT

Treatment of chronic bronchitis has two general goals: (1) to treat any superimposed acute medical problem such as congestive heart failure (CHF), pneumonia, or bronchospasm; and (2) to attempt to slow the progress of the chronic bronchitis. Treating a superimposed medical problem initially requires identification of the problem. Once identified, the physician can begin appropriate treatment (e.g., Lasix for CHF or antibiotics for pneumonia). This alone may significantly improve the clinical condition of the patient.

Long-term care is aimed at smoking cessation and medications such as bronchodilators to improve lung function. The best way to affect the course of chronic bronchitis favorably is to stop smoking. Smoking cessation appears to improve lung function significantly, even if the patient stops later in life.[2] The risk of smoking-related diseases such as lung cancer is reduced with smoking cessation and continues to drop as abstinence is maintained.[9] For these reasons, the patient should be strongly encouraged to quit smoking. The patient is more likely to stop smoking if the health care professionals provide counseling and support in addition to warning the patient about the health hazards associated with smoking.[10] Appropriate use of nicotine polacrilex (nicotine gum) and transdermal nicotine patches can be helpful in decreasing symptoms of smoking withdrawal but must be combined with counseling to obtain maximum results.[10]

Antibiotics, sympathomimetics, xanthines (theophylline), and corticosteroids may prove useful when infection and acute bronchospasm are present. Postural drainage may be useful when sputum retention is a problem. Oxygen is useful during exacerbations of chronic bronchitis to correct acute hypoxemia. Long-term supplemental oxygen therapy is needed when the patient's PaO_2 is below 55 mm Hg while breathing room air during stable condition. Evidence of cor pulmonale (e.g., jugular venous distention) also suggests that home oxygen therapy may be of benefit. Monitoring the patient for improvement in dyspnea, wheezing, vital signs, and breathing pattern will indicate the effectiveness of the therapy.

Case Study

HISTORY

JL is a 54-year-old white man currently employed as machinist. He was seen in the pulmonary outpatient clinic for the first time complaining of shortness of breath with exertion and a productive cough. JL stated that his coughing had increased recently and was productive of thick yellow sputum. He stated that his cough had been present for several years but was "usually not a problem." His cough was usually productive of clear to white sputum, mostly in the morning. He had recently noticed more than usual shortness of breath and was now dyspneic at rest. JL did admit to feeling warm at times during the past few days but had not taken his temperature with a thermometer. He denied chest pain, hemoptysis, sinusitis, weight loss, allergies, or recurrent lung diseases such as asthma.

JL admitted to smoking 2½ packs of cigarettes per day for the past 30 years. He attempted to stop on several occasions but was successful for no longer than 3 or 4 months. His machinist work has exposed him to many potentially toxic fumes. His family history is positive for lung disease, as his father died of emphysema at age 64 years, 12 years earlier. His mother is alive and well at age 75. His sister is healthy at age 47; his brother has diabetes at age 51.

Questions

1. What medical problems are suggested by the medical history and what is (are) the key symptom(s) to explore?
2. What is the significance of the patient's sputum color?
3. What is JL's smoking history in pack-years?
4. What is the significance of the family and occupational history?
5. What should the physical examination accomplish at this point in the assessment of the patient?

Answers

1. The patient's medical history suggests chronic bronchitis exacerbated by a respiratory infection such as acute bronchitis, flu, or pneumonia. Congestive heart failure is a less likely cause for the exacerbation. JL's shortness of breath needs evaluation. The interviewer should determine the severity of the dyspnea by asking about the degree to which the dyspnea

limits JL's daily routine. The changes in JL's dyspnea over the past years and factors that trigger the dyspnea are important in evaluating prognosis and avoiding exacerbation of the disease.

2. Uncomplicated chronic bronchitis most often causes clear or opaque sputum. Infection will most often cause the sputum to turn colored, but allergic reactions may also result in thick yellow-green sputum.

3. JL's smoking history in pack-years is 75 pack-years (2.5 packs per day $\times$ 30 years = 75 pack-years).

4. JL's family history is significant, given that his father died of emphysema. It appears that the tendency for COPD is genetically transferable from parent to child.[8] The occupational exposure to irritant gases as a machinist may have also increased his risk for lung disease.

5. The physical examination should help determine whether pulmonary dysfunction is present; the cause of the symptoms, the severity of JL's current pulmonary dysfunction, and the presence specifically of cyanosis, cor pulmonale, pneumonia, bronchospasm, and CHF. The clinician can accomplish this by assessing the patient's vital signs, sensorium, breath sounds, respiratory pattern, heart sounds, ankle edema, and other parameters.

PHYSICAL EXAMINATION

General   *JL is alert and oriented but in moderate respiratory distress. His speech is presented in choppy sentences because of his dyspnea and frequent coughing, which is productive of thick yellow sputum.*

Vital Signs   *Temperature is 38.1°C; respiratory rate 26/minute; blood pressure 144/90 mm Hg; pulse 120/minute.*

HEENT   *Tongue and mucous membranes slightly cyanotic; pupils equal, round, and reactive to light and accommodation (PERRLA); sinuses nontender to palpation*

Neck   *Trachea midline and mobile; transmitted wheezes present but no stridor present; carotid pulses + + bilaterally with no bruits; jugular venous distension (JVD) noted with head of bed elevated to a 45-degree angle; accessory muscles in the neck tense with each inspiratory effort*

Chest   *AP diameter large and chest wall excursion small; chest percussion reveals decreased resonance over the right lower lobe; auscultation over lungs reveals bilateral expiratory polyphonic wheezes louder on the right side; over right lower lobe coarse crackles and bronchial breath sounds present*

Heart   *Regular rhythm with rate of 120; no murmurs or rubs noted. Auscultation over the pulmonic area reveals an S_3 gallop and a loud P_2; systolic heave is noted at the left sternal border: the PMI located in fifth intercoastal space at midclavicular line on left*

Abdomen   *Soft, nontender; hepatomegaly present and hepatojugular reflex positive; no evidence of paradoxic breathing*

Extremities   *No evidence of cyanosis or clubbing; pedal edema present and 2+ bilaterally in the lower extremities up to knee level; extremities warm to touch*

Questions

6. How do you interpret the vital signs?
7. What is indicated by cyanosis of the tongue and mucous membranes?
8. What are the possible causes of the expiratory polyphonic wheezes heard bilaterally and the bronchial breath sounds heard over the right lower lobe?
9. What is suggested by the loud P_2?
10. What pathophysiology could be causing the JVD, hepatomegaly, hepatojugular reflex, and pedal edema?
11. How is the hepatojugular reflex identified?
12. How is the severity of the pedal edema characterized?
13. What is the significance of the systolic heave located at the left sternal border?
14. What is indicated by use of the accessory respiratory muscles of the neck tensing with each inspiratory effort?

Answers

6. The patient's body temperature is slightly elevated. Infections, either viral or bacterial, may cause fever. Fever increases the patient's oxygen consumption and places an increased demand on the cardiac and respiratory systems to meet this extra demand. The respiratory and heart rates are slightly elevated which may be related to the fever or to the hypoxemia, or to both. Tachycardia and tachypnea help meet the increased need for oxygen consumption and CO_2 excretion associated with fever and help compensate for hypoxemia when present.
7. Cyanosis of the tongue and mucous membranes of the mouth indicates central cyanosis. Central cyanosis is caused by hypoxemia, which turns the arterial blood dark. Polycythemia makes cyanosis more visible, and anemia makes it difficult to recognize.
8. The expiratory polyphonic wheezes may be produced by bronchospasm, mucosal edema, and/or excessive airway secretions. Intrathoracic airways tend to narrow slightly on exhalation owing to the additive effects of positive intrathoracic pressure and the retractile forces of elastic fibers within the airway walls. When the airways are obstructed because of bronchospasm, edema, or secretions, exhalation may cause severe narrowing that results in expiratory wheezes. Polyphonic wheezes suggest partial obstruction of many small airways rather than one large upper airway.
   The bronchial breath sounds suggest consolidation in the right lower lobe. Normal lung tissue acts as a filter to sound, allowing only low-pitched sounds to pass. Consolidated lung allows the turbulent flow sounds of the larger airways to pass through the lung without significant alteration. In such cases, the normal vesicular breath sound is replaced with a louder, higher-pitched, bronchial type of breath sound over the area of the consolidated lung.
9. The loud P_2 suggests pulmonary hypertension. The pulmonary circulation pressures increase as the capillary smooth muscle constricts in response to hypoxemia. Eventually collagen tissue replaces the muscle, causing irreversible pulmonary hypertension. The increase in pulmonary artery pressure causes the pulmonic valve to close more loudly than it would under normal conditions. A loud P_2 is best heard in the pulmonic area, which is located at the second left intercostal space near the sternal border (Fig. 3–2).

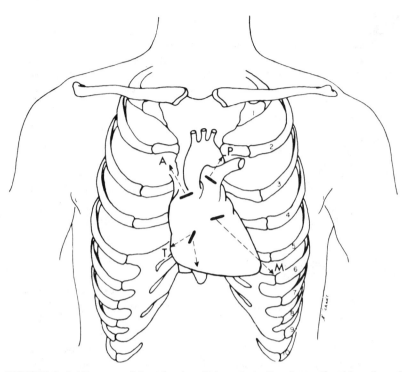

FIGURE 3–2 Diagram of the chest wall demonstrating the optimal locations for auscultating the various components of the heart sounds. The pulmonic valve is best heard over the second left intercostal space near the sternum and is known as the pulmonic area. The aortic valve is best heard in the second intercostal space on the right near the sternal border. This area is known as the aortic area. The mitral and tricuspid valves are loudest over the apex of the heart. (From Prior, JA and Silberstein, JS: Physical Examination: The History and Examination of the Patient, ed 6. CV Mosby, St Louis, 1982, p 267, with permission.)

10. JVD, hepatomegaly, pedal edema, and the hepatojugular reflex are typically caused by right heart failure. Right heart failure may be the result of left heart failure, acute severe pulmonary embolism, or chronic hypoxemia. Right heart failure allows filling pressures of the right heart to increase and all venous pressures rise. High venous pressures result in distended neck veins, an engorged swollen liver, and an accumulation of fluid in the lower extremities.

11. Right heart failure increases venous pressure and causes liver engorgement. If pressure in the neck veins appears to increase while the physician is pressing gently but firmly on the right upper quadrant of the patient's abdomen, the hepatojugular reflex is present. The presence of this reflex is consistent with right heart failure.

12. The severity of the edema is graded on a scale of 1+ through 4+ on the basis of pitting produced by sustained, light pressure applied by the examiner over the tissue being examined.[11] Minimal pitting edema is indicated as 1+, whereas 4+ suggests severe pitting edema that weeps when the examiner presses on the edematous tissue. In this case, 2+ pitting edema indicates a moderate degree of ankle edema. The level to which the edema extends up the lower extremities also indicates the severity of the right heart failure. In this case the edema is at the level

of the knees, which implies moderate disease. When the edema extends higher, more severe heart failure is present.

13. A heave at the left sternal border is usually produced by contraction of an enlarged right ventricle. Right ventricular hypertrophy often occurs when the right heart pumps against high pressures for many months (much like the biceps of a compulsive weight lifter). The heave at the sternal border along with the JVD, hepatomegaly, loud P_2, and pedal edema are evidence of cor pulmonale.[12] The right ventricular heave and loud P_2 may be difficult to identify when significant hyperinflation of the lungs is present and the AP chest diameter is large. These findings of right heart failure suggest that the patient has had hypoxemia for many months or years.

14. Use of the accessory muscles of respiration indicates that the patient has great difficulty breathing. This is a common finding in patients with acute or chronic obstructive lung disease and provides an objective parameter to monitor the patient's response to therapy because the accessory muscles become less active as the airway obstruction resolves. In cases of airway obstruction not responsive to therapy (e.g., emphysema), the use of accessory muscles will continue despite therapy.

LABORATORY EVALUATION ============

Chest Radiograph: *(Fig. 3–3)*

Arterial Blood Gases (ABGs):   *pH 7.41*
PaCO$_2$ 44 mm Hg
PaO$_2$ 45 mm Hg on room air
Bicarbonate 28 mEq
P(A-a) o$_2$ 53 mm Hg
O$_2$ content 16.4 mL

CBC

	Observed	Normal
White blood cells	16,100	4–11,000/cu mm
Red blood cells	5.7	4.1–5.5 million/cu mm
Hemoglobin	17.5	14–16.5 g
Hematocrit	56%	37–50%
Segmented neutrophils	77%	38–79%
Bands	10%	0–7%
Lymphocytes	10%	12–51%
Eosinophils	1%	0–8%
Monocytes	1%	0–10

Chemistry: All within normal limits except for the CO$_2$, which is slightly elevated at 34 mEq/liter.

Questions

15. How significant is the chest radiograph in determining the cause of the patient's symptoms? What does it show to be the underlying condition of the patient's respiratory system?

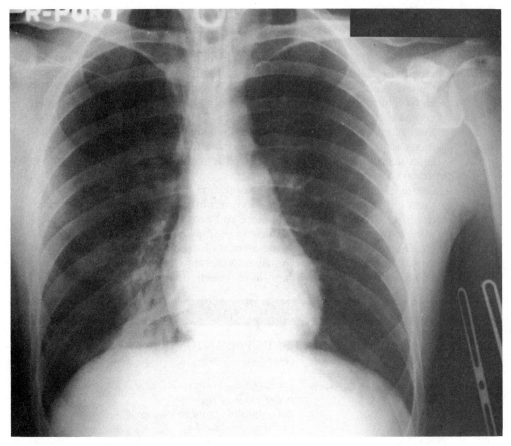

FIGURE 3–3 Chest radiograph taken a few hours after admission.

16. How do you interpret the ABGs?
17. Should complete pulmonary function testing be done at this point?
18. How do you interpret the CBC? What could be causing the elevated white cell count? What is the most likely cause of the elevated red cell count?
19. What is the tentative diagnosis, and should the patient be admitted?
20. What other diagnostic procedures should be ordered at this point?
21. What therapy should the physician order for the patient?

Answers

15. The chest radiograph is very significant, as it demonstrates an infiltrate typical of pneumonia in the right lower lobe. Respiratory infections are a common cause of exacerbation in patients with COPD.[13]
16. The ABG measurements reveal moderate hypoxemia on room air. This is a common finding in COPD patients, especially when an infection is present. The acid-base status shows both respiratory acidosis and metabolic alkalosis. Because the body never completely compensates for an acid-base disturbance and the pH is 7.41, there must be two simultaneous primary disturbances. It is possible that this patient's "normal" Pa_{CO_2} is above 45 mm Hg and is compensated for by an elevation of blood bicarbonate. When an acute problem such as pneumonia occurs, significant hypoxemia may drive the patient's respiratory system to

increase ventilation. This may result in a relative hyperventilation, with the Pa_{CO_2} decreasing back to a more normal range. This causes an acute respiratory alkalosis (even though the P_{CO_2} is normal) superimposed on a chronic respiratory acidosis. If the patient had vomiting associated with his other symptoms, he may also have developed an acute metabolic alkalosis.

17. This is not a good time to have the patient perform additional pulmonary function testing, as he is acutely ill. After his condition has stabilized, complete pulmonary function testing will provide a better indication of his pulmonary disease.

18. The CBC reveals elevated white and red cell counts. The leukocytosis is probably in response to the infiltrate seen on the chest radiograph. The elevation of the bands is known as a left shift, which indicates that immature white blood cells are being released by the bone marrow in response to the acute infection. The elevated red cell count indicates that polycythemia is present. This abnormality may be secondary to a chronically low oxygen tension in the arterial blood. Polycythemia helps to compensate for the hypoxemia by increasing the carrying capacity of the blood for oxygen. Unfortunately, it also increases cardiac work by increasing blood viscosity. Many pulmonary physicians will phlebotomize patients to a hematocrit of 55 percent to decrease right heart workload and to prevent red blood cell slugging and arteriolar obstruction.

19. The tentative diagnosis is acute exacerbation of chronic bronchitis caused by pneumonia and right heart failure. The patient should be admitted for close monitoring, intravenous (IV) bronchodilators, steroids, antibiotics, and possible phlebotomy.

20. Sputum analysis with a Gram's stain and culture may be helpful in determining the cause of the pneumonia. An ECG may be helpful in ruling out cardiac ischemia.

21. Appropriate therapy for the patient at this point would include oxygen, antibiotics, bronchodilators, and steroids.

The patient was admitted to the pulmonary care unit. The physician wrote orders for the following:

1. *Oxygen by nasal cannula 2 liters/minute*
2. *Medication nebulizer with albuterol (Ventolin/Proventil) 0.5 mL in 3.0 mL of normal saline every 4 hours*
3. *Solu-Medrol 125 mg IV every 6 hours*
4. *Aminophylline 1000 mg in 250 mL of normal saline with a rate of 10 to 15 mL/hour*
5. *Ampicillin 500 mg IV piggyback every 6 hours*
6. *ECG*
7. *Daily theophylline blood levels*
8. *Sputum Gram's stain, culture, and sensitivity*

Questions

22. What is the goal of oxygen therapy in this case? What level of arterial oxygenation is appropriate? How should the oxygen therapy be evaluated? Once this patient is stable and ready to go home, should he be sent home with a regimen of oxygen therapy?

23. What abnormalities on the ECG demonstrate right-axis deviation? What does this abnormality indicate?
24. What type of bronchodilator is albuterol, and what are the possible side effects of this medication?
25. What parameters should the respiratory care practitioner (RCP) monitor before, during, and after administration of the medication nebulizer treatments? Should the RCP recommend metered-dose inhaler to the physician for the patient's use in place of the medication nebulizer? Why or why not?
26. How should the overall effectiveness of the bronchodilators be evaluated?
27. What should the RCP do to improve the chances of obtaining an appropriate sputum sample for analysis?
28. What is the most important advice this patient's physician could give him with regard to his long-term respiratory health?

Answers

22. The goal of oxygen therapy is to correct the hypoxemia. A Pao_2 of 55 to 65 mm Hg is an appropriate level of oxgyenation in this case. The hemoglobin is more than 90 percent saturated under most conditions at a partial pressure of about 60 mm Hg. Elevating the Pao_2 above 65 mm Hg does not add significant oxygen content to the arterial blood but does slightly increase the risk of oxygen-induced hypoventilation.

    The RCP should evaluate the oxygen therapy by using a combination of parameters. Pulse oximetry is useful when changes in ventilation and therefore Pco_2 are not likely. The patient's mild hypoventilation makes it important to titrate the Fio_2 to result in an Sao_2 of 90 percent and to check ABGs to evaluate ventilatory and acid-base status. The patient's clinical condition also can provide clues regarding the effectiveness of oxygen therapy. Correcting the hypoxemia may cause the patient to feel less dyspnea and may improve the cyanosis, tachycardia, and tachypnea.

    The clinical findings consistent with cor pulmonale strongly suggest that this patient would benefit from home oxygen therapy. If the patient's resting room air Pao_2 is less than 55 mm Hg at the time of discharge, home oxygen should be arranged. If the patient's resting Pao_2 is just above 55 mm Hg, nocturnal desaturation may be demonstrated by nocturnal pulse oximetry monitoring and would indicate the need for oxygen during sleep.
23. The negative deflection of the P and QRS waves in lead I is consistent with right-axis deviation. This finding is typical for patients with cor pulmonale.[14] Normally the mean axis of electrical activity for the heart is between 0 and +90 degrees. With pulmonary hypertension, enlargement of the right side of the heart causes the mean axis to shift to the right somewhere between +90 and +180 degrees (Fig. 3–4).
24. Albuterol (Ventolin) is a sympathomimetic bronchodilator that has fewer side effects than isoproterenol.[15] It is available in oral, IV, or aerosol forms. When administered by aerosol it produces significant bronchodilatation within 15 minutes and continues to cause bronchodilatation for 3 to 4 hours.[16] Although cardiovascular side effects such as tachycardia, tremors, nervousness, and palpitations are possible with all β-agonists, they are less common in patients using this medication.
25. RCPs should monitor the patient's vital signs, breath sounds, sensorium, breathing pattern, and symptoms before, during, and after the treatment.

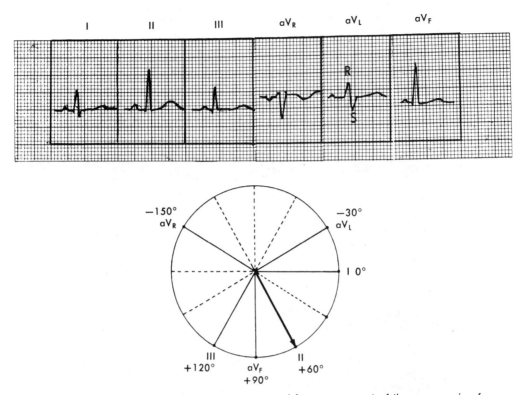

FIGURE 3–4 Hexaxial reference system used for assessment of the mean axis of electrical activity of the heart. Normal axis is between 0 and +90 degrees. Left-axis deviation exists when the mean axis is between 0 and −90 degrees. Right-axis deviation is present when the axis is between +90 and +180 degrees. To identify the axis, examine the limb leads to identify the lead with the largest (either positive or negative) deflection from baseline. Next use the hexaxial reference system to identify the position in the circle of the lead with the largest QRS complex. If the QRS complex is upright (positive) in the lead with the most voltage, the mean axis must be very close to the position of this lead on the circle. If the QRS complex is downward (negative), the mean axis must be located in the opposite direction from the location of this lead on the hexaxial circle. In this example the axis is located at +60 because lead II displays the most voltage and is upright. (From Goldberger, AL and Goldberger, E: Clinical Electrocardiography, ed 3. CV Mosby, St Louis, 1986, p 62, with permission.)

Changes in these parameters will help assess the effectiveness of therapy and the onset of complications.

26. The patient's dyspnea should improve if the bronchodilators are proving beneficial. Changes in his breath sounds that indicate bronchodilatation include a decrease in the pitch, length, and intensity of the wheezing.[17] Changes in the patient's breathing pattern with less use of accessory muscles and a shorter expiratory time also indicate improvement.

27. The RCP obtaining the sputum sample should explain the procedure to the patient, emphasizing that a true sample of phlegm from the lungs is needed. Asking the patient to rinse his mouth and brush his teeth just before obtaining the sample is a useful way of reducing the contamination of the sputum by oral bacteria. The sample should be collected in a sterile sputum cup and then transported to the laboratory with the

lid tightly in place. The patient's name and identification number must be secured to the container.

28. The best advice health care personnel can give this patient is to *stop smoking!* This advice is easy to give but not as easy for the patient to follow. Many patients may, however, stop smoking upon the firm recommendation of their physician. The physician should explain to JL that if he stops smoking, significant improvement in lung function may be attained.[2] The American Lung Association and American Cancer Society have excellent smoking cessation programs.

Over the next several days JL steadily improved. His initial ABG analysis revealed a Pao$_2$ of 66 mm Hg on 2 liters/minute of oxygen by nasal cannula. His dyspnea improved to the point that he could walk around the unit without significant difficulty by the third hospital day. On the fifth day, he was discharged with a regimen of oral antibiotics and oxygen. The attending physician requested an appointment with JL at the pulmonary outpatient clinic in 1 week.

REFERENCES

1. Snider, GL: Chronic bronchitis and emphysema. In Murray, JF and Nadel, JA: Textbook of Respiratory Medicine, WB Saunders, Philadelphia, 1988, pp 1069–1106.

2. Camilli, AE, et al: Longitudinal changes in forced expiratory volume in one second in adults. Am Rev Respir Dis 135:794, 1987.

3. Beaty, TH, et al: Risk factors associated with longitudinal change in pulmonary function. Am Rev Respir Dis 129:660, 1984.

4. Samet, JM: The relationship of smoking to COPD. In Cherniak, NS (ed): Chronic Obstructive Pulmonary Disease. WB Saunders, Philadelphia, 1991, pp 249–258.

5. Thurlbeck, WM: Pathology of chronic airflow obstruction. In Cherniak, NS (ed): Chronic Obstructive Pulmonary Disease. WB Saunders, Philadelphia, 1991, pp 3–20.

6. Wiedemann, HP and Matthay, RA: Treatment overview: Chronic hypercapnia and cor pulmonale. In Cherniak, NS (ed): Chronic Obstructive Pulmonary Disease. WB Saunders, Philadelphia, 1991, pp 429–442.

7. Wiedemann, HP and Matthay, RA: Cor pulmonale in chronic obstructive pulmonary disease: Circulatory pathophysiology and new concepts of therapy. In Simmons, DH (ed): Current Pulmonology, Vol 8. Year Book Medical, Chicago, 1987, pp 127–162.

8. Redline, S: The epidemiology of COPD. In Cherniak, NS (ed): Chronic Obstructive Pulmonary Disease. WB Saunders, Philadelphia, 1991, pp 225–234.

9. Samet, JM: Health benefits of smoking cessation. In Samet, JM and Coultas, DB (eds): Clinics in Chest Medicine: Smoking Cessation. WB Saunders, Philadelphia, 1991, p 669.

10. Schwartz, JL: Methods for smoking cessation. In Samet, JM and Coultas, DB (eds): Clinics in Chest Medicine: Smoking Cessation. WB Saunders, Philadelphia, 1991, p 737.

11. Judge, RD, Zuidema, GD, and Fitzgerald, FT: Clinical Diagnosis, ed 4. Little, Brown, Boston, 1982, p 223.

12. Georgopoulos, D and Anthonisen, NR: Symptoms and signs of COPD. In Cherniak, NS (ed): Chronic Obstructive Pulmonary Disease. WB Saunders, Philadelphia, 1991, pp 357–362.

13. Reynolds, HY: Antibiotic treatment of bronchitis and chronic lung disease. In Cherniak, NS (ed): Chronic Obstructive Pulmonary Disease. WB Saunders, Philadelphia, 1991, pp 456–460.

14. Donahoe, M and Rogers, RM: Laboratory evaluation of the patients with COPD. In Cherniak, NS (ed): Chronic Obstructive Pulmonary Disease. WB Saunders, Philadelphia, 1991, pp 373–385.

15. Peters, JA and Peters, BA: Pharmacology for respiratory care. In Scanlon, CL, Spearman, CB, and Sheldon, RL: Egan's Fundamentals of Respiratory Care, ed 5. CV Mosby, St Louis, 1990, pp 445–482.

16. Weiner, N: Norepinephrine, epinephrine, and the sympathomimetic amines. In Gilman, AG, et al (eds): Goodman and Gilman's The Pharmacological Basis of Therapeutics, ed 7. Macmillan, New York, 1985, pp 145–180.

17. Baughman, RP and Loudon, RG: Quantification of wheezing in acute asthma. Chest 86:718, 1984.

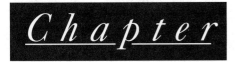

4

Kenneth D. McCarty, MS, RRT

EMPHYSEMA

INTRODUCTION

Pulmonary emphysema, from the Greek *emphysan* (to inflate), is an obstructive pulmonary disease characterized by dilation and destruction of lung units from the terminal bronchioles to the alveoli. Onset of the symptoms typically occurs after the age of 50 and affects men approximately four times as often as women. Technically, confirmation of the pathology can be made only by a lung biopsy or postmortem examination; however, certain clinical and diagnostic findings are highly suggestive of the disease.

Emphysema can be classified according to its anatomic location of the pathology. Panlobular (panacinar) emphysema involves enlargement of all airspaces distal to the terminal bronchioles including the respiratory bronchioles, alveolar ducts, and alveoli, and is most commonly caused by a deficiency in α_1-protease inhibitor (α_1PI). Conversely, centrilobular emphysema primarily involves the central acinar respiratory bronchioles, thus sparing distal lung units.[1]

ETIOLOGY

The two main etiologic factors identified in the progression of pulmonary emphysema are cigarette smoking and a genetic predisposition for the development of the disease. The most common factor associated with the development of emphysema is a history of cigarette smoking.[2] The exact mechanism and role that cigarettes play in the development of the disease is unknown; however, the inhalation of cigarette smoke does increase protease activity, which destroys the terminal bronchioles and alveolar walls. Smoking also decreases mucociliary transport, leading to retention of secretions and increased susceptibility to pulmonary infections. Whereas smoking appears to be the chief cause of emphysema in the majority of cases, a small number of individuals develop pulmonary emphysema with minimal or no smoking exposure as a result of a deficiency of the enzyme α_1PI.[3]

Normally the liver produces 200 to 400 μg/dL of this serum protein, which was previously called α_1-antitrypsin. α_1PI is responsible for the inactivation of elastase, an enzyme released from polymorphonuclear leukocytes (PMNs) and macrophages that breaks down elastin during an inflammatory response. Therefore, a deficiency in α_1PI results in elastase-induced destruction of lung tissue, producing panlobular pulmonary emphysema. This occurs as a result of a genetically inherited homozygous trait that is present in approximately 1 percent of emphysema cases, initially symptomatic in the third to fourth decade of life. Cigarette smoking also exacerbates the problem encountered in α_1PI deficiency.[3,4]

Chronic respiratory infections during childhood may result in the development of obstructive pulmonary disease later in life,[5] and inhaled pollutants such as sulfur dioxide and ozone may cause higher morbidity in patients with lung disease.[5,6] Although the exact role inhaled pollutants play in the etiology of pulmonary emphysema is not clear, exacerbations of the disease may result when pollutant levels are high. Hence, patients should avoid infections and inhaled irritants in order to prevent exacerbations of their condition.

PATHOPHYSIOLOGY

Because of the tissue destruction and loss of elastic recoil that occurs in pulmonary emphysema, limitations in exhaled flow and abnormalities in gas exchange exist. Impairment in expiratory flow results from the loss of elastic recoil by the lung tissue which results in a decreased driving pressure for exhaled gas, increased lung compliance, and an increase in collapsibility of the airway walls. These elements lead to air trapping during forced exhalation and an increase in functional residual capacity, residual volume, and total lung capacity.[3,7]

Destruction of the alveolar capillary bed results in reduced surface area, and airway dilation increases the distance for gaseous diffusion. Both of these impair the efficiency of external respiration. These abnormalities cause ventilation-perfusion ratio ($\dot{V}/\dot{Q}$) mismatching with large areas of dead space ventilation and contribute to the increase in the work of breathing.

CLINICAL FEATURES

Medical History

Findings of emphysema usually occur in conjunction with those of chronic bronchitis. However, for purposes of this discussion, the signs and symptoms of a "pink puffer," emphysematous patient will be described in order to differentiate between the two disease processes. As stated previously, an official diagnosis can only be made after pathologic examination of the patient's lung tissue; however, the medical history, physical examination, and diagnostic findings will often provide adequate information to confirm a clinical diagnosis of pulmonary emphysema. The patient often complains of shortness of breath increasing during exertion. Dyspnea at rest occurs relatively late in the disease process. Exacerbations of the disease typically occur after viral or bacterial respiratory tract infections, as a result of exposure to dust or pollutants or in association with congestive heart failure (see Chapter 8). A history of cigarette smoking should alert the clinician to the probability that the patient may develop not only emphysema but also other smoking-related respiratory diseases such as chronic bronchitis (see Chapter 3). A family history of α_1PI deficiency should also alert the clinician that signs and symptoms of emphysema may occur early in life.[3,5,8,9]

Physical Examination

The physical examination may provide key information in establishing a clinical diagnosis of pulmonary emphysema. Inspection of the patient with pulmonary emphysema will frequently demonstrate tachypnea with a prolonged exhalation, tachycardia, use of accessory muscles of breathing, increased anteroposterior (AP) diameter of the chest, and perhaps pursed-lipped breathing on exhalation. Patients also often assume a body position in which they lean forward with their hands braced on their knees or their elbows braced on a table. This provides more optimal mechanical advantage for their respiratory musculature. Palpation usually reveals decreased tactile and vocal fremitus, while percussion reveals flattened, immobile hemidiaphragms and increased resonance over the lung fields. Auscultation reveals decreased breath sounds as well as decreased transmission of heart and voice sounds.[9]

Laboratory Evaluation

Evaluation of the chest radiograph shows hyperlucent, hyperexpanded lung fields with low, flattened diaphragms, and a small, vertically oriented heart (Fig. 4–1). The lateral chest radiograph frequently demonstrates an increased retrosternal airspace.[8-11]

Pulmonary function studies, although not routinely done during an acute exacerbation, reveal increased residual volume (RV), functional residual volume (FRC), and total lung capacity (TLC) due to air trapping. Forced vital capacity (FVC), forced expiratory volume in 1 second (FEV_1), and FEV_1/FVC decrease because of airflow obstruction.[3,5,7] Decreases in D_{LCO} reflect the loss of surface area from alveolar and pulmonary vascular bed destruction.[7,12]

Arterial blood gases (ABGs) of the emphysematous patient typically do not reflect the severity of the pathologic process. Changes that are common include respiratory alkalosis with moderate hypoxemia in mild to moderate emphysema and the development of respiratory acidosis with more severe hypoxemia, which generally occurs during the terminal stage of the disease.[5,9]

Although assessment of the electrocardiogram (ECG) is not diagnostic for emphysema, it does provide valuable information about the patient. The more vertical position of the heart associated with marked hyperinflation of the lungs and flattening of the diaphragm causes a rightward shift of the P and QRS axes in the frontal plane. Tall, peaked P waves may be present and indicate atrial enlargement (P pulmonale). Lung hyperinflation also reduces the amplitude (voltage) of the limb leads.[9]

TREATMENT

Treatment of pulmonary emphysema includes both acute and supportive care. Therapy during the acute phase should decrease the work of breathing and provide optimal oxygenation and ventilation. Long-term care is designed to decrease morbidity and to increase patient autonomy and quality of life.

Advantages of a pulmonary rehabilitation program for the emphysematous patient include an opportunity for the patient to learn about his or her disease and a framework for long-term care. Careful long-term pulmonary management reduces symptoms and decreases in-hospital days. It also increases exercise tolerance and ease of performing activities of daily living, reduces anxiety and depression, and improves the quality of life.[13] Clinicians should counsel patients on the importance of smoking cessation and the avoidance of respiratory infections and irritants. The physician should encourage the patient to obtain an annual influenza shot, as an attack of the flu will often precipitate an exacerbation requiring admission to the hospital.[14] Proper nutritional status must also be emphasized, as it directly affects the patient's respiratory status and ability to perform the activities of daily living.

Supplemental oxygen therapy is useful when the resting room air Pao_2 is less than 55 mm Hg. Adequate oxygenation can usually be accomplished with a nasal cannula at a flow rate of less than 3 liters/minute in patients with emphysema. If an acute exacerbation is precipitated by an acute pneumonia or congestive heart failure, hypoxemia may be severe and require more significant elevation of Fio_2.

Treatment of the acute exacerbation involves stabilization of the patient's respiratory status and treatment of the exacerbating source. Sympathomimetic and methylxanthine bronchodilators are important agents for the treatment of bronchospasm when associated with exacerbation of emphysema.[3,5,14] Methylxanthines

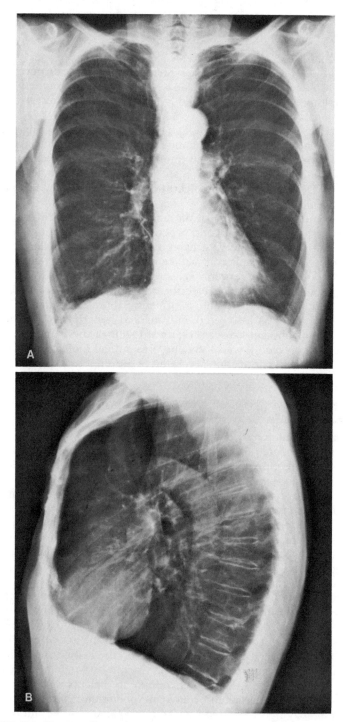

FIGURE 4–1 Chest radiograph typical for emphysema. A, Posteroanterior (PA) view demonstrates hyperinflation of the lungs and a small narrow heart. B, Lateral view demonstrates a large retrosternal airspace and low, flat hemidiaphragms.

also increase diaphragm contractility (see case study below). Steroids decrease inflammatory response in the airway and appear to be most effective in patients with a reversible airway obstruction component. In addition, anticholinergic bronchodilators are especially useful in the treatment of bronchospasm owing to an increase in parasympathetic tone.[15] The administration of antibiotics is indicated when a respiratory tract infection is present, typically seen as a change in sputum quantity, color, or consistency.[14] Diuretics are useful when congestive heart failure is complicating the patient's clinical condition.

If secretion clearance becomes a problem during acute exacerbation, caregivers should employ techniques for improving pulmonary hygiene such as chest physiotherapy and bland mist aerosol administration.[3,5] Acute respiratory failure may require the institution of continuous mechanical ventilation (CMV) to maintain adequate management of the patient's ventilatory status.[3] CMV is most reasonable when the acute respiratory failure is the result of a reversible problem superimposed on the patient's chronic obstructive pulmonary disease (COPD).

In patients suffering from $\alpha_1 PI$ deficiency, intravenous replacement can be provided with Prolastin.[16] Although this is a new, exciting, and expensive therapy available for patients with $\alpha_1 PI$ deficiency, the benefits of long-term therapy have not yet been demonstrated.[14]

Case Study

HISTORY

Mrs. DG is a 52-year-old white woman who came to the emergency room because of complaints of increasing shortness of breath. She stated that she had had the flu approximately 1½ weeks earlier and that her breathing had been more difficult since that time. Her ankles had been swollen for the first time and sleeping during this time had required "two pillows to support" her. She stated that occasionally she awakened in the middle of the night very short of breath. These episodes of nocturnal dyspnea were relieved by sitting up for several minutes. She had been producing ¼ cup of yellow sputum daily since the onset of the flu. Her exercise tolerance had been one block but was now 20 feet. Mrs. DG stated that 7 years ago her family physician had told her that she had pulmonary emphysema. She had started smoking at age 12 and smoked approximately 2 packs of cigarettes a day until she quit 2 years ago. Mrs. DG took the following home medications: small-volume nebulizer (SVN) with Metaproterenol four times a day, Theo-Dur 200 mg two times a day, and continuous oxygen via nasal cannula at 1 liter/minute.

Questions

1. What symptoms should be explored in greater detail?
2. How many pack-years has this patient smoked, and how is this significant in terms of producing pulmonary symptoms?
3. What is the most likely cause of the patient's pulmonary emphysema?
4. What is the most likely cause of the patient's exacerbation?
5. What is the pathophysiologic significance of the patient's orthopnea and paroxysmal nocturnal dyspnea (PND)?

Answers

1. The key symptoms include increasing shortness of breath, exercise intolerance, orthopnea, PND, and sputum production. Because pulmonary emphysema is a progressive and chronic disease, gradual worsening of the pathology is expected. However, a sudden decline in respiratory status indicates an acute problem that is exacerbating the COPD. This patient

should be questioned about her salt intake, including foods such as olives, pickles, and potato chips; exposure to known respiratory irritants; evidence of infection; and compliance with her treatment program. She should be questioned about subjective evidence of changes in her cardiac status to determine the presence of chest pain, palpitations, or fainting spells.

2. A 96–pack-year smoking history is present (48 years × 2 packs per day). Usually, a smoking history greater than 20 pack-years is required before symptoms or dyspnea and obstructive lung disease begin to occur.[9]

3. The most likely cause of the patient's pulmonary emphysema is cigarette smoking. Although men have historically outnumbered women in the development of smoking-related diseases, the increase in the number of female smokers since World War II has led to a related rise in the number of smoking-related diseases in women.

4. The patient's exacerbation is probably a result of her recent bout with influenza. Any acute illness frequently acts to further compromise an already borderline respiratory status in COPD patients. They should be encouraged to get annual vaccinations such as flu shots to minimize the chance of infection-induced exacerbations.[14] This patient's dyspnea appears to be exacerbated by congestive heart failure (requiring several pillows for respiratory comfort at night).

5. Orthopnea and PND are usually caused by congestive heart failure.[9] These symptoms occur as pulmonary vascular congestion increases in the reclining position. The congestive heart failure may be caused by ischemic heart disease or cardiomyopathy.

PHYSICAL EXAMINATION

General The patient is an alert, cachectic, white woman in moderate respiratory distress, sitting on the edge of her bed and leaning forward with her elbows braced on the bedside table. She appears to have difficulty talking secondary to dyspnea and pursed-lip breathing.

Vital Signs Temperature 37.8°C orally; respiratory rate 28/minute; pulse 108/minute; and blood pressure 142/80 mm Hg

HEENT Unremarkable

Neck Trachea midline without stridor or masses. Carotid pulses are ++ without bruits; no lymphadenopathy or thyromegaly present; patient using her sternocleidomastoid muscles during inspiration; no jugular venous distension (JVD) present

Chest Increased AP diameter with large supraclavicular fossae present and mild abdominal paradox during respiratory efforts; significant protrusion of the ribs with moderate retractions present during inspiration; chest expansion of 3 cm at the eighth thoracic vertebra and a diffuse reduction in tactile fremitus on palpation; point of maximum impulse (PMI) not identified with palpation; increased resonance bilaterally on percussion

Heart Heart sounds are very distant with regular rate and rhythm (RRR) of 108/minute without murmurs

Lungs	*Bilateral reduction in breath sounds anteriorly and posteriorly with a prolonged expiratory phase on auscultation; occasional scattered expiratory wheezes also present*
Abdomen	*Soft, nondistended, and nontender with bowel sounds present; no masses or organomegaly present*
Extremities	*No cyanosis, clubbing, or peripheral edema present*

Questions

6. Why is the patient pursed-lip breathing, and what is the physiologic effect that it produces?
7. Why is the patient leaning forward on her elbows to breathe?
8. What is the significance of the abdominal paradox during respiratory efforts?
9. What pathophysiology accounts for the patient's increased resonance, decreased tactile fremitus, and decreased heart sounds?
10. Why is the patient's PMI not felt? What is indicated when the PMI is in the epigastric area?
11. What is the significance of the chest expansion measurement?
12. What is the cause of the patient's decreased breath sounds?
13. What findings indicate the need for hospitalization?

Answers

6. Pursed-lip breathing provides a positive intra-airway pressure, which is thought to decrease airway closure and air trapping and aid gas exchange.[9] Patients often discover this maneuver on their own or learn it through formal instruction by health care providers, although the exact benefit of this technique has not been established.
7. Leaning forward on the elbows provides a more optimal mechanical advantage for the accessory respiratory muscles by stabilizing the shoulder girdle to which they are attached. This makes the accessory muscles more efficient and may improve ventilation for patients with poor diaphragmatic function.
8. Paradoxic abdominal movement during breathing indicates diaphragmatic muscle fatigue.[9,17] When the diaphragm is tired, accessory muscles of respiration create a negative intrathoracic pressure that pulls the fatigued diaphragm slightly upward and into the chest cage, allowing the abdominal wall to sink inward rather than rise during inspiration.
9. The patient's increased resonance, decreased tactile fremitus, and decreased heart sounds are a result of the increased intrathoracic volume. The tissue destruction and hyperinflation caused by emphysema lead to poor sound transmission through the chest.[9]
10. Normally the PMI is located along the left midclavicular line at the level of the fourth or fifth intercostal space. In emphysematous patients the loss of lung recoil allows the natural tension of the diaphragm to go unopposed and results in flattening of the diaphragms. As a result, the mediastinal structures are elongated and the PMI assumes a more centrally located position lower in the chest or in the epigastric area. The lung hyperinflation in emphysema may reduce the examiner's ability to feel the PMI.

11. Chest expansion as measured by palpation is normally 6 to 10 cm. In the case of emphysema, loss of elastic recoil causes chronic hyperinflation which increases AP diameter to near maximum, resulting in the reduced ability of the chest cage to expand during inspiration.[9]
12. Decreased breath sounds in patients with pulmonary emphysema result from both decreased sound production and decreased sound transmission. Loss of elastic recoil results in reduced expiratory flow rates, which minimizes turbulent flow sounds during exhalation. The inspiratory sounds are effectively filtered by the relatively large distal airspaces in emphysema and results in poor sound transmission to the chest wall.[18,19]
13. The need for hospitalization of this patient is indicated by the signs of respiratory distress: (1) respiratory rate greater than 24/minute; (2) paradoxic breathing pattern; and (3) use of accessory muscles. In addition, the peripheral edema (ankle swelling) indicates compromise of right heart function.

LABORATORY EVALUATION

CHEST RADIOGRAPH

(Figs. 4–2 and 4–3)

ABGs ON 1 LITER/MINUTE

pH	7.32
Pa_{CO_2}	62 mm Hg
Pa_{O_2}	50 mm Hg
HCO_3^-	30 mEq/liter
base excess (BE)	+5
Hb	13.1 g/100 mL
Sa_{O_2}	85.5 percent
Ca_{O_2}	15.2 vol%

PULMONARY FUNCTION TESTS (PFTs)

(from a previous admission when patient was stable)

FVC	1.90 liters	(58 percent of predicted)
FEV_1	1.02 liters	(39 percent of predicted)
Forced expiratory flow (FEF) 25–75 percent	0.74 liters/sec	(31 percent of predicted)
TLC	5.87 liters	(117 percent of predicted)
RV	3.97 liters	(226 percent of predicted)
FRC	4.33 liters	(170 percent of predicted)
D_{LCO}	6.4 mL/minute per mm Hg	(26 percent of predicted)

CLINICAL LABORATORY STUDIES

Complete Blood Count (CBC): Results pending
Chemistry: Results pending
Theophylline level: Results pending

ECG FINDINGS

Sinus tachycardia with decreased voltage in the limb leads; tall narrow P waves; occasional premature ventricular contractions

Questions

15. What chest radiograph findings suggest hyperexpansion?
16. What is the significance of the decreased vascular markings on the chest radiograph?
17. What is the patient's acid-base and oxygenation status?
18. What is the cause of the decreased voltage and tall P waves in the limb leads, as noted on the ECG findings?
19. How do you interpret the PFT results?
20. What pathology accounts for the decreased D_{LCO}?
21. What is your initial assessment of the patient's condition?

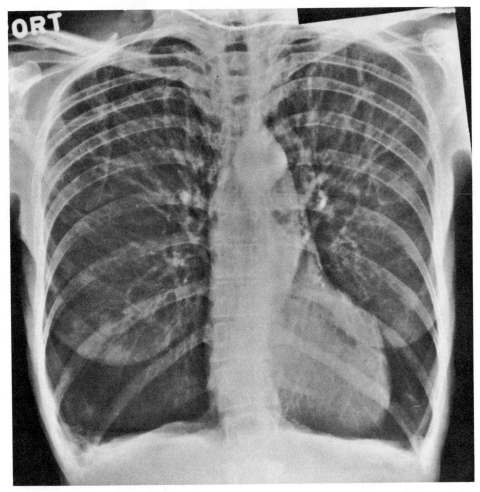

FIGURE 4–2 Anteroposterior (AP) chest radiograph showing hyperinflation and flat hemidiaphragms in pulmonary emphysema.

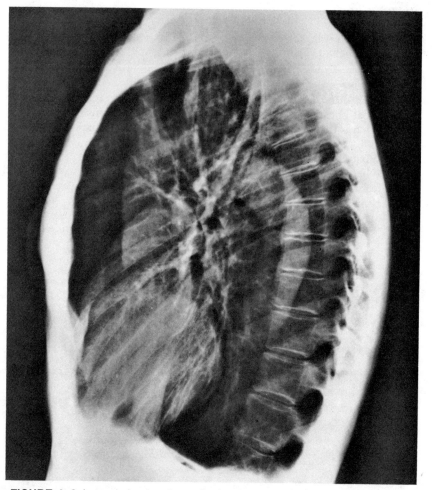

FIGURE 4–3 Lateral chest radiograph showing increased retrosternal airspace, flat hemidiaphragms, and increased AP diameter.

22. What treatment do you suggest?
23. Should the patient be monitored for any special adverse reactions to therapy?
24. Should high oxygen concentrations be administered to this patient if necessary?

Answers

15. Hyperexpansion can be assessed by counting the number of ribs seen on the posteroanterior chest radiograph. More than 11 fully visualized posterior ribs or seven anterior ribs indicates hyperexpansion.[20] In addition, flattened diaphragms, increased intercostal spaces, and increased radiolucency indicate hyperexpansion. The lateral chest radiograph demonstrates a flattened diaphragm and a large retrosternal airspace.

16. Decreased vascular markings on the chest radiograph occur as a result of the pulmonary parenchymal destruction involving not only terminal airspaces but also pulmonary capillary vasculature. Excessive vascular tapering suggests a more severe case of emphysema.

17. The elevated Pa_{CO_2} and HCO_3^- indicate partially compensated respiratory acidosis. The patient has moderate hypoxemia on 1 liter/minute, and other indices of oxygenation are abnormally low. Because Ca_{O_2} takes into account saturation, Hb level, and Pa_{O_2} it can be used to assess oxygen-carrying capacity. The Ca_{O_2} of 15.2 vol% (normally 16 to 20 vol%) is slightly reduced primarily owing to the low Sa_{O_2}.

18. Lung hyperinflation and flattening of the diaphragm result in a more vertical position of the heart and a clockwise rotation along its longitudinal axis. This may cause a rightward shift of the QRS axis, as measured by the limb leads. The mean QRS axis is also directed posteriorly and perpendicular to the frontal plane in emphysema. Electrical activity that is perpendicular to the frontal plane is not detected by the limb leads, which measure activity only in the frontal plane. As a result of the posterior shift of the mean QRS axis, the limb leads will reveal decreased amplitude. Hyperinflation also reduces the electrical conductivity of the lung, which adds to the decreased voltage seen in the limb leads of the ECG. Tall narrow P waves (P pulmonale) indicate right atrial enlargement and are characteristic of severe pulmonary disease.[21]

19. The PFT results are consistent with a diagnosis of pulmonary emphysema. The loss of airway elasticity results in collapsible airways and air trapping. The air trapping results in large lung volumes and capacities. The combination of a large intrathoracic volume, slow expiratory flow rates, and reduced diffusion capacity are typical for pulmonary emphysema.

20. The decreased D_{LCO} is caused by the loss of pulmonary vascular bed resulting from tissue destruction and dilation of the terminal lung units. This results in a loss of alveolar surface area for diffusion.

21. The initial assessment of this patient is acute exacerbation of pulmonary emphysema secondary to influenza.

22. Immediate treatment should consist of oxygen therapy at 1 to 2 liters/minute via nasal cannula in an attempt to increase the patient's Pa_{O_2} to approximately 60 to 65 mm Hg. Aerosolized adrenergic bronchodilators may prove beneficial to relieve any airway obstruction caused by reactive airways, thus reducing the patient's work of breathing. These can be administered with a metered-dose inhaler (MDI) or SVN if the patient can spontaneously take a deep breath (greater than 15 mL/kg).[20] Intermittent positive-pressure breathing (IPPB) is rarely needed but may be beneficial if the patient is unable to take a deep spontaneous breath. Intravenous (IV) aminophylline and corticosteroids may also prove useful if a reversible airway obstruction component is present. In this patient the scattered wheezing suggests that bronchodilators may be beneficial. Sputum collection for Gram's stain and culture and sensitivity is warranted in light of the yellow sputum and low-grade fever. Other measures that might prove beneficial should the patient have trouble clearing secretions include bland aerosol therapy, chest physical therapy, and aerosolized acetylcysteine (Mucomyst).

23. Yes, the caregivers should monitor the patient for certain side effects. The possible side effects of sympathomimetic bronchodilators include tachycardia, arrhythmias, tremor, nervousness, and anxiety.[22] Aminophylline may cause nausea, tachycardia, tremor, and possible seizures. Because the patient is a chronic CO_2 retainer, the respiratory therapist should administer oxygen therapy carefully to avoid depressing the patient's hypoxic respiratory drive and increasing hypoventilation. The use of fixed performance oxygen delivery devices that can administer

discrete oxygen percentages often can be used to titrate oxygen delivery carefully and minimize the chance of oxygen-induced hypoventilation.

24. High concentrations of oxygen may be lifesaving in certain situations. Although oxygen should be administered judiciously to patients who are chronic CO_2 retainers depending on hypoxic respiratory drive, oxygen should never be withheld for fear of dulling that drive at the expense of tissue oxygenation. Should the patient's drive to breathe diminish and result in an elevated $Paco_2$ to the point that the pH is less than 7.25 or the patient's sensorium is abnormal, mechanical ventilation should be used to support ventilation until the patient's respiratory status improves.

Patient was admitted to the respiratory intensive care unit (ICU) and started on the following medications: oxygen therapy at 2 liters/minute via nasal cannula, aminophylline drip, Solu-Medrol 120 mg IV every 6 hours, SVN with 0.5 mL of 0.5 percent albuterol and 2.50 mL 0.9 percent saline every 4 hours. Sputum for Gram's stain and culture and sensitivity, theophylline level, and ABGs on 2 liters/minute were ordered.

Results of the sputum Gram's stain showed +2 pus cells, no epithelial cells, and a few very small gram-negative rods; the culture eventually grew predominantly Haemophilus influenzae *sensitive to ampicillin. Theophylline level was 8.1 µg/mL. ABG results on 2 liters/minute were pH 7.33, $PaCO_2$ 65 mm Hg, Pao_2 66 mm Hg, HCO_3^- 31 mEq/liter, BE +4, Hb 13.0 g/100 mL, Sao_2 91.2 percent, Cao_2 16.2 vol%.*

Questions

25. What is the significance of the sputum Gram's stain and culture?
26. What antimicrobial agent is indicated?
27. What is the significance of the theophylline level?
28. How do you interpret the patient's acid-base and oxygenation status on 2 liters/minute or O_2?
29. Are any other changes in the patient's therapy indicated at present?
30. By what mechanism other than bronchodilation might theophylline be beneficial in the treatment of emphysema?

Answers

25. The presence of pus cells in the sputum indicates inflammation or infection. The designations 0, +1, +2, are used to indicate the number of segmented neutrophils found by the medical technologist during microscopic analysis. An average score of 0 indicates a lack of infection or contamination with saliva, whereas a score of +1 or +2 indicates active inflammation.[23] In addition, the absence of epithelial cells indicates a specimen that was not contaminated by oral secretions. Gram's stain and culture are used to identify specific microbe characteristics and to allow selective antimicrobial treatment. *H. influenzae* is a common cause of infection among patients with obstructive lung disease. The sensitivity to ampicillin means that the infection should be easy to treat.

26. Ampicillin is a broad-spectrum antibiotic commonly used for the treatment of sensitive strains of *H. influenzae*. It is inexpensive and has few side effects. Chloramphenicol can also be used to treat *H. influenzae*.[24]

27. The therapeutic theophylline level is 10 to 20 µg/mL of plasma and a

value of 8.1 µg/mL indicates that increasing the aminophylline drip might be helpful in relieving dyspnea. The serum level should be evaluated periodically after changes in aminophylline administration to avoid toxicity and ensure therapeutic serum levels.

28. The patient's ABGs show a partially compensated respiratory acidosis. The administration of oxygen has improved the patient's plasma oxygenation and oxygen-carrying capacity (Cao_2) to an acceptable level, considering the patient's age and disease state. Further increases in Pao_2 potentially run the risk of depressing the patient's respiratory drive without improving the patient's Cao_2 significantly.

29. The frequency of the patient's SVN treatments could be increased to every 2 or 3 hours to increase the bronchodilator effect if her pulse rate is not greater than 120/minute. Another method to increase the bronchodilator response would be the administration of an anticholinergic agent such as ipratropium bromide (Atrovent) in conjunction with the sympathomimetic therapy.[25]

30. In addition to bronchodilation, theophylline causes diaphragmatic stimulation[26,27] and an increase in central respiratory drive,[14,28] both of which increase ventilation.

The patient was started on a regimen of ampicillin and her aminophylline was increased. The frequency of the SVN treatments was changed to every 3 hours and prn, with an Atrovent MDI ordered to follow. Over the day the patient's respiratory status improved and she felt more comfortable. SVN and MDI were changed to every 4 hours when awake and prn at night. Subsequent follow-up revealed a therapeutic serum theophylline level of 13.5 µg/mL. Over the next 2 days (days 2 and 3) the patient's oxygen was reduced to 1 liter/minute, and her aminophylline was changed to Theo-Dur. At this time her breath sounds were clear, although decreased bilaterally, and her cough produced only opaque white secretions. The patient was discharged to home on day 5 with the following medications: Theo-Dur 200 mg twice a day, oxygen via nasal cannula at 1 liter/minute, Ventolin via MDI 2 puffs every 4 hours and prn for dyspnea, with an Atrovent MDI to follow and antibiotics. The patient was also encouraged to enter a pulmonary rehabilitation program to help manage her COPD optimally.

REFERENCES

1. Snider, GL, et al: The definition of emphysema (Report of National Heart, Lung and Blood Institute, Division of Lung Diseases Workshop). Am Rev Respir Dis 132:182, 1985.

2. US Surgeon General: The Health Consequences of Smoking: Chronic Obstructive Lung Disease. DHHS Publ No 84-50205. Washington, DC, US Dept of Health and Human Services, 1984, p 363.

3. Weinberger, SE: Chronic obstructive pulmonary diseases. In Weinberger, SE: Principles of Pulmonary Medicine. WB Saunders, Philadelphia, 1992, p 87.

4. Morrison, HM: The protease-antiprotease therapy of emphysema: Time for reappraisal? Clin Sci 72:151, 1987.

5. Des Jardins, TR: Emphysema. In Des Jardins, TR: Clinical Manifestations of Respiratory Disease. Year Book Medical, Chicago, 1990, p 91.

6. Sherrill, DL, Lebowitz, MD, and Burrows, B: Epidemiology of chronic obstructive pulmonary disease. In Hodgkin, JE (ed): Clinics in Chest Medicine. WB Saunders, Philadelphia, 1990, p 375.

7. West, WW, et al: The National Institutes of Health intermittent positive pressure breathing trial: Pathology studies. III. The diagnosis of emphysema. Am Rev Respir Dis 135:123, 1987.

8. Clausen, JL: The diagnosis of emphysema, chronic bronchitis, and asthma. In Hodgkin, JE (ed): Clinics in Chest Medicine. WB Saunders, Philadelphia, 1990, p 405.

9. Wilkins, RL, Sheldon RL, and Krider, SJ: Clinical Assessment in Respiratory Care. CV Mosby, St Louis, 1990.

10. Nicklaus, TM, et al: The accuracy of the roentgenologic diagnosis of chronic pulmonary emphysema. Am Rev Respir Dis 93:889, 1966.

11. Burki, NK: Roentgenologic diagnosis of emphysema. Chest 95:1178, 1989.

12. Morrison, NJ, et al: Comparison of single breath carbon monoxide diffusing capacity and pressure volume curves in detecting emphysema. Am Rev Respir Dis 139:1179, 1989.

13. Hodgkin, JE: Pulmonary rehabilitation. In Hodgkin, JE (ed): Clinics in Chest Medicine. WB Saunders, Philadelphia, 1990, p 447.

14. Ziment, I: Pharmacologic therapy of obstructive airway disease. In Hodgkin, JE (ed): Clinics in Chest Medicine. WB Saunders, Philadelphia, 1990, p 461.

15. Tashkin, DP, et al: Comparison of the anticholinergic bronchodilator ipratropium bromide with metaproterenol in chronic obstructive pulmonary disease—a 90 day multicenter study. Am J Med 81:81, 1986.

16. Wewers, MD, et al: Replacement therapy for alpha$_1$-antitrypsin deficiency associated with emphysema. N Engl J Med 316:1055, 1987.

17. Cohen, CA, et al: Clinical manifestations of inspiratory muscle fatigue. Am J Med 73:308, 1982.

18. Ploysongsang, Y, Pare, JA, and Macklem, P: Lung sounds in patients with emphysema. Am Rev Respir Dis 124:45, 1981.

19. Kramen, SS: The relationship between airflow and lung sound amplitude in normal subjects. Chest 86:225, 1984.

20. Krider, TM, Meyer, R, and Syvertsen, WA: Master Guide for Passing the Respiratory Care Credentialing Exams. ERC Press, Claremont, CA, 1989, p 100.

21. Goldberger, AL and Goldberger, E: Clinical Electrocardiography. CV Mosby, St Louis, 1986, p 74.

22. Rau, JL: Respiratory Care Pharmacology. Year Book Medical, Chicago, 1989, p 101.

23. Koneman, EW, et al: Diagnostic Microbiology. JB Lippincott, New York, 1988, p 38.

24. Kacmarek, RM, Mack, CW, and Dimas, S: The Essentials of Respiratory Therapy. Year Book Medical, Chicago, 1985, p 527.

25. Gross, NJ, et al: Dose response to ipratropium as a nebulized solution in patients with chronic obstructive pulmonary disease. Am Rev Respir Dis 139:1185, 1989.

26. Supinski, GS, Deal, EG, and Kelsen, SG: The effects of caffeine and theophylline on diaphragm contractility. Am Rev Respir Dis 130:429, 1984.

27. Aubier, M, et al: Aminophylline improves diaphragmatic contractility. N Engl J Med 305:249, 1981.

28. Murciano, D, et al: A randomized, controlled trial of theophylline in patients with severe chronic obstructive pulmonary disease. N Engl J Med 320:1521, 1989.

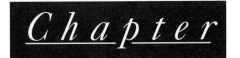

Chapter 5

N. Lennard Specht, MD

CYSTIC FIBROSIS

INTRODUCTION

Cystic fibrosis is an inherited disease that affects primarily whites of European descent. The disease is the most common lethal genetic disease in the United States, affecting as many as 1 in 2000 white children born in this country.[1] The disease is typically diagnosed in childhood and causes many organs of the body to malfunction (Table 5–1). The principal problems associated with the disease are bronchiectasis (abnormal dilation of a bronchus), pancreatic exocrine insufficiency, and an elevated sweat electrolyte concentration. Pulmonary disease causes the greatest problems for patients with cystic fibrosis and is the leading cause of mortality.[2]

Cystic fibrosis was first formally portrayed in 1936 when Fanconi and colleagues[3] described two children with "cystic fibrosis of the pancreas and bronchiectasis." Cystic fibrosis was probably just as frequent and lethal centuries before Fanconi published his landmark article. In 18th- and 19th-century European literature there are numerous references to children with abnormalities suggestive of cystic fibrosis. Most of these reports noted a correlation between a child's salty taste when kissed and the likelihood the child would die at a very young age.[4]

ETIOLOGY

Cystic fibrosis occurs primarily in individuals of European descent. The inheritance pattern is autosomal recessive. Patients affected by the disease have two genes for cystic fibrosis (one gene given by each parent). Those who have only one gene for cystic fibrosis are called carriers. Carriers show no evidence of cystic fibrosis and live normal lives. However, if two carriers have a child, chances are one in four that the child will have cystic fibrosis. It is estimated that between 1 in 16 to 1 in 25 white Americans carry the cystic fibrosis gene. The frequency of the cystic fibrosis gene in Orientals and blacks is much less than in whites. As a result, the disease occurs in nonwhites with much less frequency.

The gene responsible for the development of cystic fibrosis has been identified on chromosome 7.[5,6] The gene may be altered (mutated) in at least 20 different ways; several of these mutations cause cystic fibrosis. The most common abnormality of the gene is deletion of three base pairs in the DNA. This three-base pair deletion leads to the loss of one amino acid from the protein coded for by the gene. This mutation is known as delta F_{508}. The delta F_{508} gene accounts for 70 to 75 percent of the genetic abnormalities responsible for cystic fibrosis. The severity of cystic fibrosis is in part related to the genetic form of the disease the patient inherits.[7]

Table 5–1 Organ Systems Involved in Cystic Fibrosis

Lungs
  Bronchiectasis
  Bronchitis
  Pneumonia
  Atelectasis
  Mucus plugging
  Respiratory failure
Pancreas
  Pancreatic exocrine insufficiency
  Recurrent pancreatitis
  Diabetes mellitus
Sweat glands
  Increased electrolyte concentration in the sweat
Upper airway
  Recurrent sinusitis
  Nasal polyps
Intestines
  Meconium plug
  Meconium ileus
  Intussusception
Liver
  Cirrhosis
  Neonatal jaundice
Gallbladder
  Cholelithiasis
Salivary glands
  Altered electrolyte concentration of secretions
Reproductive system
  Obstructed vas deferens
  Decreased female fertility

The cystic fibrosis gene contains the code for a large protein that regulates the flow of ions (salt) through glands that secrete fluids (exocrine glands).[8,9] As a result cystic fibrosis patients are unable to regulate the salt composition of their secretions as a normal person would.[10] This malregulation of secretion is responsible for most if not all of the problems that these patients experience.

PATHOLOGY AND PATHOPHYSIOLOGY

Cystic fibrosis is characterized as a generalized exocrinopathy. To some degree virtually all exocrine glands of the body are affected by the disease. Cystic fibrosis is described as having a classic triad of exocrine abnormalities. These abnormalities are exocrine pancreatic insufficiency, chronic recurrent pulmonary infections, and an elevated sweat electrolyte concentration.

In very young patients with cystic fibrosis the pancreas appears normal. As the disease progresses the pancreas becomes smaller and fibrotic. Microscopic examination of the pancreas reveals obstruction of the pancreatic ducts and ductules. This is followed by dilation of the glandular lumen and, eventually, the replacement of the exocrine glands with fibrous connective tissue.

Lung disease creates the greatest morbidity and mortality for patients with cystic fibrosis. The three most common pulmonary problems faced by patients with cystic fibrosis are recurrent pulmonary infections, bronchiectasis, and bronchial hyperactivity. These problems may be mild in young children, but their frequency and severity increase as the disease progresses.

In the earliest stages of cystic fibrosis the lungs often appear normal. As patients mature, the lungs show progressive increase in the size and number of the bronchial goblet cells (mucous glands) and inflammation in the peribronchial tissue. The mucosa of the airway changes from normal epithelium to stratified squamous epithelium in a process called **squamous metaplasia.** In patients who have had pulmonary symptoms for several years, these findings are more widespread and severe. Emphysematous changes are frequently seen, and hemorrhage can be found within the lung. Mucus plugging is seen in small airways, and bronchiectasis is a universal finding.

During the end stages of the disease, obstructive emphysema is frequent but destruction rarely involves more than 10 percent of the lung.[11] Mucus plugging is pronounced and abscesses are found distal to these plugs. Lymph nodes in the hilum of the lung are enlarged.[12]

CLINICAL FEATURES

Medical History

Cystic fibrosis is usually first recognized during infancy or childhood; however, a small number of patients are diagnosed as young adults. Cystic fibrosis patients frequently first present with recurrent pulmonary infections.[13] Children with cystic fibrosis have more frequent and prolonged respiratory infections than normal children. Most infants with cystic fibrosis have a chronic cough and wheezing. As the disease progresses, symptoms of bronchiectasis and bronchial hyperactivity become more prominent. Clubbing of the digits and dyspnea on exertion are also seen. Fevers are at most mild during exacerbations of bronchiectasis but may be very high during episodes of pneumonia. In advanced stages of the disease complications of lung involvement include hemoptysis, which is occasionally massive, pneumothorax, atelectasis, cor pulmonale, and respiratory failure.

Pancreatic involvement with cystic fibrosis causes pancreatic exocrine insufficiency. The lack of pancreatic enzymes leads to maldigestion and malabsorption. Pancreatic exocrine insufficiency is associated with diarrhea and stools that contain large amounts of fat. These symptoms are frequently associated with crampy abdominal pain, malnutrition, and failure to maintain a normal growth rate.[14] Other less common gastrointestinal symptoms include meconium plug, intussusception (slipping of one part of the intestine into another part), rectal prolapse, intestinal obstruction, prolonged neonatal jaundice, hepatic cirrhosis, cholelithiasis (bilestones in gallbladder), recurrent pancreatitis, and diabetes mellitus.

Abnormalities of sweat production result in excessive concentrations of salt in sweat. This increase in salt lends a salty taste to the skin and the development of salt crystals on the skin or within clothing, particularly shoes and boots. Loss of electrolytes during warm months of the year may lead to heat intolerance, heat prostration, electrolyte depletion, and dehydration.

Upper respiratory symptoms associated with cystic fibrosis include recurrent sinusitis and the development of nasal polyps. Almost all men and most women with cystic fibrosis are sterile. If a woman with cystic fibrosis becomes pregnant she is not likely to carry the infant to term. The infant will either have cystic fibrosis or be a carrier of the cystic fibrosis gene.

Physical Examination

The physical examination of affected patients is nearly always abnormal within a few years after the diagnosis is established. Cystic fibrosis patients are typically thin children or young adults. If respiratory distress is present, accessory muscles of respiration will be used. A productive cough is an almost universal finding. Examination of the extremities may disclose clubbing of the digits. The upper airway may reveal nasal polyps or tenderness over the sinuses. The chest will appear to have a barrel configuration. The lungs usually have diffuse coarse crackles and wheezes.

In advanced disease cyanosis around the mouth is associated with hypoxemia. Auscultation of the heart may disclose a loud pulmonic component of the second heart sound, implying that pulmonary hypertension is present. Distention of the jugular neck veins and pedal edema are associated with the development of right heart failure (cor pulmonale).

Laboratory Evaluation

Arterial blood gases (ABGs) are nearly normal early in the disease with only an increase in the alveolar-arterial oxygen gradient. Hypoxemia on room air increases as the disease progresses. Hypercapnia and severe hypoxemia occur only with very advanced lung disease.

Serum chemistries and blood counts have no abnormalities unique to cystic fibrosis. However, elevation of serum bicarbonate is seen, as a result of chronic respiratory failure, and elevations of the hematocrit may reflect chronic hypoxemia. Acute bronchopneumonia may lead to an elevation of the white blood count with an accompanying shift to more immature granulocytes. Serum protein and albumin concentrations may be low if malnutrition is present.

The chest radiograph characteristically shows hyperinflation, seen as a flattening of the hemidiaphragms and an increase in the retrosternal airspace (Fig. 5–1). Bronchial wall thickening is commonly seen as parallel lines radiating out from the hilum. They are called "tram tracks" (Fig. 5–2). Small rounded opacities can be seen in the periphery of the lung, which may represent small abscesses distal to impacted airways. These areas usually clear, leaving a small cyst as residue from the infection. Other abnormalities seen on chest radiographs include atelectasis, fibrosis, hilar adenopathy, acute bronchopneumonia, and pneumothorax (Fig. 5–3).

Pulmonary function testing is very useful to evaluate the extent of lung disease and to follow the rate of disease progression. Following progression of the disease allows the clinician to increase therapy if lung function deteriorates unexpectedly. Spirometry typically shows evidence of airway obstruction with a reduction in forced expiratory volume in 1 second (FEV_1). Loss of forced vital capacity (FVC) is seen in advanced disease. Both of these changes may improve after the administration of bronchodilators. Residual volume increases early in the course of the disease and can be best measured using a body plethysmograph.

Sweat electrolyte measurement has been the standard technique for confirming the diagnosis of cystic fibrosis. Sweat secretion is stimulated and sweat is collected under an airtight seal. After collection of about 0.1 mL of sweat the electrolyte concentration is measured. In children, a sweat chloride concentration greater than 60 mEq/liter is consistent with the diagnosis of cystic fibrosis.[15] A sweat chloride concentration greater than 80 mEq/liter is usually required to confirm the diagnosis of cystic fibrosis in adults.[16] If the sweat chloride is equivocal (between 50 and 80 mEq/liter), repeat measurement of sweat chloride concentration will usually resolve the question. Although the sweat electrolyte concentration is useful for confirming the diagnosis of cystic fibrosis, it must be performed with meticulous attention to detail or the results may be misleading.[17]

Patients with cystic fibrosis typically have pathogenic organisms in their sputum. The three organisms most commonly found are *Staphylococcus aureus, Haemophilus influenzae,* and *Pseudomonas aeruginosa.* The strain of *P. aeruginosa* found in patients with cystic fibrosis typically produces mucin. This mucoid form of *P. aeruginosa* is nearly unique to cystic fibrosis. This strain is found almost

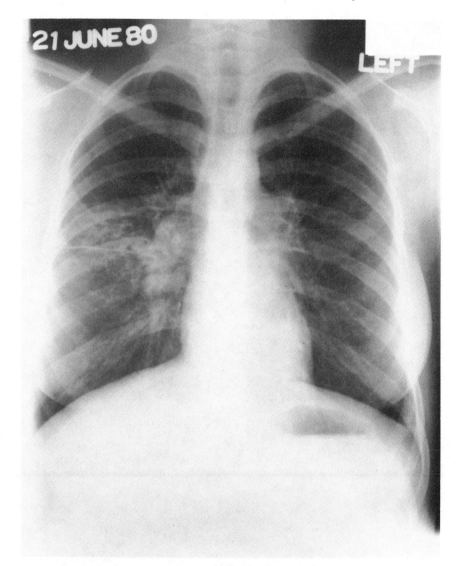

FIGURE 5–1 Chest radiograph of a patient with cystic fibrosis.

exclusively in the airways of patients with advanced cystic fibrosis. Severe exacerbations may be caused by several different strains of mucin-producing *P. aeruginosa.*

Discovery of the cystic fibrosis gene has made diagnostic testing for some of the genetic abnormalities associated with cystic fibrosis possible. Testing for just the delta F_{508} gene will identify about 70 percent of the abnormal genes or about 50 percent of affected patients. Testing for all currently known cystic fibrosis genes will identify about 80 percent of the abnormal genes responsible for cystic fibrosis. Because the test cannot identify 100 percent of the cystic fibrosis genes, it is best reserved for evaluation of patients with suspected cystic fibrosis who have equivocal results from sweat chloride testing or of subjects who require genetic counseling because they are at high risk for having children with cystic fibrosis.[18]

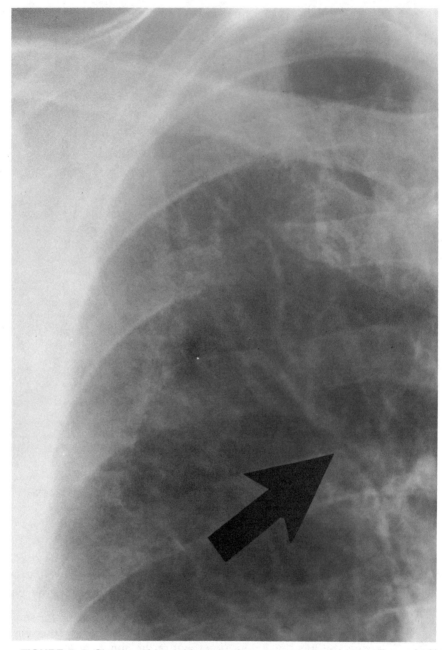

FIGURE 5–2 Closeup of bronchiectatic airway as seen on chest radiograph. Note that the thickened bronchial wall appears as parallel white lines, popularly called "tram tracks."

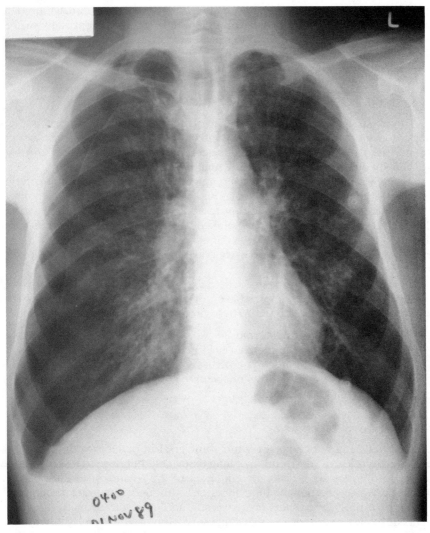

FIGURE 5–3 Chest radiograph of a patient with cystic fibrosis and a right pneumothorax. Note the pleural line visible in the right chest and the absence of lung markings beyond the line.

TREATMENT

Reversal of the Defect

Cystic fibrosis lung disease is caused by the dysfunction of a protein that regulates electrolyte movement. Several strategies are being attempted to reverse the defective electrolyte transport in the lungs of patients with cystic fibrosis.

Replacing defective lungs with normal lungs is one such approach. Heart lung transplantation and bilateral lung transplants have been used successfully to treat patients with end-stage lung disease due to cystic fibrosis. Transplantation reverses the physiologic abnormalities that characterize cystic fibrosis lung disease[19] but requires immunosuppression that may lead to opportunistic infections.[20]

Another approach to reversing the defect of cystic fibrosis is to give drugs that eliminate some or all of the abnormal electrolyte transport. Inhalation of aero-solized amiloride[21,22] or triphosphate nucleotides[23] show potential to overcome some of the ion transport abnormalities present in cystic fibrosis. Early trials on the use of these substances have shown promise; however, it is not known if these treatments alter the course of cystic fibrosis.

Respiratory Secretions

The most significant health threat to patients with cystic fibrosis is the ten-dency to develop recurrent respiratory infections. These infections are associated with increased production of mucinous secretions and the tendency to obstruct small and medium-sized bronchi with mucus plugs. Postural drainage and chest physiotherapy assist patients in clearing mucus plugs. Following administration of chest physiotherapy, there is an acute improvement in a number of pulmonary function measurements.[24,25] In addition to chest physiotherapy a number of other techniques have been successfully employed to assist in bronchial clearance. These techniques include aerosolized deoxyribonuclease (DNase),[26,27] regular aerobic exercise, autogenic drainage,[28] voluntary coughing,[29] and the use of a positive expi-ratory pressure (PEP) mask.[30]

Other treatments have been used to assist patients with cystic fibrosis clear secretions. Most of these therapies have not been shown to be clearly beneficial, and have not been widely adopted. These procedures include the following:

1. Administration of mists and aerosols of saline or water to help hydrate secretions and make them easier to expectorate
2. Administration of mucolytic aerosols to liquefy mucus plugs
3. Bronchoscopy with bronchoalveolar lavage to clear mucus plugs from intermediate and small airways

Respiratory Infections

Repeated lung infections are almost universal in patients with cystic fibrosis. These infections lead to destruction of lung tissue and therefore to loss of pulmonary function. Antibiotics are a critical component of the treatment of these infections and therefore preservation of lung function. Although the exact timing for the initiation of antibiotics remains controversial, antibiotics are usually started when patients develop new symptoms that suggest respiratory infection. These symptoms may include change in cough, new onset of cough, change in character or consis-tency of sputum, sudden deterioration in pulmonary function, fever, chest radio-graph changes, or lack of expected weight gain. The initial choice of antibiotics should be effective against those organisms that commonly infect patients with cystic fibrosis. The antibiotic coverage is adjusted once the sputum culture discloses a predominant organism. Serious infections may require intravenous (IV) antibiot-ics. Prolonged courses of IV antibiotics usually begin in the hospital but may be continued at home after the patient or family has learned to administer the antibiotics.

Oral antibiotics are frequently used for less severe respiratory infections. Flu-orinated quinolones belong to a potent new class of oral antibiotics, many of which have acceptable activity against *P. aeruginosa*. These new oral antibiotics are highly effective at controlling exacerbations of cystic fibrosis, but antibiotic resistance in the organisms may become a significant problem.

Inhaled antibiotics are occasionally used to suppress airway infections. The greatest experience with inhaled antibiotics has been with gentamicin. The dose of inhaled gentamicin typically varies from 20 to 80 mg two to four times daily.[31,32]

Bronchial Hyperactivity

A large number of patients with cystic fibrosis have bronchial hyperactivity similar to asthma (see Chapter 2). These symptoms are usually treated like asthma. Treatment includes the administration of inhaled or oral β-agonists and theophylline. Anti-inflammatory agents such as cromolyn sodium and inhaled or oral corticosteroids have been helpful in some cases.

Pancreatic Insufficiency

Patients with cystic fibrosis frequently develop malnutrition. This risk is in large part due to pancreatic exocrine insufficiency but also is related to inadequate food intake[33] and to the high metabolic demands associated with infection.

Pancreatic enzyme replacement is standard therapy to relieve the symptoms of pancreatic exocrine insufficiency. The enzymes are usually given as capsules or pills before every meal and are adjusted to relieve steatorrhea (fatty stools). In addition, fat-soluble vitamins (A, D, E, and K) are routinely supplemented. Patients should be encouraged to eat a balanced diet and avoid excessive fat intake.[34]

PROGNOSIS

The prognosis for patients with cystic fibrosis is steadily improving. At one time most patients would not live beyond their 10th birthday. Now with aggressive treatment of this multisystem disease most patients with cystic fibrosis live to age 25.[35]

Case Study

HISTORY

MB is a 26-year-old woman who presented to the pulmonary clinic for the first time with complaints of dyspnea on exertion and a productive cough. She had had a productive cough for many years and periodically developed yellow or green sputum and occasional hemoptysis. These symptoms were attributed to bronchiectasis. When she was a child, her parents were told she had asthma. She also had many childhood respiratory infections requiring hospitalization. At age 11 she was told she had bronchiectasis. Since that time her therapy included inhaled metaproterenol and occasional antibiotic therapy. She had no regular pulmonary hygiene program.

Three weeks before admission she developed an increasing cough producing greenish sputum. She also noticed increasing dyspnea on exertion, and wheezing. Her family physician gave her a prescription for ciprofloxacin 750 mg twice daily but her symptoms progressed despite this therapy. Her current symptoms increased to such a degree that she requested sick leave from her job as a secretary.

This was the third such episode MB experienced in the last year. Her previous episodes were successfully treated with oral ciprofloxacin. She chronically heard wheezing and crackles with breathing, particularly when she went to bed at night. She also had difficulty maintaining weight and felt she was far below her ideal weight. She did not have fever, chills, pharyngitis, coryza (clear nasal discharge), or purulent nasal discharge. She had no problems with steatorrhea (fatty stools), nasal polyps, or sinus infections.

MB never smoked. She had two younger sisters who had cystic fibrosis and an older brother who was healthy. Her father had a chronic problem with bronchiectasis that began as a teenager. MB had been tested for cystic fibrosis using a sweat chloride concentration when she was first diagnosed with bronchiectasis at age 11. Her sweat chloride concentration was 57 mEq/liter.

Questions

1. What features of this patient's history support the diagnosis of cystic fibrosis?
2. Which parts of MB's history suggest that she does not have cystic fibrosis?
3. Does her sweat chloride concentration help to clarify whether or not she has cystic fibrosis?
4. What findings would you expect to find on physical examination if this patient has cystic fibrosis?
5. What additional testing would be appropriate to support or refute the diagnosis of cystic fibrosis?

Answers

1. A number of features in the history support the suspicion that this woman has cystic fibrosis. The development of bronchiectasis at a young age, particularly in an area of the world where antibiotics are readily available, would suggest the diagnosis of cystic fibrosis. Children with cystic fibrosis are occasionally misdiagnosed in infancy as having asthma. Weight loss and inability to maintain a normal body weight also suggest the diagnosis of cystic fibrosis. Symptoms of asthma and recurrent pulmonary infections in childhood should lead one to consider the diagnosis of cystic fibrosis. Perhaps the most important feature in the history of this patient is the presence of siblings with cystic fibrosis. If one child in a family has cystic fibrosis, each sibling has a one in four chance of also having the disease.
2. This patient lacks certain characteristics one would normally expect to find with cystic fibrosis. She does not have diarrhea or symptoms of malabsorption that suggest pancreatic exocrine insufficiency. She also lacks a history of sinus difficulties or nasal polyps that would occur in most patients who have cystic fibrosis.
3. No, a sweat chloride value of between 50 and 80 mEq/liter is considered equivocal.
4. You would expect to find that this patient is a thin, underweight woman with an increased anteroposterior (AP) dimension of her chest. Her fingers would show clubbing, and, if the lung disease was very advanced, she may have some cyanosis. Lungs would disclose inspiratory crackles and expiratory wheezing. If cor pulmonale were present, one would see distended neck veins and edema in the lower extremities.
5. The result of the sweat chloride test this patient had as a child was equivocal. A repeat sweat chloride test should be performed. If the repeated sweat electrolyte concentrations are equivocal, then gene probes may be useful to determine if she is homozygous for the cystic fibrosis genes.

PHYSICAL EXAMINATION

General *A thin young white woman with a productive cough; uses accessory muscles of respiration but appears to be breathing comfortably and can converse without apparent dyspnea*

Vital Signs *Temperature 37.2°C; pulse 71/minute; respiratory rate 19/minute; blood pressure 105/72 mm Hg*

HEENT	*Nasal polyp seen in left nares; no sinus tenderness noted; oral examination normal and mucous membranes moist; eye and ear examinations normal*
Neck	*Trachea in midline position; both carotid impulses normal in contour and intensity; no jugular venous distention*
Chest	*AP dimensions of chest increased; diffuse inspiratory and expiratory crackles with polyphonic expiratory wheezing heard over both lungs; hyper-resonance noted with chest percussion*
Heart	*Regular rate with loud P$_2$ component of second heart sound noted on cardiac auscultation; no murmurs or gallops noted; point of maximum impulse (PMI) difficult to appreciate but located in the 5th interspace 2 to 3 cm lateral to sternal border*
Abdomen	*Bowel sounds active, with no guarding or tenderness; liver 8 cm wide in the midclavicular line; no masses palpated*
Extremities	*Digital clubbing but no cyanosis or edema; pulses equal and symmetric*

Questions

6. This patient does not have a fever at the time of examination or a history of fever before this visit. Does the lack of fever indicate the patient does not have a significant exacerbation of her lung disease?
7. What is the significance of this patient's underweight appearance?
8. What is a nasal polyp, and what respiratory problems may it create?
9. What is indicated by an increase in the AP dimension of the chest?
10. What is the significance of the crackles heard over the lungs?
11. The second heart sound has two components, an aortic (A$_2$) and a pulmonic (P$_2$) sound. Describe the source of these heart sounds and the meaning of a loud P$_2$.
12. Why does this patient have a cardiac PMI that is decreased in intensity and displaced from the normal position?
13. This patient demonstrates clubbing of the digits. Describe what clubbing of the fingers looks like and what it may indicate.
14. What laboratory work should be ordered at this time?

Answers

6. No. Patients with exacerbations of bronchiectasis typically complain of copious, grossly purulent secretions and dyspnea; however, fever is infrequent during bronchiectatic exacerbations. The best guide to determine the severity of a bronchiectatic exacerbation is the nature and severity of the symptoms. Fever is commonly found with pneumonia or viral respiratory infections. If MB had a fever, one should suspect pneumonia or viral illness.
7. The underweight appearance is suggestive of cystic fibrosis. Three reasons people with cystic fibrosis may develop malnutrition are (1) malabsorption due to pancreatic exocrine insufficiency, (2) a lower than normal caloric intake, and (3) increased metabolic demands due to respiratory effort and recurrent infections.

8. A nasal polyp is an overgrowth of mucosa in the nose that leads to a fingerlike growth in the nose. Patients with cystic fibrosis have a tendency to form nasal polyps. These polyps may become so numerous or large that they completely block the nasal passages.

9. When the lungs become hyperexpanded because of air trapping the chest enlarges, particularly in the AP dimension. This increase in chest diameter is associated with emphysema, chronic bronchitis, asthma, and cystic fibrosis.

10. Crackles are associated with increased pulmonary secretions. In advanced cases of cystic fibrosis, the lung examination will almost always disclose crackles. The presence of crackles in this case does not necessarily represent pulmonary edema or pneumonia.

11. The second heart sound (S_2) has two components. One is created when the aortic valve closes (A_2) and the other is produced when the pulmonic valve closes (P_2). Normally, A_2 is louder than P_2. If P_2 becomes louder than A_2, this suggests pulmonary hypertension.

12. As the lungs hyperexpand because of obstructive lung disease, the heart is forced to assume a more vertical and central position in the chest. This change in position can be seen on physical examination by a movement of the PMI centrally and toward the epigastrium.

13. Clubbing is enlargement of the tips of the fingers and toes; it is associated with convexity of the nails and is often seen in patients with chronic lung disease. The exact reason people with chronic lung disease develop clubbing is unclear.

14. Several questions need to be clarified before the optimum treatment program can be initiated. These questions include the following: (1) Does she have pneumonia or just an exacerbation of her bronchiectasis? (2) Is her dyspnea due in part to hypoxemia? and (3) Is her nutrition adequate?

> To evaluate for pneumonia a chest radiograph and white blood count and differential should be ordered. Hypoxemia can be identified by ABG analysis. If chronic hypoxemia is present, there is usually an elevation of the hemoglobin concentration or the hematocrit. Malnutrition can be evaluated by measurements of serum proteins such as albumin or protein.

LABORATORY EVALUATION

CHEST RADIOGRAPH:

(Fig. 5–4)

ABGs

(on room air)

pH	7.42
$Paco_2$	34 mm Hg
Pao_2	67 mm Hg
Bicarbonate	21 mEq
$P(A-a)o_2$	39 mm Hg
O_2 content	17.5 mL/dL

COMPLETE BLOOD COUNT

	Observed	Normal
White blood cells/μL	12,400	4,000–11,000
Red blood cells M/μL	4.7	4.1–5.5
Hemoglobin (g/dL)	14.2	14–16.5
Hematocrit (%)	43	37–50
Differential		
Segmented neutrophils	72%	38–79%
Band neutrophils	12%	0–7%
Lymphocytes	13%	12–51%
Monocytes	1%	0–10%
Eosinophils	1%	0–8%
Basophils	1%	0–2%

CHEMISTRY

	Observed	Normal
Sodium (mEq/liter)	138	136–146
Potassium (mEq/liter)	4.6	3.5–5.1
Chloride (mmol/dL)	106	98–106
Bicarbonate (mm/L)	20	22–29
Blood urea nitrogen (BUN) (mg/dL)	13	7–18
Creatinine (mg/dL)	0.7	0.5–1.1
Calcium (mmol/liter)	2.1	2.1–2.55
Phosphate (mg/dL)	2.7	2.7–4.5
Uric acid (mg/dL)	3.4	4.5–8.2
Albumin (g/dL)	3.1	3.5–5.0
Protein (g/dL)	6.0	6.4–8.3

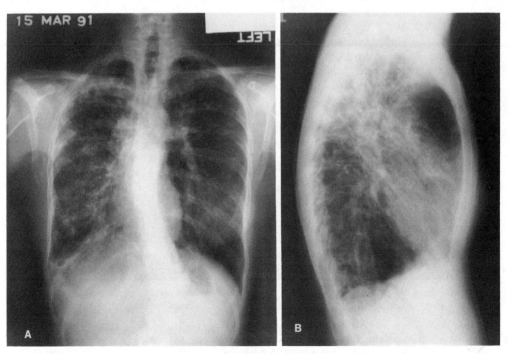

FIGURE 5–4 Chest radiograph from patient M.B. A, PA film; B, lateral view.

Questions

15. Read the chest radiograph and correlate it with this patient's condition (see Fig. 5–4).
16. How do you interpret the ABGs?
17. Why are the white blood count and the number of band neutrophils elevated?
18. What do a low albumin and total protein level indicate?
19. Name additional diagnostic tests that would be important to perform on this patient.
20. If the physician decides to admit this patient to the hospital, what respiratory therapy orders would you suggest?

Answers

15. Scoliosis is noted in the thoracic and lumbar spine. The lungs are hyperexpanded with diffuse reticular nodular opacities throughout both lungs. Numerous cystic airspaces are seen, as are occasional thickened bronchial walls.

    This radiograph is consistent with a patient with bronchiectasis or cystic fibrosis. Although the disease is more pronounced in the right lung, no focal areas of pneumonia are seen. This woman appears very thin with no excessive soft tissue shadows.
16. MB has a chronic respiratory alkalosis and a widened alveolar-to-arterial (A-a) gradient. Mild hypoxemia is present.
17. An acute infection of any type may elevate the white blood count and lead the bone marrow to release immature neutrophils (bands) into the blood to help fight the infection. In this case the elevation is most likely due to either pneumonia or an exacerbation of bronchiectasis.
18. Both of these serum proteins are likely to be depressed in the setting of malnutrition.
19. With any infection, selection of the appropriate antibiotic is easiest if the physician knows the offending organism. It is important to culture the sputum to determine, if possible, which organism is causing her infection. Identifying the infecting organism in this case is very important, because MB has already failed to respond to one course of antibiotics.
20. Respiratory therapy should aim to reverse bronchospasm and assist in the clearance of secretions. Inhaled β-agonists will help reverse bronchospasm. The optimum method of delivering β-agonists is not clearly defined. Either a metered-dose inhaler (MDI) or a nebulized solution would be appropriate. To help clear secretions, chest physiotherapy and postural drainage should also be started. Other therapies, such as mist tents, bland aerosol therapy, and N-acetyl-L-cysteine have been used to assist cystic fibrosis patients clear pulmonary secretions but have not proven effective.

Because MB failed to improve on oral antibiotics her physician admitted her to the medicine service for more aggressive treatment. The admitting orders included the following:

1. *Supplemental vitamins A, D, E, and K*
2. *Aminophylline 1 g in 0.25 liter normal saline: an initial IV infusion of 5 mg/kg over 30 minutes, then constant infusion at a rate of 0.5 mg/kg per hour*

3. *Piperacillin IV 1 g every 6 hours*
4. *Amikacin 225 mg IV every 8 hours*
5. *Medication nebulizer treatments with 0.3 mL of metaproterenol (Alupent) in 3 mL normal saline every 6 hours*
6. *Chest physiotherapy and postural drainage every 6 hours*
7. *Theophylline level for the second hospital day*
8. *Amikacin level before and after the third dose of amikacin*
9. *Sputum Gram's stain and culture*
10. *Sweat chloride concentration*
11. *Gene probe for the delta F_{508} gene*

Questions

21. The admitting physician believes that MB may have cystic fibrosis. Why did the physician prescribe the supplemental A, D, E, and K vitamins?
22. What is metaproterenol? What side effects may the patient experience while you administer this treatment?
23. Is the chest physiotherapy and postural drainage the physician ordered important for this patient, or should you recommend it be discontinued? Why?
24. What is the most important thing that you as a respiratory care practitioner could teach this patient to help in her long-term health?
25. If this patient has cystic fibrosis, what organisms would you expect to find on the sputum culture?
26. One of the microorganisms that patients with cystic fibrosis commonly have as a respiratory pathogen has a unique characteristic. Describe what is unique about the *Pseudomonas aeruginosa* found in cystic fibrosis patients.
27. If MB has cystic fibrosis, what are the odds that she will have both copies of the delta F_{508} gene?

Answers

21. MB appears mildly malnourished on physical examination and on her admitting laboratory work. If she has cystic fibrosis she may have difficulty absorbing fat and the fat-soluble vitamins. To overcome the vitamin deficiency, patients are generally given supplemental fat-soluble vitamins A, D, E, and K.
22. Metaproterenol is an inhaled β-agonist. The purpose of giving it to this patient is to reverse bronchospasm, which is the cause of her wheezing and some of her dyspnea. The primary side effects of metaproterenol are tachycardia, tachyarrhythmias, and tremors.
23. Chest physiotherapy is very important for patients with bronchiectasis and cystic fibrosis. Mucus plugs in the distal airways may obstruct these airways and cause right-to-left shunting and lead to small distal abscesses. Therefore, clearance of mucus plugs is very important for patients with cystic fibrosis. Chest physiotherapy and postural drainage will help move these mucus plugs from the distal airways to the large central airways, from which they can be coughed out.
24. MB has had no program to assist bronchial hygiene. She should be instructed in postural drainage and a family member taught to perform chest physiotherapy. Other therapies that may assist bronchial hygiene include regular exercise and the use of PEP by mask or mouthpiece.
25. The three organisms most commonly found in the tracheal secretions of patients with cystic fibrosis include: *Haemophilus influenzae, Staphylococcus aureus,* and *Pseudomonas aeruginosa.*

26. The *P. aeruginosa* organism that infects patients with cystic fibrosis differs from the vast majority of *P. aeruginosa* isolates in that it produces mucin. This can be seen in the appearance of the colony on a culture plate.

27. The delta F_{508} gene accounts for about 70 percent of the abnormal genes that cause cystic fibrosis. To have the disease, the affected individual must have two genes that cause cystic fibrosis. The chance that an individual with cystic fibrosis has both delta F_{508} genes is $0.7 \times 0.7 \times 100 = 49$ percent.

MB is hospitalized for 5 days. During this time she receives antibiotics, bronchodilators, and chest physiotherapy. Her symptoms are greatly improved with a marked reduction in her cough and dyspnea. She now produces far less sputum, and the color is a light yellow. She has been trained to administer her own IV antibiotics and to perform postural drainage; her husband has been trained to deliver chest percussion. The sputum culture grew a mucinous strain of P. aeruginosa that was resistant to ciprofloxacin. Her sweat chloride concentration was 103 mEq/liter. The gene probe revealed that MB had only one copy of the delta F_{508} gene.

Question

28. Does MB have cystic fibrosis?

Answer

28. Yes, the elevation of sweat chloride to 103 mEq/liter confirms that MB, like her sisters, has cystic fibrosis. The gene probe found that MB was heterozygous for the delta F_{508} gene. However there are several mutations of the gene other than delta F_{508} that may lead to cystic fibrosis. The delta F_{508} gene accounts for only 70 percent of the genes causing cystic fibrosis. It is thus not surprising that MB has only one of the delta F_{508} genes yet still has cystic fibrosis.

MB is not unusual for older patients with cystic fibrosis. Her presentation contained many classic features of the disease but also lacked a significant number of common abnormalities. Pancreatic exocrine insufficiency is one typical finding she does not have. Patients with normal pancreatic exocrine function have a better prognosis than those with pancreatic dysfunction.[36]

REFERENCES

1. Conneally, PM, Merritt, AD, and Yu, P: Cystic fibrosis: Population genetics. Tex Rep Biol Med 31:639, 1973.

2. Levison, H and Tabachnik, E: Pulmonary physiology. In Hodson, ME, Norman, AP, and Batten, JC: Cystic Fibrosis. Baillière Tindall, London, 1983, pp 52–81.

3. Fanconi, G, Uehlinger, E, and Knauer, C: Das coeliakiesyndrom bei angeborener zysticher pankreasfibromatose und bronchiektasien. Wein Med Wchnschr 86:753, 1936.

4. Taussig, LM: Cystic Fibrosis. Thieme-Stratton, New York, 1984.

5. Riordan, JR, et al: Identification of the cystic fibrosis gene: Cloning and characterization of the complementary DNA. Science 245:1066, 1989.

6. Rommens, JM, et al: Identification of the cystic fibrosis gene: Chromosome walking and jumping. Science 245:1059, 1989.

7. Kerem, E, et al: The relation between genotype and phenotype in cystic fibrosis of the most common mutation (delta F_{508}). N Engl J Med 323:1517, 1990.

8. Rich, DP, et al: Expression of cystic fibrosis transmembrane conductance regulator corrects defective chloride channel regulation in cystic fibrosis airway epithelial cells. Nature 347:358, 1990.

9. Anderson, MP, et al: Generation of cAMP-activated chloride currents by expression of CFTR. Science 251:679, 1991.

10. Quinton, PM and Bijman, J: Higher bioelectric potentials due to decreased chloride absorption in the sweat glands of patients with cystic fibrosis. N Engl J Med 308:1185, 1983.

11. Esterly, JR and Oppenheimer, EH: Observations in cystic fibrosis of the pancreas. Part III: Pulmonary lesions. Johns Hopkins Med J 122:94, 1968.

12. Bedrossian, CWM, et al: The lung in cystic fibrosis. A quantitative study including prevalence of pathologic findings among different age groups. Hum Pathol 7:195, 1976.

13. Rosenstein, BJ and Langbaum, TS: Diagnosis. In Taussig, LM: Cystic Fibrosis. Thieme Stratton, New York, 1984.

14. Shwachman, H: Gastrointestinal manifestations of cystic fibrosis. Pediatr Clin North Am 22:787, 1975.

15. Gibson, LE and Cook, RE: A test for concentration of electrolytes in sweat in cystic fibrosis of the pancreas utilizing pilocarpine iontophoresis. Pediatrics 23:545, 1959.

16. Report of the committee for a study for evaluation of testing for cystic fibrosis. National Academy of Sciences, Washington, DC, 1975.

17. Rosenstein, BJ, et al: Cystic fibrosis: Problems encountered with sweat testing. JAMA 240:1987, 1978.

18. Statement from the National Institutes of Health workshop in population screening for the cystic fibrosis gene. N Engl J Med 323:70, 1990.

19. Alton, EW, et al: Effect of heart lung transplantation on airway potential difference in patients with and without cystic fibrosis. Eur Respir J 4:5, 1991.

20. Higenbottam, TW, et al: Mortality and morbidity following heart-lung transplantation for cystic fibrosis. Am Rev Respir Dis 141:605, 1990.

21. App, EM, et al: Acute and long term amiloride inhalation in cystic fibrosis lung disease: a rational approach to cystic fibrosis therapy. Am Rev Respir Dis 141:605, 1990.

22. Knowles, MR, et al: A pilot study of aerosolized amiloride for treatment of lung disease in cystic fibrosis. N Engl J Med 322:1189, 1990.

23. Knowles, MR, Clarke, LL, and Boucher, RC: Activation by extracellular nucleotides of chloride secretion in the airway epithelia of patients with cystic fibrosis. N Engl J Med 325:533, 1991.

24. Desmond, KJ, et al: Immediate and long term effects of chest physiotherapy in patients with cystic fibrosis. J Pediatr 103:538, 1983.

25. Maxwell, M and Redmond, AO: Comparative trial of manual and mechanical percussion technique with gravity-assisted bronchial drainage in patients with cystic fibrosis. Arch Dis Child 54:542, 1979.

26. Hubbard, RC, et al: A preliminary study of aerosolized recombinant deoxyribonuclease I in the treatment of cystic fibrosis. N Engl J Med 326:812, 1992.

27. Aitken, ML, et al: Recombinant human DNase inhalation in normal subjects and patients with cystic fibrosis. JAMA 267:1947, 1992.

28. Partridge, C, Pryor, J, and Webber, B: Characteristics of the forced expiration technique. Physiotherapy 75:193, 1989.

29. Zinman, R: Cough versus chest physiotherapy: A comparison of the acute effects on pulmonary function in patients with cystic fibrosis. Am Rev Respir Dis 129:182, 1984.

30. Steen, HJ, et al: Evaluation of the PEP mask in cystic fibrosis. Acta Paediatr Scand 80:51, 1991.

31. Hodson, ME, Penketh, ARL, and Patten, JC: Aerosol carbenicillin and gentamicin treatment of *Pseudomonas aeruginosa* infection in patients with cystic fibrosis. Lancet 2:1137, 1981.

32. Nolan, G, et al: Antibiotic prophylaxis in cystic fibrosis: Inhaled cephaloridine as an adjunct to oral cloxacillin. J Pediatr 101:626, 1982.

33. Hubbard, VS and Mangrum, PJ: Energy intake and nutritional counseling in cystic fibrosis. J Am Diet Assoc 80:127, 1982.

34. Dodge, JA: Nutrition. In Hodson, ME, Norman, AP, and Batten, JC: Cystic Fibrosis. Baillière Tindall, London, 1983, pp 132–141.

35. Patient Registry, Cystic Fibrosis Foundation, through 1985.

36. Gaskin, K, et al: Improved respiratory prognosis in patients with cystic fibrosis with normal fat absorption. J Pediatr 100:857, 1982.

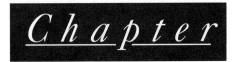

Chapter 6

Robert L. Wilkins, MA, RRT
James R. Dexter, MD, FCCP

HEMODYNAMIC MONITORING and SHOCK

INTRODUCTION

The circulatory system comprises the heart, blood vessels, and blood. Each component plays a vital role in the process of circulation. The heart serves as the pump that provides the power to move blood throughout the blood vessels (**perfusion**). The blood vessels direct the blood from the heart to the tissues through arteries and back to the heart through veins. The arteries are endowed with smooth muscle that provides variable resistance to flow to help maintain the blood pressure needed for perfusion. Blood serves as the medium in which the oxygen and other nutrients are carried to the tissues.

Supplementary organs involved in circulation include the lungs, which provide oxygen; the bone marrow, which provides red blood cells; the liver, which processes nutrients from the digestive tract; and the nervous system, which regulates muscle tone in the arteries.

The circulatory system can be divided into two major parts: the pulmonary system and the systemic system. The pulmonary circulation is made up of the right side of the heart (right atrium and right ventricle), pulmonary arteries, and pulmonary veins. The pulmonary arteries direct blood from the right ventricle to the lungs for gas exchange. The pulmonary veins conduct the oxygenated blood from the lungs back to the left side of the heart. The systemic system is made up of the left side of the heart (left atrium and left ventricle), the arteries, and the veins. The systemic arteries carry oxygenated blood from the left heart to the different organ systems, where oxygen and nutrients are given up to the tissues and metabolic waste products are removed. The veins return the partially deoxygenated blood back to the right side of the heart.

Because the purpose of circulation is to provide the organs of the body with oxygen and other vital nutrients, circulatory failure is defined in terms of vital organ system dysfunction. When circulation is not sufficient to meet the metabolic needs of vital organs such as the brain, heart, kidneys, and so on, the patient is suffering from circulatory failure or **shock.** Although many parameters may indicate that circulation may not be optimal (e.g., hypotension), shock is present only when there is evidence of vital organ dysfunction (e.g., abnormal sensorium, decreased urine output).

77

WHAT IS CARDIAC OUTPUT?

The pumping function of the left ventricle is very important because it moves the oxygenated blood to all areas of the body in order to maintain life. The quantity of blood pumped out of the left ventricle each minute is the **cardiac output.** Normally the adult cardiac output is approximately 4 to 8 liters/minute. Because normal cardiac output depends on the size and metabolic rate of the patient, clinicians must interpret it in relation to the patient's body mass and metabolic rate. A cardiac output of 3.5 liters/minute might be acceptable for a petite, afebrile, resting woman, whereas this same value could represent a circulatory crisis for a large man with a fever.

Cardiac index (cardiac output/body surface area) is a useful parameter because it accounts for the variations in body size. The patient's body surface area in square meters can be determined from standard nomograms and is divided into the cardiac output to determine cardiac index. Normal cardiac index is 2.5 to 4.0 liters/minute per m^2.

WHAT DETERMINES CARDIAC OUTPUT?

Cardiac output is the product of heart rate and **stroke volume** (the volume of blood ejected by the ventricle with each contraction). Heart rate is strongly influenced by the sympathetic and parasympathetic nervous systems. Activation of the sympathetic nervous systems leads to tachycardia and usually increases cardiac output, except at extremes. Stimulation of the parasympathetic nervous system promotes bradycardia, and profound bradycardia may reduce cardiac output.

Stroke volume is a function of three important factors: filling volume of the ventricle **(preload),** arterial resistance to flow out of the ventricle during contraction **(afterload),** and cardiac **contractility** (Fig. 6–1). Bedside clinicians must evaluate all three factors in patients suffering from circulatory insufficiency.

Preload

The strength of myocardial muscle contraction is directly related (within limits) to the amount of stretch applied to the muscle before contraction. This precontraction stretch is known as preload and is primarily a function of venous pressure, which determines the volume in the ventricle just before contraction. Up to a certain point the more the ventricle is stretched during ventricular filling (diastole), the greater the force of the subsequent contraction and the greater the stroke volume (Fig. 6–2). If the filling of the ventricle is minimal (as in hypovolemia), the subsequent contraction will result in a reduced stroke volume. Excessive overfilling of the ventricle will also lead to a reduced stroke volume due to overstretching of the myocardium. The point at which optimal filling of the heart occurs varies from patient to patient, depending on the compliance of the ventricles.

At the bedside, clinicians look at the patient's neck veins and measure central venous pressure (CVP) to evaluate right heart filling pressure. Clinicians measure the pulmonary capillary wedge pressure (PCWP) to assess preload for the left ventricle. Physicians place a balloon-tipped catheter into the pulmonary artery to obtain this measurement (Fig. 6–3). Indications for the use of a pulmonary artery catheter are described later, in the section on treatment. Normal CVP is 2 to 6 mm Hg and normal PCWP is 4 to 12 mm Hg.[1]

Afterload

The tension created by the cardiac muscle fibers during contraction to overcome impedance to flow out of the ventricle is known as afterload. Because ven-

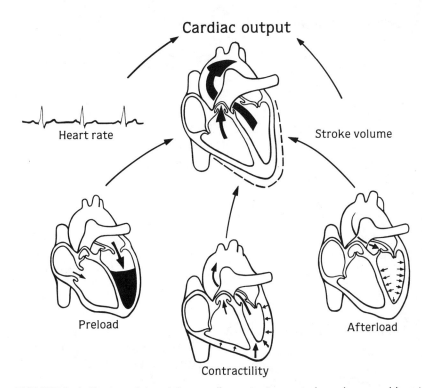

FIGURE 6–1 Factors determining cardiac output are stroke volume and heart rate. Stroke volume is determined by preload, afterload, and contractility. (From Wilkins, RL, Sheldon, RL, and Krider, SJ: Clinical Assessment in Respiratory Care. Mosby-Yearbook, St Louis, 1990, with permission.)

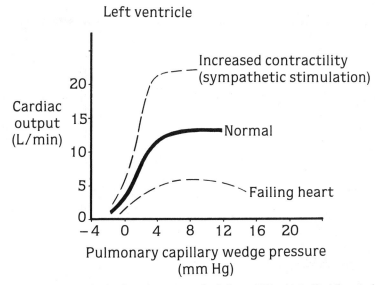

FIGURE 6–2 Ventricular function curves for left ventricle. Note that the stroke volume increases with a rise in filling pressure, up to a certain point. Overfilling of the ventricle results in a decrease in stroke volume, especially in the failing heart. (From Wilkins, RL, Sheldon, RL, and Krider, SJ: Clinical Assessment in Respiratory Care, Mosby-Yearbook, St Louis, 1990, with permission.)

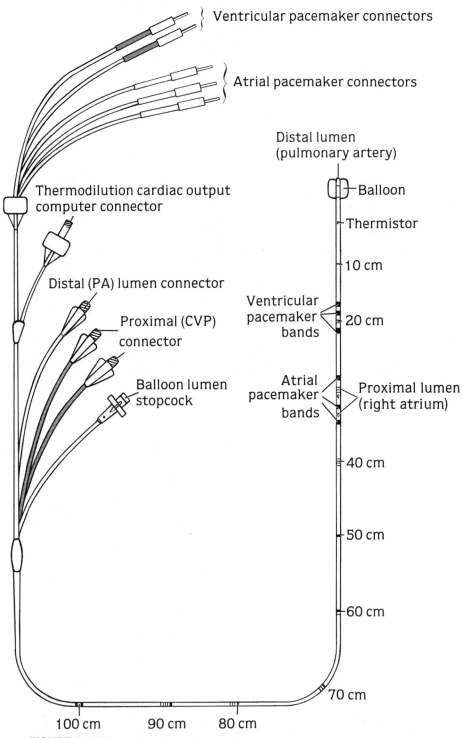

FIGURE 6–3 Illustration of a pulmonary artery catheter. (From Wilkins, RL, Sheldon, RL, and Krider, SJ: Clinical Assessment in Respiratory Care. Mosby-Yearbook, St Louis, 1990, with permission.)

Table 6-1 Hemodynamic Parameters

Parameter	Normal Range	Indication
Cardiac output	4–8 L/min	Total blood flow
Cardiac index	2.5–4.0 L/min/m²	Blood flow for size of patient
CVP	0–6 mm Hg	Right ventricle preload
PCWP	6–12 mm Hg	Left ventricle preload
SVR	900–1400 dynes/sec/cm²	Left ventricle afterload
PVR	200–450 dynes/sec/cm²	Right ventricle afterload
MAP	80–100 mm Hg	Perfusion pressure
P$\bar{v}O_2$	35–45 mm Hg	Tissue oxygenation
PAP	20–30/6–15 mm Hg	Pulmonary artery pressure

PAP = Pulmonary artery pressure

tricular wall tension is very difficult to measure, other parameters are used to reflect afterload. Systemic vascular resistance (SVR) reflects afterload for the left ventricle. Pulmonary vascular resistance (PVR) indicates afterload for the right ventricle (see Table 6-1 for normal values). Afterload for the left ventricle increases with systemic vasoconstriction and decreases with peripheral vasodilatation. Afterload increases for the right ventricle with pulmonary vasoconstriction and decreases with pulmonary vasodilatation. The interaction between cardiac output and afterload determines blood pressure.

The calculation of resistance requires measurement of the driving pressure across the circuit. For SVR this driving pressure is the difference between mean arterial pressure (MAP) and CVP; for PVR the driving pressure is the difference between mean pulmonary artery (PA) pressure minus left atrial pressure (PCWP). Once the driving pressure is determined, the resistance can be calculated by dividing the cardiac output into the pressure difference:

$$SVR = \frac{MAP\ (mm\ Hg) - CVP\ (mm\ Hg)}{Cardiac\ output\ (liter/minute)} \times 80*$$

$$PVR = \frac{PA\ (mm\ Hg) - PCWP\ (mm\ Hg)}{Cardiac\ output\ (liter/minute)} \times 80*$$

An appropriate level of afterload for the left ventricle is essential to maintain adequate perfusion pressures throughout the body. Decreases in afterload (peripheral vasodilatation) will cause the blood pressure to drop. The decrease in blood pressure will stimulate the heart to increase cardiac output in an effort to maintain circulation. If the drop in afterload is excessive and the compensatory mechanisms are inadequate, blood pressure may be inadequate for perfusion of vital organs (shock).

Contractility

The forcefulness of myocardial contraction is known as contractility. Even if the ventricle is adequately filled and resistance to outflow optimal, cardiac output will not be adequate if contractility is poor. Common vascular responses to decreased cardiac contractility include an increased afterload (elevated SVR) and

*Used to convert the units to dynes/second per cm − 5

increased preload (elevated CVP and PCWP). Factors that reduce cardiac contractility are called negative **inotropes** and include hypoxemia, acidosis, and medications such as β-adrenergic blocking agents. Damage to the myocardium as occurs with myocardial infarction will also reduce cardiac contractility. Factors that increase contractility are called positive inotropes and include certain β-adrenergic agents (e.g., Isuprel) and parasympatholytics (e.g., atropine).

ETIOLOGY

Circulatory shock results from inadequate cardiac contractility, failure of vascular tone (inadequate afterload), or hypovolemia (inadequate preload). For example, myocardial infarction may cause inadequate cardiac contractility and shock (see Chapter 8). Sepsis (infection in the bloodstream) may cause vasodilatation with decreased afterload and shock. Bleeding, trauma, or surgery and dehydration may result in significant hypovolemia (a decrease in circulating blood volume). This can precipitate hypovolemic shock when the circulating blood volume is inadequate to meet the metabolic needs of the body. This typically requires a loss of more than 20 to 25 percent of the circulating blood volume.[2] Other causes of shock include those that obstruct the flow of blood (e.g., massive pulmonary embolism, which causes high afterload for the right heart and inadequate preload to the left heart), and those that cause inadequate contractility by restricting the function of the heart (e.g., constrictive pericarditis and pericardial tamponade).

The most complex forms of shock are those that are caused by maldistribution of blood flow. This category of circulatory failure includes **septic shock, toxic shock, anaphylactic shock,** and **neurogenic shock.** In each case perfusion of vital organs is diminished owing to loss of peripheral resistance from vasodilatation and hypotension. Of these different types of shock due to failure of vascular tone, septic shock is the most common.[3] Septic shock produces a syndrome that affects the heart, vascular system, and most organs of the body. Although gram-negative bacteria are the most common cause of septic shock, a vast number of microorganisms can cause it by releasing toxins into the blood.[2]

The role of metabolism in the evaluation of patients with circulatory failure is important to consider. Anything that increases the metabolic rate of the patient will potentially increase the incidence and severity of the shock. For example, fever increases oxygen consumption and may result in shock in the patient with marginal cardiac function.

PATHOPHYSIOLOGY

The majority of organ systems in the body are affected by circulatory failure. Reduced perfusion to the brain initially results in diminished cognitive function and alertness, followed eventually by coma. The kidneys will reduce urine output in response to inadequate circulation. The skin typically becomes cool and clammy to the touch as peripheral circulation is reduced in an effort to preserve blood flow to the vital organs. Shock may even impair the blood clotting system and lead to disseminated intravascular coagulation (DIC),[4] a complex medical problem that results in hemorrhage caused by the consumption of platelets and clotting factors.

The lungs are also affected when circulatory failure is present. The type of shock present determines the effect of the circulatory problem on the lungs. When the left ventricle is unable to pump effectively (decreased contractility), blood backs up into the pulmonary circulation causing pulmonary edema; this is known as congestive heart failure (see Chapter 8). When the shock is due to loss of vascular tone or hypovolemia, pulmonary consequences are minimal except under the most severe circumstances when underperfusion of the lungs leads to adult respiratory distress syndrome (ARDS) (see Chapter 11).

CLINICAL FEATURES

Shock typically produces a similar clinical picture in most patients, regardless of its cause. Patients in shock usually have hypotension, tachypnea, and tachycardia. The peripheral pulses are typically weak or "thready" owing to the reduced stroke volume associated with shock. Signs of organ dysfunction are present and include oliguria (diminished urine output), altered sensorium, and hypoxemia.[5] The skin often becomes cool and clammy as epinephrine is released, causing peripheral vasoconstriction in an attempt to compensate for the hypotension.

Severe shock often leads to metabolic acidosis, which indicates the occurrence of an anaerobic metabolism due to the lack of oxygen delivery to the tissues.[2] This is often (but not always) accompanied by a decrease in mixed venous oxygen tension ($P\bar{v}o_2$) and an increase in serum lactate, which is a product of the anaerobic metabolism. The decrease in $P\bar{v}o_2$ occurs as tissues extract more than usual amounts of oxygen from the slowly passing blood to compensate for the reduced cardiac output.

Evaluation of the serum electrolytes is useful in patients with shock because significant defects (e.g., low potassium) may contribute to the cardiovascular compromise and can be easily corrected. The electrolytes are also useful in calculation of the anion gap for detecting the onset of lactic acidosis due to lactic acid production from anaerobic metabolism. To calculate the anion gap the chloride (Cl^-) and bicarbonate (HCO_3^-) values are added together and the total subtracted from the sodium (Na^+). Normal values are 8 to 16 mEq/liter. An anion gap higher than 16 mEq/liter in the patient with shock indicates that the shock is more severe and is resulting in lactic acidosis.

For patients with failure of vascular tone (e.g., septic shock, toxic shock), fever or hypothermia and leukocytosis are typically present.[6] Because the patient with maldistribution shock has peripheral vasodilation, the extremities may remain warm and pink despite poor circulation to the vital organs. Hemodynamic monitoring of the patient with septic shock reveals an increased cardiac output, reduced systemic vascular resistance, and a low to normal PCWP in the hyperdynamic phase of this syndrome (Table 6–2). $P\bar{v}o_2$ may be normal despite inadequate tissue oxygenation. The normal $P\bar{v}o_2$ in patients with septic shock is probably due to decreased peripheral use of oxygen and peripheral arteriovenous shunts.[1] Later the myocardium often becomes depressed as part of the septic shock syndrome, and cardiac output decreases.

Table 6–2 Assessment of the Type of Shock

Parameter	Hypovolemic	Septic	Pump Failure
Cardiac output/CI	Decreased	Increased*	Decreased
CVP	Decreased	Normal to low	Increased
PCWP	Decreased	Normal to low	Increased
SVR	Increased	Decreased	Increased
MAP	Normal/low	Decreased	Decreased
$P\bar{v}o_2$	Decreased	Normal	Decreased

*Cardiac output/CI is often increased in the early phase of septic shock but may decrease later.

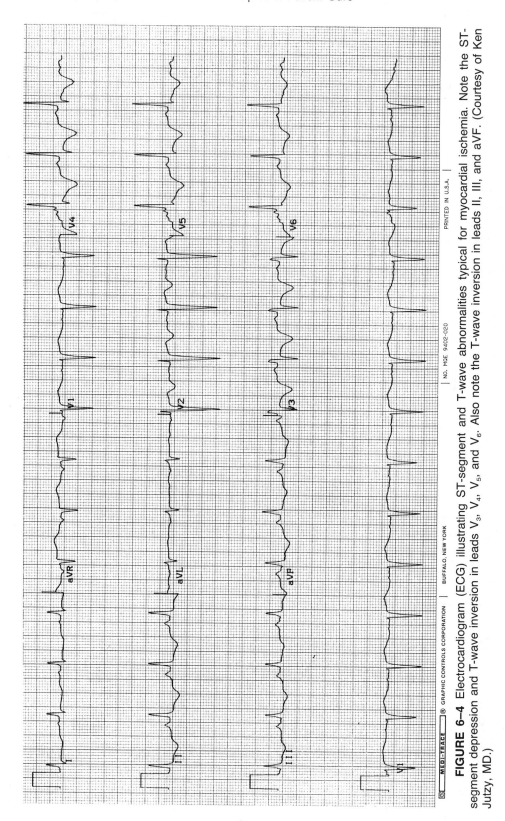

FIGURE 6-4 Electrocardiogram (ECG) illustrating ST-segment and T-wave abnormalities typical for myocardial ischemia. Note the ST-segment depression and T-wave inversion in leads V_3, V_4, V_5, and V_6. Also note the T-wave inversion in leads II, III, and aVF. (Courtesy of Ken Jutzy, MD.)

Patients with hypovolemic shock typically have poor perfusion to the extremities, which results in a slow capillary refill, peripheral cyanosis, and cool digits. Hemodynamic monitoring reveals reduced filling pressures of the heart (low CVP and PCWP), low cardiac output, and high systemic vascular resistance. Urine output decreases with hypovolemic shock as the kidneys try to conserve body fluids.

The electrocardiogram (ECG) most commonly shows tachycardia although abnormal rhythms may be seen when coronary perfusion is inadequate. When coronary artery perfusion is inadequate, the ECG will demonstrate ST-segment elevation or depression or T-wave inversion, or both (Fig. 6–4).[2] When considering the use of a vasopressor to correct hypotension, the presence of abnormal ST segments or T waves on the ECG suggests that the patient's heart may not tolerate the strain on it associated with an increased afterload from the vasopressor.

Chapter 8 reviews the clinical findings typical for cardiogenic shock resulting from left heart failure.

TREATMENT

A few general guidelines apply to treating all patients with shock. Oxygen therapy is needed to treat hypoxemia and maximize efficiency of circulation. Oxygen may need to be given in high concentrations (more than 40 percent) initially, especially if pulmonary edema is present. Endotracheal intubation is required when the patient's sensorium is depressed to the point that aspiration of gastric contents might occur.[2]

Mechanical ventilation is often needed to treat the patient in shock, as this will reduce the oxygen consumption of the respiratory muscles and circulatory demands as well as treat the respiratory failure. Mechanical ventilation is most helpful when a quick recovery from the shock is not likely (e.g., septic shock) and when respiratory failure occurs. The use of positive end-expiratory pressure (PEEP) may be needed when the Pao_2 is less than 60 mm Hg on a Fio_2 greater than 0.50. Close monitoring of the patient in an intensive care unit (ICU) is very important. The physician may need to place a PA catheter to allow accurate assessment of the cause of the circulatory problems and to monitor the patient's response to therapy. In general, the PA catheter is used when measurement of PA pressures, cardiac output, or mixed venous Po_2 are needed to assess the patient and monitor treatment. A list of the hemodynamic parameters useful in monitoring patients in shock is provided in Table 6–1.

For patients with hypovolemic shock, rapid replacement of circulating blood volume is crucial. As a general rule, fluid resuscitation is needed whenever the systolic blood pressure is below 90 mm Hg and there are signs of vital organ dysfunction (e.g., abnormal sensorium).[2] When the patient has lost large amounts of blood it is ideal to use blood as the replacement. When there is no time to type and cross-match blood, rapid infusion of a volume expander (e.g., normal saline, hetastarch) supports circulation until definitive treatment is available.

Administration of antibiotics and volume expanders is essential treatment for patients with septic shock. The potential source of the infection should be sought and may include surgical sites, wounds, and indwelling catheters and tubes. Volume expansion may prove useful to improve the blood pressure by filling the void created by the peripheral vasodilatation associated with sepsis. Vasopressors such as dopamine or norepinephrine improve hypotension by partially reversing the vasodilatation caused by sepsis and by stimulating cardiac contractility and thus improving cardiac output. (See Chapter 8 for a discussion about the treatment of heart failure.)

Case Study

HISTORY

Mr. E is a 46-year-old white man brought to the emergency room by ambulance following a gunshot wound to the abdomen. The patient was found by the emergency medical technicians outside a local bar lying on his side in a pool of blood. At the scene of the shooting, the patient was semiconscious with a pulse rate of 128/minute, a breathing rate of 32/minute, and a blood pressure of 95/60 mm Hg. The single gunshot wound was stabilized by the ambulance crew and an intravenous (IV) infusion of normal saline was initiated before his transfer to the hospital. At the emergency room Mr. E's vital signs revealed pulse thready at 130/minute; respiratory rate 34/minute; and blood pressure 80/50 mm Hg. Mr. E was semiconscious and disoriented. His skin was cool and clammy to the touch, with peripheral cyanosis noted. Breath sounds and heart sounds were normal. His abdomen was distended, and bowel sounds were absent. Neurologic status was grossly intact. Past medical and family history was not available.

Questions

1. What is indicated by the cool cyanotic extremities? What is suggested by the thready pulse?
2. What is indicated by the abnormal sensorium?
3. Is oxygen therapy indicated, and if so, at what F_{IO_2}?
4. What is your assessment of the patient's condition? Is shock present? If so, what is the most likely cause?
5. Should the patient be intubated and mechanically ventilated?
6. What is the patient's most urgent need for care at this point?

Answers

1. Cool cyanotic extremities indicate poor perfusion. Peripheral vasoconstriction is a compensatory mechanism in which the body attempts to preserve blood flow to the central, vital organs whenever blood pressure falls below a crucial level. This results in the patient's feet and hands feeling cool to the touch. Peripheral cyanosis occurs when the tissues extract excessive amounts of oxygen from the slowly passing blood, leaving it very desaturated. The thready pulse indicates that this patient's stroke volume is abnormally low.
2. The abnormal sensorium may indicate that the brain is not receiving optimal oxygenation. In this case this is probably the result of inadequate perfusion to the brain, which occurs when the mean arterial pressure drops below 90 mm Hg.[2]
3. Oxygen therapy is useful whenever a patient demonstrates the signs of circulatory or respiratory failure. An F_{IO_2} greater than 0.40 would be most appropriate.
4. There is evidence of vital organ dysfunction (an abnormal sensorium), most likely as a result of poor circulation. The patient is most likely suffering from hypovolemic shock caused by blood loss from the gunshot wound (Table 6–2).
5. Mechanical ventilation is not indicated at this point, as there is no evidence of respiratory failure and the patient may respond rapidly to treatment. Intubation may be useful if the patient's mental status deteriorates to the point where he may aspirate if vomiting occurs.

6. The patient's most urgent need is replacement of the blood lost by hemorrhage. A blood sample should be obtained immediately for cross-matching so that the appropriate blood type can be given. Large amounts of a volume-expanding fluid must be given until the cross-matching has been completed. Additionally the patient will need to be taken to the operating room to repair internal injuries related to the gunshot wound.

The patient was given oxygen via simple face mask and a follow-up arterial blood gas (ABG) analysis revealed pH 7.41, P_{CO_2} 34 mm Hg, P_{O_2} 98 mm Hg. A CVP catheter was placed, demonstrating a reading of 2 cm H_2O. The patient was taken to the operating room, where the inferior vena cava and portions of the small bowel were repaired. A total of 4 units of whole blood and 3 liters of normal saline were given to the patient.

Upon return to the ICU the patient assessment revealed blood pressure 125/75 mm Hg, pulse 96/minute, respiratory rate 14/minute via mechanical ventilation, with a tidal volume of 1000 cc and an F_{IO_2} of 0.45. ABGs show pH 7.47, P_{CO_2} 33 mm Hg, and a Pa_{O_2} of 110 mm Hg. CVP reading was 6 cm H_2O and the patient's body temperature rectally was 36.5°C. A urinary catheter was in place and urine output was 50 mL for the 2 hours of surgery. The patient was nonresponsive owing to the effects of general anesthesia. His peripheral pulses were normal and his hands and feet were warmer than they had been before surgery.

Questions

7. What is your assessment of Mr. E's circulatory status following the surgery?
8. Interpret the ABG findings after surgery. What changes in the ventilator settings do you recommend?
9. When should weaning from the mechanical ventilation begin?
10. What complications of circulatory shock might occur in this patient?

Answers

7. Mr. E's circulatory status following surgery appears to be improved, based on the fact that his peripheral pulses, blood pressure, CVP, and urine output are adequate and his extremities warmer.
8. Analysis of ABGs reveals respiratory alkalosis with supernormal oxygenation on an F_{IO_2} of 0.45. This suggests that the F_{IO_2} and the minute volume could be decreased. The minute volume can be lowered by decreasing the tidal volume or the ventilator rate. Keeping the tidal volume at 10 to 15 cc/kg helps to reduce the incidence of atelectasis. For this reason, reducing the ventilator rate would probably be the best choice in this case.
9. Weaning from mechanical ventilation can begin as soon as the patient recovers from the effects of the general anesthesia. Evidence of recovery includes increased mental acuity, ability to follow commands, and a return of reflexes (e.g., gag reflex). As there is no evidence of prior respiratory disease, the patient will probably not need the ventilator after he wakes up from the anesthesia.
10. The patient is at risk for ARDS (see Chapter 11), DIC, renal failure, sepsis, and postoperative atelectasis (see Chapter 13).

Mr. E was weaned from mechanical ventilation without difficulties during the next 3 hours. ABGs on an F_{IO_2} of 0.35 via entrainment mask demonstrated pH 7.43, P_{CO_2} 36 mm Hg, and P_{O_2} 88 mm Hg. Because of the injury to his intestinal tract, Mr. E was fed intravenously to meet his nutritional needs. Mr. E's only complaint at this time was abdominal pain related to the gunshot and subsequent surgery. The pain was controlled by IV morphine.

Over the next 3 days Mr. E continued to improve. His hemodynamic status was stable with normal sensorium, blood pressure, urine output, and vital signs. At the end of the third hospital day Mr. E began to complain of intermittent fever, chills, and general malaise. He subsequently became restless and somewhat confused. A physical examination was performed, revealing the following findings.

PHYSICAL EXAMINATION

General *Patient awake but slow to respond and confused; appears to be in mild respiratory distress*

Vital signs *Temperature 38.5°C, respiratory rate 32/minute, pulse 124/minute, and blood pressure 85/50 mm Hg*

HEENT *Normal findings*

Neck *Trachea midline, mobile, with no stridor; carotid pulses ++ with no bruits; no lymphadenopathy, thyromegaly, or jugular venous distension noted; accessory muscles of breathing not being used*

Chest *Normal anteroposterior (AP) diameter and bilateral expansion noted with breathing; resonance to percussion normal bilaterally*

Heart *Regular rhythm with a rate of 124/minute; no murmur or heave noted; point of maximum impulse (PMI) not palpable*

Lungs *Rapid, shallow breathing noted; breath sounds normal in middle and upper lung regions but diminished in the bases posteriorly with end-inspiratory crackles*

Abdomen *Slightly distended, tender, and no bowel sounds noted; no masses or organomegaly noted*

Extremities *No clubbing, cyanosis, or edema; pulses weak but present bilaterally; extremities warm to the touch*

Because of the concern for Mr. E's hemodynamic status, a PA catheter was inserted. Hemodynamic and clinical measurements at this time revealed:

Cardiac output 6.0 liters/minute
Urine output 15 mL/hour
Plasma lactate 3.5 mg/dL
Arterial pH 7.32
Pa_{O_2} 70 mm Hg on F_{IO_2} of 0.35
Pa_{CO_2} 26 mm Hg
Plasma bicarbonate 16 mEq/liter
SVR 675 dynes/second per cm
PCWP 7 mm Hg
CVP 4 mm Hg

Questions

11. Is circulatory failure evident? If so, what evidence suggests circulatory failure?
12. What do the ABG findings suggest? Are the ABG findings consistent with the circulatory picture? If so, how? Does the acid-base status influence cardiac performance?
13. How do you interpret the systemic vascular resistance? What could cause this finding?
14. How do you interpret the PCWP?
15. How would you classify this type of circulatory problem?
16. What therapy is indicated at this time?
17. What laboratory tests would you suggest at this time?
18. If Mr. E's body surface area is 1.7 m², what is his cardiac index? If cardiac output is 6.0 liters/minute and heart rate 124/minute, what is the stroke volume?

Answers

11. Circulatory failure is present despite the normal cardiac output. Evidence to support this is found in the abnormal sensorium, reduced urine output, and elevated plasma lactate.
12. The ABG results suggest metabolic acidosis partially compensated for by hyperventilation. The patient also suffers from mild hypoxemia on 35 percent oxygen. The metabolic acidosis and hypoxemia are consistent with circulatory failure. Lactic acidosis due to anaerobic metabolism is common in circulatory failure and suggests a more severe case. Metabolic acidosis has a negative inotropic effect on the heart. Hypoxemia is common in patients with shock and in those bedridden following surgery; in this case it is probably the result of atelectasis and shunting.
13. The systemic vascular resistance is markedly reduced. The peripheral vasodilatation is probably due to the release of chemical mediators (endotoxins) into the circulation from an infecting microorganism.
14. The PCWP is at the lower end of normal limits. Most patients will have a better stroke volume if the PCWP is in the 12 to 16 mm Hg range.
15. This type of clinical picture suggests circulatory failure due to sepsis or septic shock. This assessment is based on the fever, low SVR, and high CO (Table 6–2).
16. Therapy should aim at improving the perfusion of vital organs. Even though the cardiac output is in the normal range, blood flow to many organs is insufficient as a result of the vasodilatation and precapillary arteriovenous shunting. Giving IV fluids could help to increase the mean arterial blood pressure and perfusion pressure by improving preload. Antibiotics are needed to treat the sepsis. Increasing the F_{IO_2} will correct the hypoxemia. A vasopressor such as dopamine may be useful to increase the perfusion pressure if the patient does not respond adequately to fluid therapy. This patient will need close monitoring, as he is at high risk for respiratory failure and would then need intubation and positive pressure breathing (see Chapter 11).
17. Laboratory tests that could be useful to assess this patient would include an ECG, chest radiograph, complete blood count, blood cultures, and electrolytes. ABGs should be repeated if evidence of respiratory problems occur.
18. Mr. E's cardiac index (CI) is 3.5 liters/minute/m². This is calculated by

dividing the body surface area (BSA) into the cardiac output as follows: CI = cardiac output ÷ BSA = 6.0 liters/minute ÷ 1.7 m² = 3.5 liters/minute per m². The stroke volume (SV) is calculated by dividing the pulse rate into the cardiac output: SV = 6000 mL/minute ÷ 124/minute = 48 mL.

LABORATORY EVALUATION

ECG

Sinus tachycardia with no evidence of ST-segment depression or elevation

CHEST RADIOGRAPH

Diminished lung volumes with normal heart size; no evidence of infiltrates or pulmonary edema

ELECTROLYTES

Na⁺ 140 mEq/L; K⁺ 3.6 mEq/L; HCO₃ 17 mEq/L; Cl⁻ 102 mEq/L

COMPLETE BLOOD COUNT

White blood cells 18,500/mm³; 60 percent segmented neutrophils; 8 percent bands

Following the administration of fluids, the patient's PCWP increased to 12 cm H_2O and cardiac output increased to 6.5 liter/minute. SVR was measured at 660 dynes/sec cm². IV gentamicin and piperacillin were started. $P\bar{v}o_2$ was measured at 42 mm Hg. The patient remained semiconscious with blood pressure 90/52 mm Hg, respiratory rate 35/minute, and pulse 130/minute. His rectal temperature was measured at 38.5°C.

Questions

19. Calculate the anion gap for this patient and state what the results indicate.
20. What are the potential sources for the infection?
21. Should the patient be intubated and mechanically ventilated?
22. How is the effectiveness of the fluid therapy evaluated?
23. What is indicated by the $P\bar{v}o_2$ of 42 mm Hg?
24. What is the significance of the patient having an elevated body temperature? How does this influence his clinical condition?
25. What therapy is needed at this point?

Answers

19. The anion gap is calculated by subtracting the HCO₃⁻ and Cl⁻ from the Na⁺ (140 − 102 − 17 = 21). An anion gap of 21 is elevated above normal and indicates the presence of metabolic acidosis caused in this case by lactic acidosis.
20. Potential sources for the infection include the abdominal wound, indwelling pulmonary artery catheter, and IV feeding line.

21. Because this patient is not expected to recover quickly and oxygenation is marginal on supplemental oxygen, this patient could benefit from intubation and mechanical ventilation.

22. The fluid therapy is evaluated with a combination of hemodynamic parameters such as PCWP, blood pressure, and cardiac output and by looking for evidence of improved organ perfusion (e.g., increased urine output). Evidence of better vital organ perfusion includes improved urine output and sensorium. In this case it appears that the fluid therapy did not improve blood pressure and vital organ perfusion, despite an increase in cardiac output. This is typical for septic shock, in which maldistribution of circulation is prevalent.

23. A $P\bar{v}o_2$ of 42 mm Hg is considered in the normal range and often indicates that tissue oxygenation is optimal. In this case, however, the normal $P\bar{v}o_2$ may be misleading owing to the fact that septic shock causes precapillary shunting and often results in an inappropriately increased $P\bar{v}o_2$. Because there is evidence that tissue oxygenation is less than optimal in this case, the $P\bar{v}o_2$ must be inappropriately elevated.

24. The elevated body temperature is significant because this results in an increased metabolic rate and adds to the problems created by circulatory failure.

25. Because volume expansion did not significantly improve blood pressure, the use of a vasopressor is needed. Dopamine or levarterenol should be given.

Over the next several days the patient slowly responded well to therapy despite the onset of respiratory failure due to ARDS (see Chapter 11). His hemodynamic status improved with the use of vasopressors and fluid therapy. He was eventually weaned from vasopressors and mechanical ventilation and transferred to the general care unit on the 12th hospital day.

REFERENCES

1. Daily, EK and Schroeder, JP. Techniques in Bedside Hemodynamic Monitoring, ed 4. CV Mosby, St Louis, 1989, pp 88–150.

2. Schuster DP and Lefrak, SS: Shock. In Civetta, JM, Taylor, RW, and Kirby, RR (eds): Critical Care. JB Lippincott, Philadelphia, 1988, pp 891–908.

3. Parillo, JE: Septic shock in humans: Clinical evaluation, pathogenesis, and therapeutic approach. In Shoemaker, WC: Textbook of Critical Care, ed 2. WB Saunders, Philadelphia, 1989, pp 1006–1023.

4. Marini, JJ and Wheeler, AP: Critical Care Medicine—The Essentials. Williams & Wilkins, Baltimore, 1989, p 31.

5. Shoemaker, WC. Shock states: Pathophysiology, monitoring, outcome prediction and therapy. In Shoemaker, WC. Textbook of Critical Care, ed 2. WB Saunders, Philadelphia, 1989, pp 977–992.

6. Marino, PL: The ICU Book. Philadelphia, Lea & Febiger, 1991, p 174.

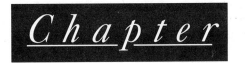

Chapter 7

Kenneth D. McCarty, MS, RRT

PULMONARY THROMBOEMBOLIC DISEASE

INTRODUCTION

Pulmonary thromboembolism, a relatively common disorder affecting approximately 500,000 persons a year in the United States, refers to the vascular obstruction (embolization) of the pulmonary vessels by blood clots (thrombi) that have traveled through the venous system to the lungs.[1] Many materials in addition to clots such as fat deposits, air, tumor fragments, and amniotic fluid can produce an embolus.[2-4] This chapter discusses the most common form of embolism, thromboembolism.

ETIOLOGY AND PATHOLOGY

Three main factors are associated with the formation of venous thrombi: hypercoagulability, damage to endothelial wall of the blood vessel, and venostasis.[1] Hypercoagulability is a factor in emboli caused by genetic deficiencies in antithrombin III, protein S, and protein C, and in patients with fibrinolytic abnormalities.[5-8] Fractures and surgical procedures along with trauma are common causes of venous blood vessel damage. Stasis of venous blood flow is common in many circumstances that promote physical immobilization such as surgery, fractures, or prolonged illness.

Risk factors for venous thrombosis include obesity, congestive heart failure, malignancy, burns, use of estrogen-containing drugs, and postoperative and postpartum states.[1]

Although thromboemboli may form at almost any site, approximately 95 percent originate in the deep veins of the lower extremities. The embolic risk increases if thrombosis occurs in veins above the knee.[9,10]

The pathologic changes in the lung are related to both the magnitude of the occlusion and the pulmonary blood supply. Small thromboemboli may cause little or no injury to the distal lung tissue, whereas large thromboemboli may disrupt blood flow enough to destroy lung parenchyma (infarction).

PATHOPHYSIOLOGY

Pulmonary vascular obstruction due to thromboembolism may affect both respiratory and hemodynamic systems.[1] Vascular occlusion by a large thrombus decreases perfusion of the affected pulmonary vascular bed and initially leads to parenchymal areas with more ventilation than perfusion (alveolar dead space). Local bronchoconstriction also typically accompanies pulmonary embolism. The release of cellular mediators such as serotonin, histamine, and prostaglandins from platelets, local areas of alveolar hypocapnia, and hypoxemia are thought to play roles in causing the bronchoconstriction, although the exact etiology is unknown.[1,11,12]

Bronchospasm may also cause hypoxemia during a pulmonary embolism by producing ventilation-perfusion ratio ($\dot{V}/\dot{Q}$) mismatching. Although the entire cause of emboli-induced hypoxemia is unclear, many factors are probably involved including venous shunting and reduced cardiac output, resulting in an increased arterial-venous oxygen difference and worsened venous admixture.[1] Obstruction of blood flow to the lung tissue results in a decrease in surfactant production about 24 hours after the embolization,[13] which leads to decreased pulmonary compliance, atelectasis, and further $\dot{V}/\dot{Q}$ mismatching and hypoxemia.

Vascular occlusion and vasoconstriction cause an increase in pulmonary vascular resistance (PVR).[1] Cardiac output is maintained only by increased right ventricular work and hence pulmonary artery pressures. If the output of the right ventricle falls, filling of the left heart diminishes, resulting in systemic hypotension and eventual cardiovascular collapse. Approximately 50 percent or more occlusion of the pulmonary vasculature, however, must occur in previously healthy individuals before sustained pulmonary hypertension develops and cardiac output falls.[14]

The severity of the hemodynamic compromise depends not only on the magnitude of the embolism but also on the patient's preexisting cardiovascular and pulmonary status.[15] Pulmonary or cardiovascular diseases that limit the pulmonary vascular reserve such as congestive heart failure, chronic obstructive pulmonary disease (COPD), and aortic or mitral valve disease, frequently result in greater than expected pulmonary hypertension compared with otherwise healthy patients.

Although pulmonary infarction is a potential consequence of thromboembolism, death of lung tissue owing to ischemia is not a common occurrence.[1] This is because there is usually some perfusion past the embolus, collateral blood flow via bronchial arteries, and oxygenation from the airways. Pulmonary infarction is more likely when COPD or left ventricular failure is present.[16] This is probably because of reduced cardiac output in patients with congestive heart failure and reduced collateral blood flow in patients with COPD.[14,17]

Natural resolution of the thromboembolus begins shortly after the clot lodges in the lung.[1,11] Fibrinolysis is the process of clot destruction in which blood-borne and vascular endothelial factors act to dissolve the clot. Clot resolution involves organization of the thrombus, attachment to the vascular wall, and return of blood flow.

CLINICAL FEATURES

Medical History

The clinical symptoms of pulmonary thromboembolism are not specific and emboli may even occur without causing symptoms.[14,17] Therefore it is important to have a high index of suspicion, especially if risk factors are present.[18]

The most common symptom associated with pulmonary embolism is transient acute dyspnea[19] (Table 7–1). Pleuritic chest pain and hemoptysis indicate pulmonary infarction and pleural involvement. Syncope, although uncommon, suggests large clots and severe hemodynamic compromise.[11] A sense of impending doom is a potential symptom and is usually associated with large emboli and hypotension.[1]

Table 7–1 Common Symptoms of
Pulmonary
Thromboembolism

Symptom	Occurrence (%)
Dyspnea	73
Pleuritic pain	66
Cough	37
Leg swelling	28
Leg pain	26
Hemoptysis	13
Palpitations	10
Wheezing	9
Anginalike pain	4

Adapted from and used by permission of
Stein, PD, et al: Clinical, laboratory, roentgenographic, and electrocardiographic findings in
patients with acute pulmonary embolism and no
pre-existing cardiac or pulmonary disease. Chest
100(3):598, 1991.

Physical Examination

Physical examination of the patient with thromboembolism most commonly reveals tachypnea, tachycardia, and fever[19] (Table 7–2). Inspection of the patient is most often normal, but if clots are large there may be findings suggesting right ventricular strain (e.g., jugular venous distension). The lower extremities are often normal but may reveal swelling and tenderness associated with deep venous thrombosis. The patient's breath sounds may be clear or may reveal localized wheezing or crackles.[19] A pleural friction rub may also be heard, particularly if infarction is present involving the pleura. Percussion of the chest wall is usually normal. Aus-

Table 7–2 Common Signs of
Pulmonary
Thromboembolism

Sign	Occurrence (%)
Tachypnea (≥20/min)	70
Crackles	51
Tachycardia (≥100/min)	30
Increased P_2	23
Diaphoresis	11
Fever	7
Pleural friction rub	3
Cyanosis	1

Adapted from and used by permission of
Stein, PD, et al: Clinical, laboratory, roentgenographic, and electrocardiographic findings in
patients with acute pulmonary embolism and no
pre-existing cardiac or pulmonary disease. Chest
100(3):598, 1991.

cultation of the heart may identify loud pulmonic valve closure (P_2) as part of the second heart sound (S_2) and S_2 splitting.[19]

Hemodynamic and Laboratory Data

The insertion of a balloon-tipped flow-directed catheter classically reveals an increased pulmonary artery pressure (PAP) and central venous pressure (CVP), and a normal or low pulmonary capillary wedge pressure (PCWP). A low PCWP occurs when significant occlusion of the pulmonary vasculature leads to inadequate filling of the left side of the heart.

The chest radiograph is often normal or shows only nonspecific abnormalities such as signs of volume loss or pleural effusion most often located in the middle to lower lung fields (Fig. 7–1).[11,19] Pulmonary vascular distension may be caused by pulmonary hypertension. A subtle localized vascular narrowing in the area of decreased perfusion distal to the emboli may be evident (Westermark's sign).[11,19]

Arterial blood gases (ABGs) commonly show an uncompensated respiratory

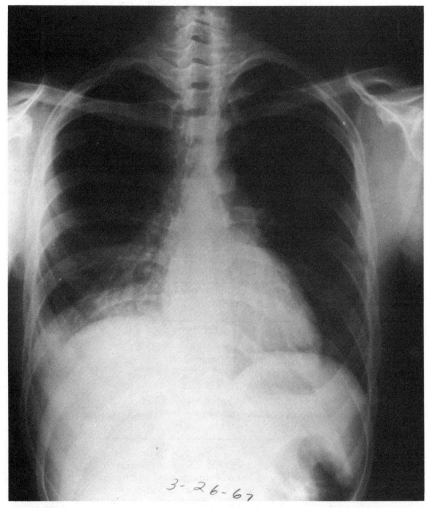

FIGURE 7–1 Chest radiograph of a patient with pulmonary embolism showing right hemidiaphragm elevation and right lower lobe radiopacity as a result of atelectasis.

alkalosis with mild to moderate hypoxemia on room air and an increased alveolar-to-arterial oxygen gradient.[1,11] The electrocardiogram (ECG) is frequently normal or reveals sinus tachycardia.[1,19] Changes indicating acute right heart strain such as right-axis deviation and P pulmonale occur relatively infrequently, whereas the presence of premature ventricular contractions is a more common finding.[11,19]

V̇/Q̇ scans demonstrate the difference between the alveolar distribution of inhaled radioactive xenon-133 and pulmonary capillary distribution of albumin radioactively labeled with iodine or technetium. Healthy patients have an even distribution of ventilation and perfusion. Typical findings with pulmonary embolus include normal ventilation and segmental or lobar defects in perfusion. Matching defects in ventilation and perfusion such as those that occur with pneumonia are nondiagnostic for pulmonary embolism. A normal perfusion scan effectively rules out thromboembolism.[20] Normal ventilation in the presence of at least two segmental defects or one lobar defect in perfusion indicates a 95 percent probability that pulmonary embolism is present.

Pulmonary angiography is the diagnostic gold standard and also demonstrates the extent of vascular involvement. A radiopaque contrast material is introduced via catheter into the pulmonary artery and radiographs are taken as it circulates. Two signs are diagnostic for pulmonary emboli: abrupt cutoff of a vessel or intraluminal filling defects.[21] Angiography requires catheterization of large veins and catheter manipulation through the right heart. Complications associated with these maneuvers make pulmonary angiography a diagnostic modality of last resort.

TREATMENT

The therapy for pulmonary thromboembolism is aimed at treating the vascular occlusion, its pulmonary and hemodynamic consequences, and preventing the recurrence of emboli.

Anticoagulant therapy using intravenous (IV) heparin is the most common initial form of treatment.[1] Heparin inactivates thrombin and clotting factor X and inhibits platelet aggregation, thereby inhibiting the formation of new thrombi.[22] Oral anticoagulants such as the coumarin derivatives, sodium warfarin (Coumadin) and dicumarol are used for long-term therapy.[23] Anticoagulation caused by heparin therapy is monitored by partial thromboplastin time (PTT), whereas anticoagulation caused by the oral anticoagulants is monitored by prothrombin time (PT).[11] Heparin is used initially and usually continued for 5 to 10 days until the PT is stabilized in the therapeutic range. Duration of coumarin therapy varies depending on the likelihood of clot recurrence. Patients with clots caused by easily identifiable insults and not associated with risk factors for recurrence are usually treated for 3 to 6 months, whereas recurrent clots may require years of therapy.

Although anticoagulants prevent new clot formation and the growth of already existing thrombi, they do relatively little to dissolve existing clots.[1] The administration of thrombolytic agents such as streptokinase and urokinase dissolve fresh clots and help restore vascular patency. Because these agents affect any recently formed clots, and therefore increase the risk of bleeding,[24] relative contraindications to their use include recent surgical procedures, ulcers, stroke, and childbirth. Thrombolytic agents are most often used in patients with thrombi causing significant hemodynamic compromise.[11] Thrombus treatment is most effective during the first 5 days after the embolus and is usually followed by heparin, and then Coumadin, therapy.

Surgical removal of massive pulmonary emboli is probably not more effective than thrombolytic therapy. Because the mortality rate following this procedure is approximately 60 percent, it is used only as a last resort.[11]

Since the advent of modern anticoagulant therapy, vena caval interruption by surgical ligation, clips, or vena caval umbrella is less frequent. These procedures limit the entry of clots into the pulmonary vasculature by blocking their path of entry from the lower extremities.[1] Vena caval interruption is most useful if emboli reccur after anticoagulation or if anticoagulant therapy is contraindicated.[11]

In addition to specific therapy patients with pulmonary thromboembolism may need additional supportive treatment. Respiratory care practitioners can administer oxygen when hypoxemia is present. The elimination of carbon dioxide is rarely a problem; however, the patient may benefit from intubation and mechanical ventilation if a massive embolus causes respiratory failure. If hypotension develops, volume expansion and dopamine can be used to maintain adequate perfusing pressure.[11]

Because pulmonary thromboembolism is a relatively common and potentially severe problem, prophylaxis is important for high risk patients. The use of standard elastic stockings and early ambulation after surgical procedures offer no proven prophylactic benefit.[1] Three methods that have proved useful in preventing thromboembolism include low-dose heparin, Coumadin (sodium warfarin), and venous compression devices.[1] Two to three doses of heparin each day administered subcutaneously is effective in many patients at risk from surgical immobilization and myocardial infarction. Likewise, sodium warfarin is commonly used after the initial heparin therapy to prevent recurring thrombosis. Use of external venous compressive devices, in which an air-filled cuff is alternately inflated and deflated, is effective in reducing thrombi formation in the lower legs. This modality is especially useful in patients with an increased risk of bleeding from anticoagulant therapy.

Case Study

HISTORY

Mr. H is a 52-year-old Asian man who presented to the emergency room. His left leg was in a cast, and he stated that 1 week earlier he had been in an automobile accident and had broken his leg. Since that time he had had difficulty "getting around" and has mostly been lying on the couch watching television. On the evening of admission he noticed a sudden onset of dyspnea and chest pain. He denied orthopnea, cough, hemoptysis, or wheezing. He routinely took iron supplements and occasionally took aspirin but no other medications. He smoked 2 packs of cigarettes a day for 19 years, but quit 3 years ago.

Questions

1. What are the key pulmonary symptom(s) that the attending physician should explore in greater detail, and what problems do these symptoms suggest?
2. What further questions should the physician ask of the patient to aid in the differential diagnosis?
3. Why is the diagnosis of pulmonary embolism most likely?

Answers

1. The key pulmonary symptoms in this case are dyspnea and chest pain. The sudden onset of the dyspnea and chest pain indicate an acute problem rather than a chronic condition. Dyspnea and chest pain occur with pulmonary thromboemboli, pneumonia, myocardial infarction, and pneumothorax (Table 7–3).[14] Differentiation among these medical problems is extremely important because they are all potentially lethal diseases with similar symptoms yet require different treatment.

Table 7–3 Differential Diagnosis of Pulmonary Thromboembolism

---

Pneumonia (bacterial or viral)
Pneumothorax
Aortic dissection
Tuberculosis
Acute pleuritis from:
    Collagen vascular disease
    Viral pleurisy
Myocardial infarction

---

2. Pertinent questions should be asked in an attempt to differentiate among the various problems that cause chest pain and dyspnea. The interviewer should identify the risk factors and other symptoms present in this patient for each of the diseases listed in the differential diagnosis. Risk factors for deep venous thrombosis include those that promote stasis, injury to blood vessels, or increased coagulability of the blood. Other symptoms associated with deep venous thrombosis include fever, leg tenderness, and hemoptysis. Risk factors for heart disease include smoking, high cholesterol, high-stress lifestyle, and lack of exercise. Other symptoms associated with heart disease include nausea, diaphoresis, radiation of the chest pain to the shoulder or jaw, and exercise-related pain. Risk factors for pneumonia include immune deficiency disorders, poor nutrition, chronic lung disease, head injuries, and chronic health problems. Other symptoms associated with pneumonia include cough, fever, and sputum production. Patients with pneumothorax may have only pleuritic chest pain and dyspnea.

3. Two factors in the patient's history that favor the diagnosis of pulmonary embolism are trauma and immobilization. Trauma damages blood vessels and releases endothelial factors that promote clotting, while immobilization predisposes the patient to blood stasis.

PHYSICAL EXAMINATION

General   *A well-nourished Asian man who is alert and oriented, anxious, and in mild respiratory distress*

Vital Signs   *Temperature 37.6°C orally; respiratory rate 26/minute; pulse 110/minute; blood pressure 134/88 mm Hg*

HEENT   *Unremarkable*

Neck   *Supple with full active range of motion; trachea midline, mobile, and without stridor or wheezes; carotid pulses are 3+, symmetric, and without bruits; no thyromegaly, jugular venous distension, or lymphadenopathy present*

Chest   *Normal configuration and expansion with breathing*

Lungs   *Right middle lobe and right lower lobe late-inspiratory crackles revealed on auscultation*

Heart	*Regular rhythm with rate of 110/minute; a slightly increased S_2 (P_2) heard at the second intercostal space at the left sternal border; systolic heave located at the fourth intercostal space near the left border of the sternum*
Abdomen	*Nondistended, soft, nontender with no masses or organomegaly*
Extremities	*No cyanosis, digital clubbing, or peripheral edema; left leg is in a cast*

Questions

4. What is the significance of the patient's anxiety?
5. What is the significance of the patient's temperature?
6. What is the significance of the systolic heave noted at the left sternal border?
7. What is the cause of the patient's crackles?
8. What pathophysiology accounts for the louder P_2 component of the second heart sound?
9. What findings, if any, indicate the presence of hypoxemia?

Answers

4. Anxiety and apprehension may be produced by any medical condition. They are relatively common symptoms of pulmonary emboli and are usually displayed by restlessness and irritability.[1,25] The etiology of these symptoms is unknown.
5. While the presence of a fever is common with infections such as pneumonia, a low-grade fever is also a common finding in pulmonary embolism[1] and may help rule out other differential diagnoses such as pneumothorax.
6. A heave is an abnormal pulsation occurring on the precordium and when palpated at the left sternal border is often caused by right ventricular hypertrophy. A right ventricular heave is indicative of pulmonary hypertension.[26] Many pulmonary vessels must be occluded before pulmonary hypertension develops. Therefore, a right ventricular heave indicates relatively severe disease.
7. Crackles are a common finding in patients with pulmonary emboli. Atelectasis is a common result of pulmonary embolism and is most likely responsible for the inspiratory crackles. In addition, atelectasis may also be the cause of the fever if infection is present.
8. The P_2 portion of the second heart sound (S_2) represents pulmonic valve closure. An increased intensity of the P_2 portion of that sound is indicative of more forceful valve closure caused by pulmonary vascular hypertension. Obstruction of the pulmonary vessels by thromboemboli causes an increase in pulmonary artery pressure, which results in the valve snapping shut with more force.[26]
9. Although the patient is not cyanotic, more subtle signs of acute hypoxemia are present. Tachycardia and tachypnea are nonspecific cardiovascular and pulmonary responses to hypoxemia. In addition, the patient's anxiety might also indicate that he is hypoxemic.[26]

LABORATORY EVALUATION

CHEST RADIOGRAPH

(Figs. 7–2 and 7–3)

ABGs

pH	7.51
$Paco_2$	30 mm Hg
PaO_2	60 mm Hg
HCO_3^-	24 mEq/liter
base excess (BE)	−1
Hb	13.1 g/100 mL
Sao_2	87.8 percent
Cao_2	15.6 vol% on room air

CLINICAL LABORATORY STUDIES

Complete Blood Count: Results pending
Chemistry: Results pending
    ECG
    Sinus tachycardia

Questions

10. What chest radiograph findings are consistent with pulmonary embolism? How do you interpret the chest films (Figs. 7–2 and 7–3)?
11. What is the patient's acid-base and oxygenation status?
12. What treatment would you suggest at this time?
13. What other diagnostic information would be useful?

Answers

10. Although the findings on the chest radiograph are frequently nonspecific for thromboembolism, hemidiaphragm elevation is common and is probably indicative of atelectasis.[1] The atelectasis is thought to occur as a result of bronchospasm, surfactant depletion, and underperfusion of alveolar spaces. Normally most of the pulmonary perfusion is to the middle and lower lung fields. Most clots follow the perfusion to these areas and, as a result, atelectasis is most often found in the middle to lower lung fields.[11]

    Figures 7–2 and 7–3 demonstrate no significant abnormality which is common for patients with pulmonary embolism.

11. The patient's acid-base status shows acute respiratory alkalosis. Moderate hypoxemia on room air is also present, which is common in patients with emboli. In addition, the arterial oxygen saturation (Sao_2) is low and the arterial oxygen content (Cao_2) slightly reduced. Because the calculation of Cao_2 includes Sao_2, Pao_2, and hemoglobin, it reflects oxy-

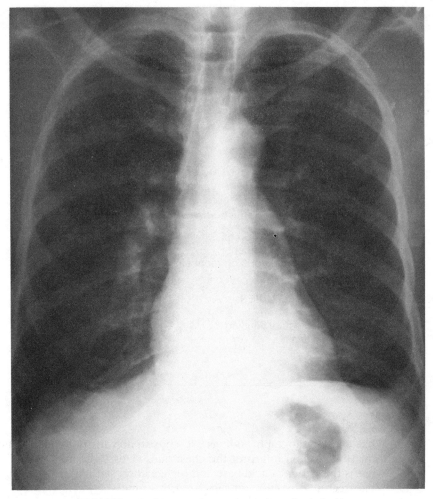

FIGURE 7–2 Chest radiograph on day of admission.

gen-carrying capacity, which in this case is mildly reduced mostly owing to the low Sao_2.

12. Treatment at this time should consist of oxygen therapy administered via nasal cannula to increase the patient's Pao_2 above 80 mm Hg. The physician should order IV anticoagulant therapy to prevent further thrombi. The use of thrombolytic agents is not indicated because of the relatively limited lung involvement and the absence of systemic hypotension. Should further embolization occur and cause hemodynamic compromise, the use of thrombolytic agents might be warranted.

13. The patient's history, physical examination, and diagnostic findings provide a presumptive diagnosis of pulmonary embolism. A $\dot{V}/\dot{Q}$ scan might be useful to confirm the presence of pulmonary thromboembolism. Pulmonary angiography would better document the exact location and extent of the embolism but is not necessary under these circumstances.

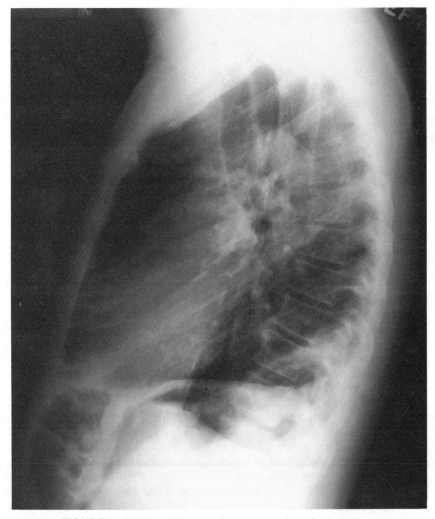

FIGURE 7–3 Lateral chest radiograph on day of admission.

A day later, after having a V̇/Q̇ scan (Fig. 7–4) and while ambulating around the unit, the patient stated that he was feeling "worse" and having trouble breathing. He was acting very agitated and was slightly confused. There was no change in the physical examination findings except that he was pale, his skin was cool and clammy, and his blood pressure was 88/45 mm Hg.

Questions

14. What is the significance of the results of the V̇/Q̇ scan?
15. Of what significance is the change in the patient's mental status?
16. What pathophysiology accounts for the patient's hypotension?
17. What therapy is indicated at this time?
18. Should the patient be admitted to the intensive care unit (ICU)?

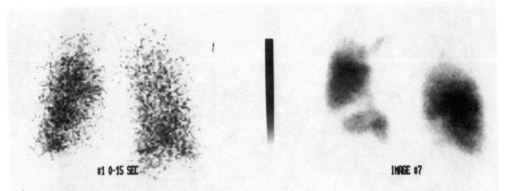

FIGURE 7–4 Ventilation-perfusion ($\dot{V}/\dot{Q}$) scan (ventilation on left, perfusion on right) 1 day after admission, showing scattered reduced perfusion compared with ventilation on the right and left sides.

Answers

14. $\dot{V}/\dot{Q}$ scans depict the relative matching of ventilation to perfusion in the lung. In this case segmental decrease in perfusion compared with ventilation in otherwise healthy lungs suggests vascular occlusion by pulmonary emboli. Unfortunately, other problems such as vasculitis, vasospasm, vessel destruction, and neoplastic vascular compression can reduce perfusion and result in similar findings during $\dot{V}/\dot{Q}$ scanning.[11]

15. Agitation, confusion, anxiety, and restlessness are all nonspecific symptoms associated with severe diseases including pulmonary embolism. The sudden change in mental status most likely indicates a deterioration in perfusion and oxygenation of the brain and in this case most likely represents the arrival of another pulmonary embolus.

16. Systemic hypotension in this case is a result of pulmonary vascular occlusion by thrombi. The vascular occlusion causes an increased pulmonary vascular resistance, reduced right ventricular output, and corresponding decrease in left ventricular filling, cardiac output, and systemic blood pressure.

17. Oxygen therapy and anticoagulant therapy are still indicated. An increased fraction of inspired oxygen (FIO_2) is useful in this case because hemodynamics are marginal. In addition, thrombolytics may be necessary to induce rapid clot breakdown and aid the maintenance of cardiovascular hemodynamics.

18. The patient should be admitted to the ICU for close monitoring and definitive therapy. Massive pulmonary emboli such as this are life threatening and require aggressive treatment.

The attending physician inserted a pulmonary artery catheter and ordered another chest radiograph and ABG analysis. The results were as follows:

PA CATHETER DATA

CVP 16 mm Hg
PAP 45/32 mm Hg

PCWP 4 mm Hg
Cardiac output 2.7 liters/minute
Cardiac index 1.6 liters/minute per m²

ABGs

pH 7.37, $Paco_2$ 30 mm Hg, Pao_2 54 mm Hg, BE -5, HCO_3^- 16 mEq/liter, Hb 13.5 g/100 mL, Sao_2 86 percent, Cao_2 15.8 vol% on 6 liters/minute O_2 by simple mask

Questions

19. What is the significance of the PA catheter measurements and why is the cardiac output low?
20. What is the patient's prognosis?
21. What could explain the metabolic acidosis shown by the ABGs?

Answers

19. The CVP and PAP are both elevated as a result of the pulmonary vascular obstruction that causes pulmonary hypertension. This leads to an acute increase in right ventricular work and predisposes the patient to right ventricular failure. Cardiac output and index are reduced as a result of acute right ventricular failure, which reduces left ventricular filling (as evidenced by the low PCWP). These measurements indicate life-threatening disease with right heart failure.
20. The patient has a life-threatening problem that requires urgent treatment. Fatalities usually occur within the first hour after the embolus occurs. If the patient survives longer than an hour and appropriate treatment is initiated, there is relatively good chance for survival.[25]
21. The metabolic acidosis is most likely due to lactic acidosis. This is common in patients who have reduced cardiac output and tissue hypoxia, which leads to anaerobic metabolism and the production of lactic acid.

The patient was admitted to the ICU and given thrombolytic therapy, low-dose heparin therapy, and high-flow oxygen therapy. Within 24 hours of initiating thrombolytic therapy the patient's hemodynamic parameters normalized. Over the next several days the patient gradually improved and on day 4 was able to maintain adequate oxygenation via nasal cannula at 3 liters/minute. The remainder of his hospital stay was uneventful, and he was discharged on a regimen of Coumadin therapy on day 7.

REFERENCES

1. Moser, KM: Pulmonary embolism. In Murray, JF and Nadel, JA (eds): Textbook of Respiratory Medicine. WB Saunders, Philadelphia, 1988, p 1299.

2. Coosling, H and Pelligrini, V: Fat embolism syndrome. Clin Orthop 615:68, 1982.

3. Moylan, J and Evenson, MA: Diagnosis and therapy of fat embolism. Annu Rev Med 28:85, 1977.

4. Morgan, M: Amniotic fluid embolism. A review. Anaesthesia 34:20, 1979.

5. Griffin, JH, et al: Deficiency of protein C in congenital thrombotic disease. J Clin Invest 68:1370, 1981.

6. Comp, PC and Esmon, CT: Recurrent venous thrombosis in patients with a partial deficiency of protein S. N Engl J Med 311:1525, 1984.

7. Egeberg, O: Inherited antithrombin deficiency causing thrombophilia. Thromb Diath Hem 13:516, 1965.

8. Wohl, RC, et al: Physiologic activation of the human fibrinolytic system: Isolation and characterization of human plasminogen variants. J Biol Chem 254:9063, 1979.

9. Havig, GO: Source of pulmonary emboli. Acta Chir Scand 478:42, 1977.

10. Moser, KM and LeMoine, JR: Is embolic risk conditioned by location of deep venous thrombosis? Ann Intern Med 94:439, 1981.

11. West, JW: Pulmonary embolism. In Wu, K (ed): Pathophysiology and Management of Thromboembolic Disorder. PGS Publishing, Littleton, MA, 1984, p 351.

12. Severinghaus, JW, et al: Unilateral hypoventilation produced by occlusion of one pulmonary artery. J Appl Physiol 16:53, 1961.

13. Chernik, V, et al: Effect of chronic pulmonary artery ligation on pulmonary mechanics and surfactant. J Appl Physiol 21:1315, 1966.

14. Moser, KM: Pulmonary embolism. Am Rev Respir Dis 115:829, 1977.

15. McIntyre, KM and Sasahara, AA: Determinants of right ventricular function and hemodynamics after pulmonary embolism. Chest 65:534, 1974.

16. Dalen, JE, et al: Pulmonary embolism, pulmonary hemorrhage, and pulmonary infarction. N Engl J Med 296:1431, 1977.

17. LeMoine, JR and Moser, KM: Leg scanning with radioisotope-labeled fibrinogen in patients undergoing hip surgery. JAMA 243:2035, 1980.

18. Dalen, JE: Clinical diagnosis of acute pulmonary embolism. When should a V̇/Q̇ scan be ordered? Chest 100(5):1185, 1991.

19. Stein, PD, et al: Clinical, laboratory, roentgenographic, and electrocardiographic findings in patients with acute pulmonary embolism and no pre-existing cardiac or pulmonary disease. Chest 100(3):598, 1991.

20. Kipper, MS, et al: Long-term follow up of patients with suspected embolism and a normal lung scan. Chest 82:411, 1982.

21. Sharma, GV and Sasahara, AA: Diagnosis and treatment of pulmonary embolism. Med Clin North Am 63:239, 1979.

22. Wessler, S and Gitel, SN: Heparin: New concepts relevant to clinical use. Blood 53:525, 1979.

23. Moser, KM and Fedullo, PF: Venous thromboembolism: Three simple decisions. Chest 83:117, 256; 1983.

24. Goldhaber, SZ, et al: Pooled analysis of randomized trials of streptokinase and heparin in phlebographically documented acute deep venous thrombosis. Am J Med 76:393, 1984.

25. Hinshaw, HC and Murray, JF: Pulmonary thromboembolism. In Hinshaw, HC and Murray, JF (eds): Diseases of the Chest. WB Saunders, Philadelphia, 1979, p 653.

26. Wilkins, RL: Techniques of Physical Examination. In Wilkins, RL, Sheldon, RL and Krider, SJ (eds): Clinical Assessment in Respiratory Care. CV Mosby, St Louis, 1990.

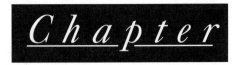

Chapter 8

George H. Hicks, MS, RRT

HEART FAILURE

INTRODUCTION

Heart failure is a condition that results in the heart's inability to pump appropriate blood flow to meet the metabolic needs of the body. An estimated more than 4 million people in the United States suffer from heart failure and its complications, with another 400,000 diagnosed annually.[1,2] Approximately 50 percent of those with heart failure die within the first 2 years following diagnosis.[3] This mortality rate is associated with multiorgan failure secondary to poor blood flow and organ congestion.

Physiologically the heart in failure is unable to maintain an adequate cardiac output. Hypoperfusion and subsequent pulmonary and/or systemic vascular congestion occur. The clinical manifestations depend on which side of the heart (left, or right, or both) is in failure. Heart failure can present in varying degrees of acute or chronic conditions as a result of the magnitude of failure and the ability for compensation.

The term congestive heart failure (CHF) is frequently used in making the diagnosis of heart failure from a large set of symptoms which result from many different causes. In general, CHF results in an accumulation of fluid in the lungs (pulmonary edema) and dependent extremities as a consequence of left heart failure. **Cor pulmonale** is the term used to describe right heart enlargement and failure as a result of primary pulmonary disease.

ETIOLOGY

The Framingham 20-year follow-up study has established that more than 60 percent of heart failure cases are caused by hypertension and coronary artery disease.[4,5] Idiopathic dilated cardiomyopathy or primary myocardial disease causes 30 to 40 percent of cases.[1] Valvular heart disease accounts for less than 20 percent.[4] Table 8–1 lists the various causes of heart failure.

Acute episodes of heart failure are caused by one or more precipitating factors that lead to cardiac decompensation. These factors interfere with one or more of the compensatory mechanisms that support appropriate cardiovascular function. Awareness of these precipitating factors may greatly improve the recognition and treatment of heart failure. The more common factors are listed in Table 8–2.

Acute cor pulmonale is most frequently associated with an abrupt elevation of pulmonary artery pressure.[6] This can be caused by massive pulmonary embolism, severe hypoxemic pulmonary vasoconstriction from acute hypoventilation, and/or

Table 8–1 Etiologic Factors of Heart Failure

Coronary artery disease
Hypertension
Primary or idiopathic dilated cardiomyopathy
Valvular abnormalities: regurgitation and stenosis
Congenital cardiac defects
Chronic pulmonary disease
Drug-induced: amphetamines, heroin, cocaine, antituberculosis combinations, high-dose
    cancer chemotherapy combinations
Infectious myocardial inflammation:
    Viral (e.g., influenza, mumps, and rabies)
    Bacterial (e.g., streptococcal, rheumatic heart disease)
    Mycotic (e.g., histoplasmosis)
Other causes
    Chronic alcohol ingestion
    Acute leukemia
    Metal poisonings (e.g., cobalt, iron, and lead)
    Metabolic defects (e.g., myxedema)
    Neurologic disorders (e.g., Duchenne's muscular dystrophy)
    Trauma (e.g., cardiac tamponade)

Source: Modified from Chesebro, JH and Burnett, JC: Cardiac failure: Characteristics and clinical manifestations. In Brandenburg, RO, Fuster, V, Giuliani, ER, and McGoon, DC (eds): Cardiology: Fundamentals and Practice. Year Book Medical, Chicago, 1987, p 646.

adult respiratory distress syndrome, as well as from mechanical constriction of the pulmonary vasculature. Chronic cor pulmonale is responsible for 10 to 30 percent of the admissions for "congestive heart failure" and is primarily caused by hypoxemia associated with chronic obstructive pulmonary diseases such as chronic bronchitis, emphysema, and cystic fibrosis.[6]

Table 8–2 Acute Precipitating Factors of Heart Failure

Patient-induced
    Failure to take medications
    Excessive sodium consumption
    High alcohol ingestion
    Physical inactivity or overactivity
    Emotional stress
Infection: Viral and/or bacterial
Arrhythmias: premature ventricular contractions (PVCs), AV block, bradycardia,
    tachycardia
Excessive fluid administration
Pulmonary embolism
High cardiac output demand: Fever, anemia, pregnancy, hypermetabolism
Acute MI or ischemia
Renal failure
Respiratory failure
Liver disease
Drug-induced failure
Environmental stress: Hyperthermia or hypothermia

Source: Developed from Chesebro, JH and Burnett, JC: Cardiac failure: Characteristics and clinical manifestations. In Brandenburg, RO, et al (eds): Cardiology: Fundamentals and Practice. Year Book Medical, Chicago, 1987, p 652.

PATHOPHYSIOLOGY

The product of cardiac pump performance is the cardiac output ($\dot{Q}_T$) or outflow in liters/minute from one ventricle. Cardiac output is primarily influenced by heart rate (HR) and stroke volume (SV). The mathematical description is the following simple product:

$$\dot{Q}_T = HR \times SV$$

Heart rate is regulated by the pacing system of the heart and influenced by the neurotransmitters (norepinephrine and acetylcholine) released by autonomic nervous systems. SV is influenced by venous return (preload pressure), downstream resistance (afterload pressure), myocardial contractility, and ventricular compliance. A more complete discussion of these factors and their inter-relationships can be found in Chapter 6.

In the normal heart, there is an exceptional degree of autoregulation of cardiac output from the right and left sides of the heart to prevent an imbalance in output. A difference of as little as 1 mL/minute can lead to venous congestion behind the failing side.[7] The smaller venous reservoir behind the left heart allows symptoms to occur with milder degrees of dysfunction when compared with the right heart. The thicker-walled left heart can sustain a greater workload than the thinner-walled right heart. The limited functional capacity of the right heart predisposes it to failure when challenged with increasing preloads or afterloads or both. As a consequence, the right heart commonly fails following primary left heart failure.[5] Interestingly, secondary right heart failure actually reduces the pulmonary congestion and preload of the failing left ventricle and thus provides a type of compensation. Rarely does primary right heart failure lead to left side failure.[5]

Myocardial Performance

The myocardial fibers in heart failure are characteristically found to have both decreased length-tension and force-velocity capabilities when stimulated to contract.[5,8] This causes the heart to have a reduced contractibility and reduced ability to generate a normal ejection fraction (the percent of end-diastolic ventricular volume pumped out in one stroke volume). The normal ejection fraction is approximately 70 percent and can fall to values of 20 percent or below in severe failure.

Three types of cardiac compensatory mechanisms improve myocardial performance during greater demands and in failure.[8]

SYMPATHETIC NERVOUS RESPONSE Release of norepinephrine stimulates the β-receptors of the cardiac pacing system and myocardium. This increases heart rate and strength of myocardial contraction which improves cardiac output. During acute heart failure there is increased sympathetic activity and greater concentrations of norepinephrine in plasma during conditions of rest and exercise.[9] This response improves cardiac performance initially but yields a diminished response over time. Later, sympathetic stimulation may provoke ischemic symptoms as the myocardium's metabolic rate exceeds the coronary circulatory capacity to supply adequate blood flow. In long-term failure, many patients develop a persistent tachycardia that lacks a parasympathetic bradycardia response. This results in a condition of reduced ability to alter heart rate from rest to exercise.[8]

FRANK-STARLING RESPONSE As the myocardial fibers are stretched by increasing the end-diastolic ventricular pressure and volume, the fibers contract with greater force.[10] Figure 8–1 illustrates this relationship in the normal heart with increased contractility (e.g., following the influence of epinephrine or digoxin) and in a heart with decreased contractility (e.g., heart failure). In the normal heart, the attendant increase in venous return and ventricular filling associated with exercise

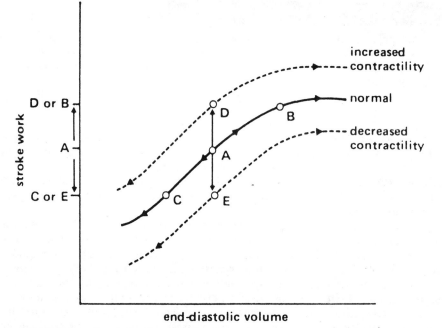

FIGURE 8–1 Frank-Starling ventricular function curves relating output (stroke work) and end-diastolic volume in three myocardial states of contractility. Output is varied along a single curve (e.g., A to B or A to C) as end-diastolic volume is altered by venous return. Output may also be changed by shifting from one curve to another (e.g., A to D or A to E) as the contractile or inotropic state of the ventricle is altered. Increased contractility can be brought about by hormonal or drug action, whereas decreased contractility is typical of heart failure. (From Katz, AM: Physiology of the Heart. Raven Press, 1977, p 225, with permission.)

or other forms of stress are easily compensated for through this mechanism. Failure of a ventricle results in a progressive increase in end-diastolic volume and ventricular dilation. To further complicate cardiac performance, an overly elevated end-diastolic volume reduces the compliance of the ventricle, which will reduce contractility and nullify or greatly reduce the Frank-Starling reflex and further contribute to congestive failure.[5,8]

VENTRICULAR HYPERTROPHIC RESPONSE Hypertrophy, an increase in myocardial muscle thickness and mass, is produced by a chronic exposure to elevated vascular pressure, greater blood volume, and increased release of neurotransmitters (e.g., norepinephrine and dopamine).[5,8] Although the hypertrophy is beneficial to improve the strength of contraction in the early stages of heart failure, this benefit is eventually offset by a decreasing ventricular compliance and increasing force necessary to compress a dilated ventricle. This condition is often further exacerbated by ischemic changes that are brought about by inadequate oxygen delivery to an enlarged and overexpanded myocardium during conditions of increased myocardial work. Hypertrophy is not necessarily permanent if produced over a short period of time and then corrected. This reversal is not uncommon, for example, following surgical prosthetic replacement of a stenotic aortic valve.

Peripheral and Pulmonary Circulation

Significant systemic redistribution of blood flow occurs in congestive failure as an important compensatory mechanism. This adjustment results in a diversion of the already reduced cardiac output away from renal and cutaneous tissues to the more important coronary and cerebral circulations.[8] These adjustments not only occur during rest but are further intensified during exercise and other forms of increased metabolism through the influence of the sympathetic nervous system.

During heart failure the systemic vascular resistance is usually increased through the vasoactive effects of an elevated plasma norepinephrine concentration and vessel wall engorgement from sodium and water absorption.[11] This results in a generalized inability of vasodilation, which limits the ability to increase oxygen transport and dissipate heat during exercise or other forms of stress. Thus, these patients are often very sensitive to heat and have reduced exercise tolerance.

Right heart failure results in systemic venous and capillary congestion and hypertension. This leads to liver engorgement, portal hypertension, reduced lymphatic drainage back to the venous system, and fluid retention in various third spaces (e.g., dependent extremities, peritoneal cavity, and pleural space).

Failure of the left heart produces pulmonary artery engorgement and hypertension. Initially, pulmonary hypertension leads to increased flow to the upper lung or nondependent zones. Further left heart failure results in greater pulmonary vascular pressures that can lead to pulmonary congestion and edema.

Fluid and Electrolyte Balance

In heart failure reduced cardiac output and generalized vasoconstriction result in renal hypoperfusion.[5] This results in reduced glomerular filtration and subsequent sodium and water retention. Systemic venous congestion during right heart failure can lead to renal venous hypertension, which can also cause reductions in glomerular filtration and increase tubular reabsorption of sodium.[12] Thus, arterial hypoperfusion or venous hypertension, or both, can lead to renal responses that compound the congestive component of failure.

In addition to the renal vascular changes brought about by norepinephrine during heart failure, a variety of other hormonal adjustments induce further changes in renal function.[12] Reduced renal perfusion triggers the kidney's production of renin, which stimulates the production of angiotensin I, which is then converted to angiotensin II following transit through the lung. Angiotensin II stimulates renal tubular sodium reabsorption, causes vasoconstriction which intensifies renal hypoperfusion, and stimulates adrenal gland secretion of aldosterone. Aldosterone induces further renal retention of sodium.

As a result of these renal changes, patients in heart failure often have increased blood volume, interstitial fluid volume, and increased total body sodium. This altered fluid and electrolyte balance coupled with poor cardiac performance can easily lead to the formation of systemic and pulmonary edema as a result of right and left heart failure, respectively.

Edema Formation

The movement of fluid through the walls of the vascular compartment into the interstitial space is a normal phenomenon. The movement of water is governed by the permeability of the capillary wall and the balance between hydrostatic pressure and the osmotic pressure. The balance of these properties and forces results in a net outward driving force of 10 mm Hg.[13] This results in the movement of approximately 150 mL of fluid into the interstitial space per hour. Normally this fluid is absorbed by the lymphatics and returned to the systemic venous circulation resulting in a stable interstitial fluid volume. When this natural drainage mechanism fails, excessive fluid collects in the interstitial space.

Edema is the clinical appearance of fluid accumulation in the interstitial spaces of the body. A variety of conditions can lead to the formation of edema:[13]

1. An increase in capillary permeability (e.g., the effects of histamine)
2. Increased capillary blood pressure

3. Reduction in blood protein concentration (e.g., hypoalbuminemia) which results in reduced osmotic retention of intravascular water

4. Lymphatic obstruction

Congestive heart failure is characterized by increased pulmonary capillary blood pressure. Pulmonary capillary pressures reaching 18 to 25 mm Hg increase the accumulation of fluid along the vessel walls, around the small airways, and in the pleural space. This initially occurs in the dependent regions of the lung where gravity dictates that capillary pressures are always the highest. As the severity of the left heart failure increases, pulmonary edema occurs in those lung regions where capillary pressures exceed 25 mm Hg.

Pulmonary Dysfunction

Pulmonary function is often disturbed during left ventricular failure (Table 8–3).[14–16] Advanced congestive failure produces marked impairment in pulmonary function whereas, in contrast, early left heart failure with its attendant mild pulmonary hypertension (e.g., pulmonary artery wedge pressure of 15 to 22 mm Hg) may actually improve gas exchange because of an increased pulmonary blood volume and improved ventilation-perfusion ($\dot{V}/\dot{Q}$) matching. As congestive failure advances and pulmonary congestion increases, lung water increases. Pulmonary edema reduces lung volume and diffusion capacity and increases airway resistance and $\dot{V}/\dot{Q}$ mismatching. Severe failure and frank alveolar flooding results in dramatic deterioration of forced vital capacity, lung compliance, and gas exchange. As a result of respiratory and cardiac failure, a mixed respiratory and metabolic acidosis often occurs. These changes cause further cardiopulmonary dysfunction and a vicious cycle of cardiac and respiratory failure.

Table 8–3 Pulmonary Dysfunction During Left Heart Failure

Severity	Pathophysiology	Pulmonary Abnormalities
Mild	Pulmonary vascular congestion	↑ Diffusing capacity of lungs for carbon monoxide (D_{LCO}) ↑ Pa_{O_2} Pa_{CO_2} and pH normal
Moderate	Pulmonary interstitial edema	↓ Forced vital capacity (FVC) or unchanged ↓ Forced expiratory volume in 1 sec (FEV_1) or unchanged ↑ Closing volume ↑ Physiologic dead space in percent of tidal volume (V_D/V_T) ↓ $\dot{V}/\dot{Q}$ matching ↓ D_{LCO} ↓ Pa_{O_2} ↓ Pa_{CO_2} and ↑ pH
Severe	Alveolar flooding	↓↓ FVC ↓↓ FEV_1 ↓↓ Compliance ↑↑ Closing volume ↑↑ V_D/V_T ↓↓ $\dot{V}/\dot{Q}$ matching ↓↓ D_{LCO} ↓↓ Pa_{O_2} ↑ Pa_{CO_2} and ↓ pH

Source: Pastore, JO: Cardiac disease in respiratory patients in the intensive care unit. In MacDonnell, KF, Fahey, FJ, and Segal, MS (eds): Respiratory Intensive Care. Little, Brown, Boston, 1987, p 377.

CLINICAL FEATURES

The major clinical manifestations of heart failure can be arbitrarily categorized into those associated with fluid retention and peripheral edema (right heart failure) and those due to pulmonary vascular congestion (left heart failure). This division is clinically useful but potentially misleading because biventricular failure often occurs as one ventricle fails and precipitates failure of the other. Early cor pulmonale is difficult to recognize because the clinical picture is almost always dominated by chronic pulmonary disease (see Chapter 3). The clinical manifestations not only vary with the major form of heart failure present but also vary as the patient's ability to compensate changes or as the patient responds to therapy.

The morbidity and mortality associated with heart failure necessitates early recognition and treatment. The historic details of having one or more of the triggering factors (see Table 8–2) are very useful in making the determination that heart failure is the primary or contributing cause of the patient's complaints or condition.

The initial impression of the patient often reveals dyspnea, generalized weakness, delirium, anxiety, and occasionally psychosis during moderate to severe failure. The increased sympathetic activity and release of norepinephrine combined with poor cardiac output leads to poor peripheral circulation, which produces cool skin, diaphoresis, cyanosis of the digits, and peripheral pallor. Distended jugular veins and pitting edema of the ankles are common hallmarks of congestive failure.

Dyspnea at rest and with minimal exertion is frequently seen during significant heart failure. The dyspnea commonly becomes worse when the patient is lying flat **(orthopnea)** and at night **(nocturnal dyspnea)**. For this reason, these patients often report that they sleep better with their head elevated by numerous pillows. Tachypnea is common and often intensifies with severe hypoxemia or metabolic acidosis or both. Cheyne-Stokes breathing may occur in patients who have severe failure. This may be related to a prolonged circulation time between the lungs and the chemoreceptors of the nervous system.[5]

Tachycardia is a common finding and represents a compensatory mechanism for maintaining cardiac output in the face of a poor SV. Alterations in the pulse amplitude from beat to beat **(pulsus alternans)** may be detected, indicating severe myocardial disease. An irregular or very rapid pulse (more than 130/minute) may contribute to the degree of heart failure and be a sign of electrolyte imbalance, hypoxemia, and drug toxicity, and indicates the need for electrocardiographic (ECG) monitoring.[5]

The compensatory sympathetic vasoconstriction may support a normal blood pressure, but in severe failure the systolic and mean arterial pressures will be reduced. The patient's peripheral skin temperature is frequently reduced whereas the core temperature may actually be elevated as a result of impaired heat dissipation.

Auscultation of the chest during left heart failure often reveals fine inspiratory crackles and polyphonic expiratory (cardiac) wheezes. Crackles occur as small airways of atelectatic regions "pop" open upon inspiration. Wheezes are caused by airflow through airways that are narrowed by fluid accumulation in the surrounding extracellular space. These findings are often heard over the lung bases of the patient in moderate failure and farther up into the midlung and apical regions of the chest as congestive failure worsens. Cardiac gallop rhythms and murmurs are common findings and become more severe with exertion.

Peripheral edema, abdominal distension, and superficial abdominal vein distension are common findings in those with chronic heart failure. Liver congestion **(hepatomegaly)** and excessive peritoneal fluid retention **(ascites)** cause abdominal distension as a result of chronic venous hypertension and impaired lymphatic drainage. In most adults, fluid retention of approximately 5 liters must occur before peripheral edema is detectable.[5] Edema fluids collect in the most dependent regions of the body such as the ankles in the upright patient. The edema formation may become so severe that pressing on the skin will leave a dent or pit. In those patients unable to get out of bed, edema collects in the posterior parts of the arms, thighs, and legs.

In right heart failure the chest radiograph is often normal unless pulmonary disease is present. Radiographic changes during left heart failure can be classified as consistent with mild, moderate, and severe failure:[5,15,17]

Mild Failure

This is defined as pulmonary venous congestion with widening of pulmonary arteries and redistribution of pulmonary blood flow to the upper lung fields.

Moderate Failure

Moderate heart failure is characterized by cardiomegaly (greater than half the diameter of the thorax); pulmonary artery engorgement; and interstitial pulmonary edema—presence of Kerley A lines (1- to 2-cm lines of interstitial edema extending out from the hilum) and Kerley B lines (short, thin streaks of interstitial edema outlining the lymphatics of a subsegmental region of lung that extends inward from the pleural surface).

Severe Failure

Severe heart failure leads to cardiomegaly, pulmonary artery engorgement, interstitial pulmonary edema, fluffy and patchy alveolar edema (often in a "butterfly" pattern that radiates out from the perihilar region), and pleural effusion.

Sinus tachycardia is the most common ECG abnormality.[5] Frequent premature ventricular contractions and atrial fibrillation may contribute to failure or be a result of it. Bundle branch blocks are common in ischemic heart failure, and axis deviation is common with cardiac hypertrophy. ST–T-wave changes are frequently present and suggest myocardial hypoxia or infarction or both. R-wave, right-axis, or right bundle branch block changes are common during right heart failure.[6]

Arterial blood gas (ABG) analysis is useful in determining the degree of gas exchange derangement and the trend of the patient's pulmonary status.[16,17] (Table 8–3). Reduced Pao_2 and an increased alveolar-arterial difference in partial pressure of oxygen $P(A-a)o_2$ or reduced Pao_2/Fio_2 may be the most practical and sensitive signs of respiratory impairment as a consequence of pulmonary edema and $\dot{V}/\dot{Q}$ mismatching. Respiratory alkalosis is frequently found in the early failure period and often continues until the patient's compensation fails. With the onset of severe left heart failure and frank pulmonary edema, ventilatory failure is likely and a combination of severe hypoxemia and respiratory acidosis will ensue. A mixed respiratory and metabolic acidosis is not uncommon in severe failure as a result of anaerobic metabolism caused by poor circulation and ventilatory failure.

Routine laboratory studies are seldom useful in establishing heart failure as the cause of the patient complaints, but some tests are useful. With chronic cor pulmonale, the hematocrit, hemoglobin concentration, and erythrocyte count are frequently elevated to 10 to 25 percent above normal values as a result of chronic hypoxia.[6] Hyponatremia and hypokalemia are often seen in patients with congestive failure and may result from excessive fluid retention or diuretic therapy.[8] Right heart failure with sufficient liver engorgement will cause bilirubin and liver enzymes to increase.[18]

Table 8–4 Hemodynamics and Physical Finding Subsets Following Heart Failure from Acute Myocardial Infarction

Subset	PAWP (mm Hg)	Cardiac Index (L/min/m²)	Mortality (percent)
I. No pulmonary congestion and no peripheral hypoperfusion	≤18	>2.2	3
II. Pulmonary congestion and no peripheral hypoperfusion	>18	>2.2	9
III. Peripheral hypoperfusion and no pulmonary congestion	≤18	≤2.2	23
IV. Pulmonary congestion and peripheral hypoperfusion	>18	≤2.2	51

PAWP = Pulmonary artery wedge pressure.

Source: Adapted from Forrester, JS, et al: Medical therapy of acute myocardial infarction by application of hemodynamic subsets. N Engl J Med 295:1404–1413, 1976.

The echocardiogram, Doppler flow, and radionuclide studies are useful in establishing the anatomic changes in heart structure and motion often found in failure. Typical findings include dilated end-diastolic ventricular dimensions, hypertrophic myocardial changes, valvular dysfunction, and reduced ventricular motion and ejection fraction.[5]

Pulmonary artery catheterization is useful in evaluating the degree of pulmonary hypertension, severity of left ventricular dysfunction, and cardiac output. It is also useful in guiding therapy in those patients with severe heart failure.[19] Table 8–4 illustrates that the combination of physical findings and hemodynamic data is useful in predicting the severity of heart failure and patient outcome following myocardial infarction.[20]

Aerobic exercise capacity is frequently diminished in the patient with chronic heart failure.[21] This impairment is associated with inadequate oxygen delivery to skeletal muscle and their subsequent shift to anaerobic metabolism and fatigue.[21,22] As heart failure increases, exercise capacity and maximum oxygen use decrease in relationship to the decreasing maximum cardiac output attainable.

The combination of physical assessment, chest radiography, ABG analysis, ECG, and hemodynamic monitoring form the core for early detection, differentiation, and management.

TREATMENT

Therapy for heart failure depends on the cause of failure, its severity, and the secondary complications. The treatment of heart failure should address the following objectives:

1. Reduction of cardiac workload
2. Control of sodium and fluid retention
3. Improvement of cardiac pump performance
4. Prevention of thromboembolism
5. Support for secondary organ dysfunction

Management of Heart Failure

Cardiac function can be improved by reducing workload and enhancing contractility. Cardiac work can be reduced through afterload reduction. Control of hypertension or afterload reduction is most often achieved with direct-acting vasodilators (e.g., nitroglycerin, nitroprusside, hydralazine, and minoxidil) or indirect neurohumoral antagonistic drugs (e.g., captopril, prazosin, and trimazosin) and calcium-channel blockers (e.g., verapamil and nifedipine), which inhibit the action of the endogenous vasoconstrictive mechanisms.[23] The individual response to drug-induced afterload reduction is quite variable and requires careful titration to avoid hypotension. Other techniques for reducing workload on the heart include reduction in physical activity, emotional stress, and body weight (if above ideal body weight). Sedation with appropriate drugs (e.g., morphine or Versed) may be necessary to reduce the anxiety and agitation and relieve the heart from autonomic stimulation.

Sodium and water retention can be corrected first by bed rest, which induces a natural diuresis by the kidney. Upright positions decrease sodium and water excretion and should be restricted until fluid and electrolyte balance is more acceptable.[23] Dietary restriction of sodium and water are the next step toward reduction of the fluid retention. Use of diuretics such as loop of Henle agents (e.g., furosemide), thiazides (e.g., metolazone), and potassium-sparing agents (e.g., spironolactone) are useful in controlling water retention.[23]

High-dose diuretic therapy is usually started at the beginning of severe congestive failure and then tapered as the patient responds. The end points of diuretic therapy are frequently the volemic status that give maximal cardiac output without causing pulmonary congestion. This usually results in a targeted pulmonary artery wedge pressure (preload) of 15 to 18 mm Hg. The disappearance of the inspiratory crackles during chest auscultation and reduced pulmonary edema on the radiograph frequently requires as much as 24 hours following "arrival" at the optimal preload pressure. Careful use of these agents is necessary to avoid overdiuresis, which could lead to electrolyte imbalance and rebound hypotension. Cautious fluid replacement and potassium therapy is almost always necessary to avoid hypokalemia and fluid imbalance.

Inotropic drugs (e.g., digitalis, dobutamine, and amrinone) are used to improve ventricular function by increasing contractility, which improves cardiac output and venous congestion.[23] Digitalis remains the most frequently prescribed inotropic agent used in heart failure and is still the drug of choice. Those patients with chronic heart failure due to systolic dysfunction are the most responsive. Digitalis intoxication can occur in up to 30 percent of patients treated with this medication.[24] The classic signs and symptoms of digitalis intoxication include nausea, vomiting, insomnia, altered color vision, and irregular cardiac rhythm (e.g., frequent ventricular premature contractions).

Patients in heart failure often have venous stasis and are at high risk for developing emboli.[25] This event can lead to devastating pulmonary embolization. Short-term heparin and long-term coumarin anticoagulant therapy reduce the risk of embolization (see Chapter 7).

Patients in severe congestive failure will require all or most of the foregoing measures to correct their condition. The actions of these agents can be seen in Figure 8–2, which shows several Frank-Starling cardiac output and left ventricular filling pressure (preload) curves. The diuretics reduce preload and venous congestion but do not directly improve cardiac output. Vasodilators reduce afterload and improve cardiac output. Inotropic agents improve contractility and reduce preload and, when used with vasodilators, further improve cardiac performance and reduce venous congestion.

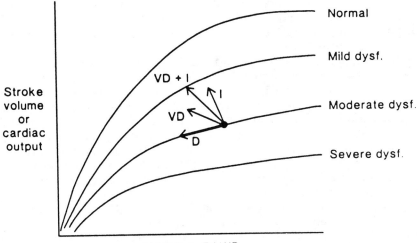

LVEDP or PAWP

FIGURE 8–2 Frank-Starling left ventricular function curves relating preload pressure (left ventricular end-diastolic pressure [LVEDP] or pulmonary artery wedge pressure [PAWP] and stroke volume or cardiac output. Curves showing normal and various degrees of dysfunction (dys) are shown. Diuretics (D) are shown to reduce preload and venous congestion without acutely improving cardiac output. Inotropic drugs (I) or vasodilators (VD), and especially the combination of these two (VD + I), act to shift heart function toward better cardiac output with reduced preload. (From Chesebro, JH: Cardiac failure: Medical management. In Brandenburg, RO, Fuster, V, Giuliani, ER, and McGoon, DC (eds): Cardiology: Fundamentals and Practice. Year Book Medical, Chicago, 1987, with permission.)

Surgical treatment of heart failure is directed toward specific repair of the cause. This would include valvular repair or replacement for valvular heart disease and coronary artery bypass grafting for coronary artery disease. However, those patients with severe left ventricular dysfunction generally have higher mortality rates postoperatively.[26] For younger patients, cardiac transplantation holds the best hope for long-term treatment of severe chronic heart disease failure (e.g., dilated cardiomyopathy).

Respiratory Care for Cardiogenic Pulmonary Edema

Initial treatment with oxygen therapy is necessary to improve arterial oxygenation, which will improve cardiac function. Low-flow oxygen therapy with a nasal cannula can be the starting point if the patient is conscious and is responding to the medical management just described. A nonrebreathing mask with adequate flow should be used in patients with severe hypoxemia or those in frank pulmonary edema.

High-flow mask continuous positive airway pressure (CPAP) has been used for heart failure induced "cardiac asthma" sporadically since its initial description more than 50 years ago.[27] More recently it has been shown that patients in cardiogenic pulmonary edema with serious tachypnea (respiratory rate greater than 25/minute) and $\dot{V}/\dot{Q}$ mismatching (Pao_2/Fio_2 less than 200) had a significant and rapid improvement in oxygenation and reductions in respiratory and heart rates with the use of mask CPAP.[28] Although hypoventilation and subsequent hypercapnia are potential contraindications to the use of mask CPAP, they have not detracted from its effective use in treating hypoxemia induced by heart failure.[29] The suggested mechanism behind the effectiveness of mask CPAP in this setting is the improved lung compliance, reduced work of breathing, improved gas exchange, and reduced vascular congestion.[28,29] Mask CPAP should be used with a nasogastric tube and avoided if the patient is at high risk for vomiting or if they have severe respiratory acidosis (pH less than 7.20).

Intubation and ventilatory support will be necessary if the patient develops respiratory acidosis or becomes hypoxemic on an elevated FIO_2 (greater than 0.60). Initial ventilator settings should be assist-control mode, 100 percent oxygen, V_T 10 mL/kg (ideal body weight), respiratory rate 12/minute, and sensitivity of -2 cm H_2O. The addition of positive end-expiratory pressure (PEEP) (5 to 15 cm H_2O) is appropriate if the oxygenation and lung mechanics remains poor despite ventilatory support with an elevated FIO_2 (e.g., greater than 0.50). Care must be given to the application of positive pressure ventilation with PEEP in these patients because of their precarious cardiac function. Use of a pulmonary artery catheter may be necessary to guide therapy and avoid decompensating the heart.[19]

Special attention to airway care will be necessary following intubation in patients with frank pulmonary edema. Edema foam will need to be cleared rapidly to improve the effectiveness of the oxygen therapy and ventilatory support. In the past, aerosolized ethyl alcohol (20 to 40 percent) was used to reduce the pulmonary edema foam but this has been abandoned because of its bronchial irritation and the more direct response to airway suctioning and application of high-dose diuretics. Aerosolized bronchodilators (e.g., albuterol) should be used in those patients who have a compounding component of asthma or bronchitis or both.

Case Study

HISTORY

Mr. N, a 64-year-old man, is a retired concession operator with a history of coronary artery disease, arrhythmia, and chronic obstructive pulmonary disease. He had a recent episode of pneumonia and a small anterior wall myocardial infarction and was in a Veterans Administration hospital for 1 month. He was discharged 4 days ago with an extensive assortment of medications to maintain his cardiac, renal, and pulmonary functions. While at home he experienced a coughing spell, which then led to increasing shortness of breath and mild substernal pressure. He became increasingly anxious and called the paramedics. He was taken to the hospital immediately because he could not "catch his breath" and that his "heart would not slow down." During transportation to the hospital he was treated with oxygen via nasal cannula at 4 liters/minute.

Questions

1. What signs and symptoms will need to be evaluated immediately upon his arrival?
2. What diagnostic techniques can be used to help determine the nature of his shortness of breath?
3. What therapeutic techniques should be readily available upon his arrival?

Answers

1. The level of consciousness, signs of delirium, signs of a patent airway, spontaneous breathing rate and chest motion, quality of breath sounds and their symmetry, pulse rate, blood pressure, and temperature should be evaluated. Clinicians should look for symptoms of respiratory distress, shock, and mental impairment.
2. The severity and origin of his shortness of breath can be evaluated by taking a rapid history, if possible, to determine the triggering factors that

led up to the sudden exacerbation. A symptom-directed physical evaluation followed by appropriate laboratory studies will be needed. The source of the dyspnea (pulmonary versus cardiac) can then be sorted out after the needed information has been collected.

3. Oxygen therapy (cannula, Venturi mask, and nonrebreathing mask), intubation equipment, manual resuscitation bag with proper mask, oxygen reservoir, venous and arterial line placement equipment, various fluids for vascular support, appropriate resuscitation drugs, and medications for pain and agitation.

PHYSICAL EXAMINATION

General Mr. N. is an obese elderly man with an approximate weight of 110 kg. who is alert and in obvious respiratory distress while sitting up, despite oxygen therapy via nasal cannula at 4 liters/minute. His wife stated, with his confirmation, that he had been a heavy smoker for 26 years and then quit 12 years ago, had a myocardial infarction (MI) 10 years ago, had had multiple hernia operations 10 years ago, has chronic lung disease, and had recently been discharged from a veterans administration (VA) hospital after treatment of pneumonia and heart disease. He indicated that he has been taking all his medications and staying on his prescribed low-salt, low-fat diet.

Vital Signs Temperature 37.5°C; respiratory rate 32/minute; blood pressure 100/70 mm Hg; pulse 160/minute; nailbed refill 5 seconds

HEENT Pupils equal and reactive to light; some nasal flaring; normal oral structures

Neck Trachea is midline; no signs of inspiratory stridor or laryngeal abnormality; carotid pulses ++ bilaterally without bruit; no signs of lymphadenopathy or thyroidomegaly; noticeable jugular vein distension; some tensing of sternocleidomastoid and scalene muscles during inspiration

Chest Normal chest configuration; no scars; some diminished motion noted; breath sounds reveal bilateral inspiratory crackles from bases midway up chest with some scattered expiratory wheezes; some thoracoabdominal paradoxic motion noted

Heart Heart tones diminished; point of maximum impulse (PMI) not palpable; no murmurs, rub, or gallop

Abdomen Obese; soft; no hepatomegaly; bowel sounds not heard clearly

Extremities Moving all extremities; +2 pulses felt throughout; +2 pitting edema in both ankles; no clubbing; skin cool and diaphoretic with some peripheral cyanosis

---

Questions

4. What are the possible causes of his respiratory distress?
5. What signs and symptoms indicate congestive heart failure?
6. How does left heart failure influence respiratory function?

7. What diagnostic techniques should be used to evaluate his cardiorespiratory distress further?

Answers

4. His respiratory distress may be caused by (1) pulmonary edema due to heart failure; (2) exacerbation of his chronic obstructive pulmonary disease (COPD); (3) MI; or (4) pulmonary infection.

5. The signs and symptoms of congestive heart failure he displays include rapid onset of dyspnea; anxiety; disproportionate tachycardia and relatively low blood pressure; inspiratory crackles in the dependent lung regions; jugular vein distension; cool, diaphoretic skin and poor peripheral circulation; and ankle edema.

6. Left heart failure can induce pulmonary hypertension, increased lung water, increased airway resistance, alveolar edema, increased work of breathing, decreasing pulmonary compliance, $\dot{V}/\dot{Q}$ mismatching, diffusion defect, hypoxemia, and respiratory failure.

7. To evaluate further his cardiorespiratory distress, ABG analysis, chest radiograph, and a 12-lead ECG with subsequent ECG monitoring are immediately needed. Continuous noninvasive monitoring of his oxyhemoglobin saturation and blood pressure will further help guide his cardiopulmonary care. Laboratory assessment of complete blood count (CBC), electrolytes, and standard blood chemistry are indicated. Assessment of his cardiac enzymes (creatine kinase [CK]) and digitalis levels would help rule out an MI and help guide digitalis therapy.

BEDSIDE AND LABORATORY EVALUATION

ECG

Supraventricular tachycardia of 158/minute; normal axis; first-degree atrioventricular (AV) block; and left bundle branch block

CHEST RADIOGRAPH

(Fig. 8–3)

ARTERIAL BLOOD GASES

pH 7.24, $Paco_2$ 51 mm Hg, Pao_2 38 mm Hg, HCO_3^- 22 mEq/liter while breathing oxygen via nasal cannula at 4 liters/minute

HEMATOLOGY

Hematocrit (Hct) 45 percent; Hb 15 g/dL; red blood cells (RBC) $5.2 \times 10^6/mm^3$; white blood cells (WBC) 15.2×10^3; platelets 262×10^3

CHEMISTRY

Results pending

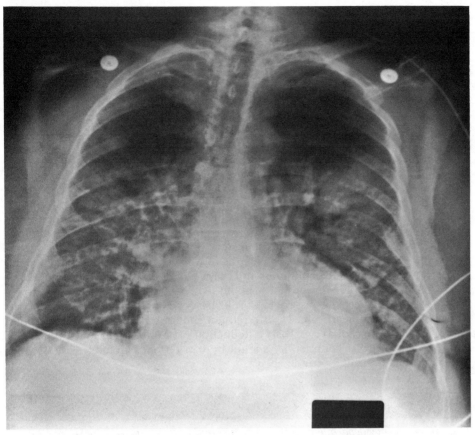

FIGURE 8–3 Portable AP chest radiograph taken at admission in the emergency department.

Questions

8. What does the ECG indicate?
9. What does the chest radiograph indicate?
10. How would you interpret the ABG data?
11. What do the hematologic data indicate?
12. What respiratory care is indicated at this time?
13. What cardiac care is indicated at this time?

Answers

8. The ECG indicates tachycardia with other cardiac conduction disturbances. This rate may be responsible for the acute congestive heart failure but is most likely a sign of the severity of the cardiac failure.

9. The chest radiograph reveals cardiomegaly; bilateral pulmonary vascular engorgement; interstitial and alveolar edema and atelectasis bilaterally; some Kerley B lines in both bases; no signs of pleural effusion or hemopneumothorax; trachea seen at midline; some scoliosis in the thoracic vertebral column; and rib cage normal

10. The ABG analysis shows severe hypoxemia. Both hypoventilation and shunting appear to be present. Hypoventilation, despite a significant tachypnea, indicates ventilatory decompensation, resulting in mixed res-

piratory and metabolic acidosis. The mild metabolic acidosis may be caused by lactic acidosis associated with poor tissue perfusion. CHF usually stimulates hyperventilation; however, in this patient the $Paco_2$ of 51 mm Hg suggests respiratory acidosis from COPD exacerbation or severe overwhelming CHF.

11. The hematologic data are relatively normal, with the exception of the slight-to-moderate elevation of the WBC count, which may be consistent with an infection or possibly induced by the stress of the illness.

12. The oxygen therapy currently in use is inadequate. The patient has significant hypoxemia and moderate ventilatory failure, and intubation and ventilatory support could be helpful at this time. Mask CPAP may be attempted as a temporary maneuver to improve ventilatory mechanics and oxygenation. If the patient's clinical status or ABGs deteriorate in spite of mask CPAP, intubation and mechanical ventilatory support would be necessary. Aerosolized bronchodilator therapy (e.g., albuterol) should be continued to optimize airway resistance given the clinical findings of wheezes and the history of COPD.

13. The supraventricular tachycardia of this magnitude requires immediate treatment and continuous ECG and blood pressure monitoring. Intravenous (IV) infusion lines should be placed for the resuscitative drugs. The underlying disorders should be corrected as soon as possible, to slow the heart rate. Fluid retention should be relieved by giving high-dose diuretics (e.g., Lasix). Reduction of afterload and improvement of myocardial contractility should be carried out carefully with IV vasodilators and inotropic agents.

In the emergency department continuous ECG and pulse oximetry were started, two peripheral IV lines were placed, and oxygen therapy was switched to a nonrebreathing mask supplied with 15 liters/minute of oxygen. A single dose of slowly administered verapamil was given with a prompt decline in heart rate to 130/minute. Lasix, Isordil, captopril, digitalis, morphine sulphate, and erythromycin were started. The patient was then transferred to the coronary care unit with the diagnosis of congestive heart failure caused by possible myocardial infarction, possible dietary indiscretion, possible noncompliance in taking his medication, and/or possible underlying pulmonary infection. Upon admission to the unit an arterial line was placed and continuous ECG and pulse oximetry monitoring continued.

BEDSIDE AND LABORATORY EVALUATION

Mr. N was alert, sitting up in his bed in obvious respiratory distress receiving high-concentration oxygen via nonrebreathing mask, and somewhat anxious. Occasionally he coughed up thick brown sputum. He stated, "I'm afraid to be taken off the oxygen." He was being given 2.5 mg of aerosolized albuterol diluted in 3 mL of saline every 2 hours and he indicated that these treatments helped to reduce his dyspnea.

VITAL SIGNS, HEMODYNAMICS, AND URINE OUTPUT

Rectal temperature 37.2°C; respiratory rate is 34/minute; pulse 132/minute; systemic arterial blood pressure is 143/97 mm Hg; Spo_2 81 percent; breath sounds continuing with bilateral inspiratory crackles, expiratory wheezes, and occasional expiratory rhonchi; urine output brisk at 500 mL over the past hour since his admission and the administration of Lasix

ECG FINDINGS

Sinus tachycardia of 130/minute; first-degree AV block; and left bundle branch block

LABORATORY FINDINGS

ABGs

pH 7.26; $Paco_2$ 51 mm Hg; Pao_2 49 mm Hg, HCO_3^- = 24 mEq/liter, $P(A-a)o_2$ 660 mm Hg; Pao_2/Fio_2 49 (assumes Fio_2 = 1.0); Sao_2 79 percent (calculated); Spo_2 81 percent (pulse oximeter)

Electrolytes and Chemistry

Na^+ 137 mEq/liter, K^+ 3.7 mEq/liter; Ca^{++} (ionized) 8.2 mg/dL, Cl^- 101 mEq/liter glucose 239 mg/dL, blood urea nitrogen (BUN) 13 mg/dL, creatinine 1.3 mg/dL

Cardiac Enzymes

Pending

Microbiology

Sputum smear and cultures pending

Questions

14. What do the bedside findings and vital signs indicate about Mr. N's response to treatment?
15. What do the laboratory findings indicate about Mr. N's status?
16. What changes in his respiratory care, if any, would you recommend?

Answers

14. His bedside findings indicate that his heart rate, blood pressure, and urine output have responded to treatment but that his respiratory status has not improved.
15. The ECG changes are encouraging and his chemistry panel results are acceptable; however, the ABG and acid-base balance show moderate hypoxemia despite very high concentrations of oxygen and continued hypoventilation with respiratory acidosis despite significant tachypnea.
16. Mr. N is now a candidate for a mask CPAP trial or intubation and mechanical ventilation. Continuation of aerosolized bronchodilators to help reduce his work of breathing is appropriate. It is not appropriate to leave the patient hypoxemic and in respiratory failure while waiting for the diuresis to reduce the pulmonary edema

Following assessment of Mr. N's condition, he was placed on a continuous high-flow mask CPAP system (Fig. 8–4) and a nasogastric tube to suction was placed. The initial settings were a flow of 60 liters/minute, Fio_2 1.0 and CPAP 5 cm H_2O. He was initially apprehensive but then became less dyspneic with his respiratory rate declining to 28/minute, pulse to 103/minute; the blood pressure remained at 140/96 mm Hg, and Spo_2 has increased to 89 percent following 30 minutes of CPAP and continued diuresis. CPAP was then increased to 7.5 cm H_2O to improve gas exchange further

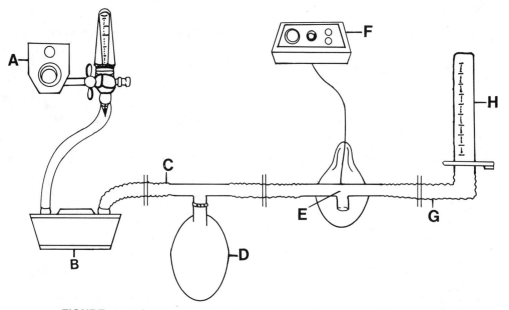

FIGURE 8–4 Continuous high-flow mask continuous positive airway pressure (CPAP) system. A, High-flow blender and flow meter; B, low-resistance, high-efficiency humidifier; C, inspiratory limb and water traps; D, 5-liter reservoir bag; E, clear plastic soft-seal patient mask; F, manometer and high-low pressure alarm; G, expiratory limb and water traps; H, threshold resistor for CPAP generation. (From Branson, RD, Hurst, JM, and DeHaven, CB: Mask CPAP: State of the art. Respir Care 30:846, 1985, with permission.)

and attempt some reduction of his F_{IO_2}. Thirty minutes later the following observations were made.

BEDSIDE FINDINGS AND LABORATORY EVALUATION _____

Mr. N was sitting up in bed, wearing a clear plastic CPAP mask; he was alert, communicative, and appeared more comfortable and less dyspneic. He continued to use his accessory muscles with some thoracoabdominal asyncrony. The F_{IO_2} had been reduced to 0.80 with orders to keep his Sp_{O_2} more than 92 percent. Chest auscultation revealed improved breath sounds throughout the lower lung zones with scattered inspiratory crackles and occasional expiratory wheezes and rhonchi.

VITAL SIGNS, HEMODYNAMICS, AND URINE OUTPUT

Temperature 37.3°C; respiratory rate 22/minute; pulse 98/minute; systemic arterial blood pressure 138/98 mm Hg; and Sp_{O_2} 96 percent; ECG shows sinus tachycardia, first-degree AV block, and left bundle branch block; urine output totaled 1.9 liters over the past 4 hours since admission

ARTERIAL BLOOD GASES

pH 7.39, Pa_{CO_2} 50 mm Hg, Pa_{O_2} 96 mm Hg, HCO_3^- 30 mEq/liter; $P(A-a)_{O_2}$ 465 mm Hg; Pa_{O_2}/F_{IO_2} 120; Sa_{O_2} 97 percent (calculated); Sp_{O_2} 96 percent (pulse oximeter)

17. How would you interpret his bedside findings and vital signs?
18. What do the ABGs indicate?
19. What would you recommend with regard to the respiratory care at this time?

17. His bedside findings and vital signs indicate mild-to-moderate respiratory distress, reduced apparent respiratory work of breathing, enhanced oxygenation, an improving cardiovascular response, and a continued brisk diuresis.
18. ABGs reveal improving oxygenation (although his F_{IO_2} requirement remains elevated) with a declining $P(A\text{-}a)O_2$. Respiratory acidosis is present, which is common in patients with a history of COPD (see Chapters 3 and 4). The rapid increase in HCO_3^- suggests diuretic-related metabolic alkalosis.
19. He is having a very good response to the mask CPAP, diuretic, vasodilators, and inotropic therapy. His treatment is on the right course and

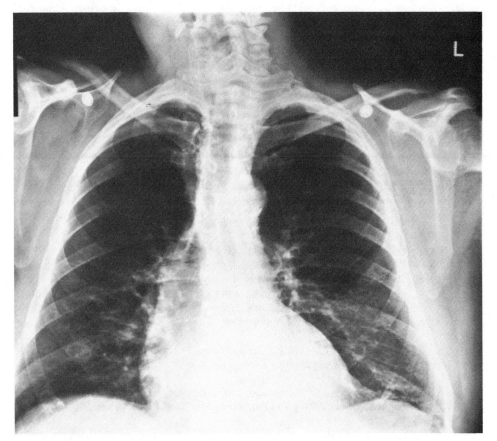

FIGURE 8–5 Portable AP chest radiograph taken 12 hours after admission to the hospital.

should allow continued reduction of the F_{IO_2} in 10 percent increments until reaching 40 percent. If his respiratory and cardiovascular status are stable or improving at that point for an hour or more and the tachypnea tapers down below 22/minute, the CPAP levels can be reduced to 5 and then 0 cm H_2O. He could then be placed on oxygen therapy via nasal cannula. Continued cardiopulmonary monitoring remains necessary.

Mr. N's respiratory status continued to improve over the next 8 hours as the F_{IO_2} was gradually reduced to 0.40. His respiratory rate remained below 20/minute and pulse in the 85 to 95/minute range; blood pressure dropped to 125/75 mm Hg, and Sp_{O_2} was maintained greater than 95 percent. Breath sounds demonstrated better aeration and scattered expiratory rhonchi. A chest radiograph (Fig. 8–5) at this time showed almost complete interval clearing with some scattered atelectasis in the right peri-hilar region and basal zones of the right and left lungs; heart size was reduced; and all other anatomic structures looked unchanged. Digitalis levels were found to be in the therapeutic range. ABGs were pH 7.37, Pa_{CO_2} 49 mm Hg, Pa_{O_2} 105 mm Hg, and HCO_3 29 mEq/liter. The CPAP level was gradually reduced to 0 cm H_2O over the next hour. This was tolerated without noticeable change in the patient's clinical state or pulse oximetry. He was then placed on a nasal cannula at 4 liters/minute, which was later reduced to 2 liters/minute. Cardiac enzyme levels (CK and lactate dehydrogenase [LDH]) and isoenzymes were found to be in the high-normal range, suggesting that the patient did not have a MI. Diuretic, vasodilator, inotropic, aero-solized bronchodilator, and oxygen therapy were continued when he was transferred to the post-coronary care unit and ambulation was begun. He was discharged 2 days later in stable condition.

REFERENCES

1. Gorlin, R: Incidence, etiology and prognosis of heart failure. Cardiovasc Rev Rep 4:765, 1983.

2. Furburg, CD, Yusuf, S, and Thom, TJ: Potential for altering natural history of congestive heart failure: Need for large clinical trials. Am J Cardiol 55:45A, 1985.

3. Smith, WM: Epidemiology of congestive heart failure. Am J Cardiol 55:3A, 1985.

4. Kannel, WB, Savage, D, and Castelli, WP: Cardiac failure in the Framingham Study: Twenty-year follow-up. In Braunwald, E, Mock, MB, and Watson, JT (eds): Congestive Heart Failure: Current Research and Clinical Applications. Grune & Stratton, New York, 1982, pp 15–30.

5. Chesebro, JH and Burnett, JC: Cardiac failure: Characteristics and clinical manifestations. In Brandenburg, RO, et al (eds): Cardiology: Fundamentals and Practice. Year Book Medical, Chicago, 1987, pp 645–665.

6. Horn, MJ: Pulmonary heart disease (cor pulmonale). In Bordow, RA and Moser, KM (eds): Manual of Clinical Problems in Pulmonary Medicine. Little, Brown, Boston, 1985, pp 262–268.

7. Rushmer, RF: Cardiovascular Dynamics, ed 4. WB Saunders, Philadelphia, 1976, pp 532–567.

8. Smith, JJ and Kampine, JP: Circulatory Physiology—the Essentials. Williams & Wilkins, Baltimore, 1980, pp 264–274.

9. Cohn, JN, et al: Plasma norepinephrine as a guide to prognosis in patients with chronic congestive heart failure. N Engl J Med 311:819, 1984.

10. Bove, AA and Santamore, WP: Mechanical performance of the heart. In Brandenburg, RO, et al (eds): Cardiology: Fundamentals and Practice. Year Book Medical, Chicago, 1987, pp 149–163.

11. Burnett, JC and Knox, FG: Renal interstitial pressure and sodium excretion during renal vein constriction. Am J Physiol 238:F279–282, 1980.

12. Dzau, VJ, et al: Relation of the renin-angiotensin-aldosterone system to clinical state in congestive heart failure. Circulation 63:645, 1981.

13. Smith, JJ and Kampine, JP: Circulatory Physiology—the Essentials. Williams & Wilkins, Baltimore, 1980, pp 129–140.

14. Light, RW and George, RB: Serial pulmonary function in patients with acute heart failure. Arch Intern Med 143:429, 1983.

15. Pastore, JO: Cardiac disease in respiratory patients in the intensive care unit. In: MacDonnell, KF, Fahey, PJ, and Segal, MS (eds): Respiratory Intensive Care. Little, Brown, Boston, 1987, pp 370–384.

16. Fuster, V, et al: The heart and lungs A. Interrelationships between disease of the heart and disease of the lung. In Brandenburg, RO, et al (eds): Cardiology: Fundamentals and Practice. Year Book Medical, Chicago, 1987, pp 1797–1810.

17. Sheldon, RL and Wilkins, RL: Clinical application of the chest radiograph. In Wilkins, RL, Sheldon, RL, and Krider, SJ (eds): Clinical Assessment in Respiratory Care. CV Mosby, St Louis, 1990, pp 107–127.

18. Kaymakcalan, H, et al: Congestive heart failure as cause of fulminant hepatic failure. Am J Med 65:384, 1978.

19. Krider, SJ: Invasively monitored hemodynamic pressures. In Wilkins, RL, Sheldon, RL, and Krider, SJ (eds): Clinical Assessment in Respiratory Care. CV Mosby, St Louis, 1990, pp 231–265.

20. Forrester, JS, et al: Medical therapy of acute myocardial infarction by application of hemodynamic subsets. N Engl J Med 295:1404, 1976.

21. Weber, KT, et al: Oxygen utilization and ventilation during exercise in patients with chronic cardiac failure. Circulation 65:1213, 1982.

22. Zelis, R, et al: A comparison of regional blood flow and oxygen utilization during dynamic forearm exercise in normal subjects and patients with congestive heart failure. Circulation 50:137, 1974.

23. Chesebro, JH: Cardiac failure: Medical management. In Brandenburg, RO, et al (eds): Cardiology: Fundamentals and Practice. Year Book Medical, Chicago, 1987, pp 666–688.

24. Beller, GA, et al: Digitalis intoxication: A prospective clinical study with serum level correlations. N Engl J Med 284:989, 1971.

25. Fuster, V, et al: The natural history of idiopathic dilated cardiomyopathy. Am J Cardiol 47:525, 1981.

26. Manley, JC, et al: The "bad" left ventricle: Results of coronary surgery and effects on late survival. J Thorac Cardiovasc Surg 72:841, 1976.

27. Branson, RD, Hurst, JM, and DeHaven, CB: Mask CPAP: State of the art. Respir Care 30:846, 1985.

28. Rasanen, J, et al: Continuous positive pressure by face mask in acute cardiogenic pulmonary edema. A randomized study. Crit Care Med 12:A325, 1984.

29. Perel, A, Wiliamson, DC, and Modell, JH: Effectiveness of CPAP via face mask for pulmonary edema associated with hypercarbia. Intensive Care Med 9:17, 1983.

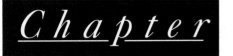

Chapter 9

George H. Hicks, MS, RRT

SMOKE INHALATION and BURNS

INTRODUCTION

Fire continues to be a major source of injury, death, and economic loss. In 1987, the 23 million fires reported in the United States were responsible for 28,200 injuries, 5800 deaths, and economic losses that exceeded $8 billion.[1] Residential fires, the most common setting for the cause of burn-related civilian injuries, produce more than 80 percent of the deaths.[1] The overall mortality rate for the general burn population is approximately 15 percent, but in the very young (less than 4 years of age) and the elderly (greater than 65 years of age) the rates are significantly higher.[1,2] These statistics make fire-related death the third most common cause of accidental death in this country, after motor vehicle accidents and accidental falls.[1] However, fire-related morbidity and mortality rates have continued to decline over the past two decades from 3.3 per 100,000 population in 1970 to 2.0 per 100,000 population in 1986.[1] These changes are most likely the result of public education, use of fire detection equipment, improved fire rescue techniques, and better established burn care.

Smoke inhalation injury dramatically increases the mortality rate for burn victims[2–5] (Fig. 9–1). Approximately 30 percent of burn victims admitted to burn centers also have smoke inhalation injuries.[2,6–9] Smoke inhalation injury coupled with a third-degree or full-thickness skin burn almost doubles the mortality rate.[2,10]

The injuries sustained by a burn victim are highly complex in that they influence or compromise most of the major organ systems and are not confined to the skin and respiratory systems. Although it is convenient to categorize these changes into various periods or phases, in reality they often overlap. Different pulmonary complications are associated with each phase of recovery.[6,11–13] The early or resuscitative phase (first 24 hours) is usually associated with complications arising from inhalation of toxic gases, or hot gases, or both. In the intermediate or postresuscitative phase (1 to 5 days), pulmonary edema, secretion retention, atelectasis, adult respiratory distress syndrome (ARDS), and hypermetabolic-induced ventilatory failure can occur. During the late phase (beyond 5 days), infectious pneumonia, sepsis syndrome, pulmonary embolism, and chronic pulmonary disease are more frequent respiratory problems.

Pathophysiologic changes associated with burns and smoke inhalation make the burn victim extremely challenging to treat. Although these changes are complex, they are relatively predictable and allow more successful preventative measures. This chapter will focus on the pulmonary problems and required treatment for smoke inhalation and burn injuries.

BURN INJURY MORTALITY

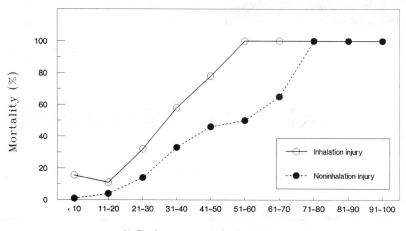

FIGURE 9–1 The distribution of mortality in 914 burn victims, as influenced by the size of the burn and the presence or absence of an inhalation injury. (Adapted from data presented in Venus, B, et al: Prophylactic intubation and continuous positive airway pressure in the management of inhalation injury in burn victims. Crit Care Med 9:519, 1981.)

ETIOLOGY

Smoke produced in a hot, hypoxic environment is a complex mixture of gaseous poisons. The nature and extent of injuries produced by smoke are a product of the heat produced and the complex chemistry of the fire environment.

Air temperatures can climb to values in excess of 550°C in less than 10 minutes in a fuel-rich environment such as the home or office.[3] As the heat builds, spontaneous combustion of other fuel sources such as carpet, furniture, wall coverings, and appliances occurs with the development of "flash over." Flash over is usually seen as a wall of fire extending down from the ceiling billowing out door or window openings. Fires associated with steam produce much more heat damage than fires associated with dry air. Steam has 500 times the heat energy content of dry gases at the same temperature and can scald greater areas of skin and cause deeper respiratory tract thermal injury.

Interior design products found in the modern residential, office, and industrial settings produce a large number of toxic combustion products. Some of the more common toxic gases produced are listed in Table 9–1. A variety of aldehydes (e.g., acrolein) and organic acids (e.g., acetic acid), which are potent respiratory tract irritants, are produced from burning wood, cotton, paper, and many acrylics.[14] As the fire continues, the carbon dioxide (CO_2) that is produced can increase beyond 5 percent, whereas the oxygen concentration can drop below 10 percent.[15] Decreased oxygen availability prevents complete combustion and results in the production of carbon monoxide (CO).[3,4] Burning polyvinyl chloride, a component of plastics found throughout homes and offices, produces more than 75 different toxic chemicals including hydrogen chloride, phosgene, chlorine, and CO.[16] The burning of polyurethane materials, such as nylon and many upholsteries, can produce the very irritating isocyanates and extremely toxic hydrogen cyanide (HCN).[17] Inhaled soot particles carrying toxic chemicals cause damage deep in the lung if

Table 9–1 Toxic Gases Found in House Fire Smoke

Substance	Source	Effect
Ammonia	Melamine resins	Inflammation
Aldehydes (acrolein, acetaldehyde, formaldehyde)	Wood, cotton, paper	Inflammation
Benzene	Petroleum products	Irritation and coma
Carbon dioxide	Organic materials	Asphyxiation and coma
Carbon monoxide	Organic materials	Asphyxiation and coma
Hydrogen chloride	Polyvinyl chloride	Inflammation
Hydrogen cyanide	Polyurethanes	Cellular asphyxia
Isocyanate	Polyurethanes	Inflammation and bronchospasm
Organic acids (acetic and formic acids)	Wood, cotton, paper	Inflammation
Oxides of nitrogen and sulfur	Nitrocellulose film	Pulmonary edema
Phosgene	Polyvinyl chloride	Inflammation

the particle diameters are from 0.1- to 5-μm.[16,18] Larger soot particles (e.g., 30-μm diameter) are filtered out in the upper airway. Chemical products of combustion can generally be divided into two categories: those that are absorbed and produce systemic toxic effects and those that produce local inflammatory changes in the mucosa.

To summarize, the nature and severity of injury is a function of the size and depth or degree of the skin burn, heat of the gases inhaled, chemical composition of the smoke, extent and duration of exposure, and the age and preexisting health status of the victim.[2,10,12,13]

PATHOPHYSIOLOGY

Early Pulmonary and Systemic Changes: 24 Hours Postburn

Exposure to the hypoxic and poisonous environment of a fire can cause rapid and severe organ dysfunction. The dysfunction is usually caused by reductions in both oxygen (O_2) transport and its use. Those tissues at particular risk are the central nervous system and myocardium. CO produced by fire in a hypoxic environment is easily absorbed into the blood where it converts oxyhemoglobin (Hbo_2) to carboxyhemoglobin (Hbco). CO does not bind to hemoglobin as quickly as oxygen but does bind much more tightly, with an affinity 200 times that of oxygen. Hbco levels can reach 15 percent in minor smoke inhalation and extend to beyond 60 percent in severe smoke inhalation. Conversion of Hbo_2 to Hbco compromises oxygen transport primarily through Hbco's inability to carry O_2. The presence of CO also results in retarding the oxygen release from hemoglobin's remaining ferrous-binding sites by a chemically induced increase in Hbo_2 affinity (i.e., shift of the oxyhemoglobin dissociation curve to the left). The hemoglobin conversion and inhibition of oxygen release results in a functional form of anemia that causes reduced oxygen transport and hypoxia despite the presence of a normal Pao_2 in the plasma. Cerebral edema can rapidly occur during severe CO poisonings as a result of impaired oxygen transport and hypotension.[19] In a small number of victims who appear to recover, neurologic dysfunction can occur 3 days to 4 weeks after a significant poisoning.[20] Lethal levels of CO poisoning are generally associated with Hbco concentrations greater than 60 percent.

Inhaled hydrogen cyanide (HCN) has been linked to both early and late death in burned patients.[17,21] Cyanide is easily transported to the tissues through the circulatory system and binds to the cytochrome oxidase enzymes of the mitochondria. This results in the inhibition of oxidative cellular metabolism and causes the tissues to shift to an inefficient anaerobic metabolism. Fatal exposure to HCN is usually associated with blood levels that exceed 1 mg/liter.[21] CO is also capable of binding to cytochrome oxidase and causing mitochondrial dysfunction.[22] Metabolic acidosis, caused by anaerobic metabolism, frequently accompanies CO and HCN exposure and is proportional to the severity of the poisoning. Thus, reduced oxygen transport and cellular metabolic dysfunction rapidly compromise the central nervous system and cardiovascular function and are the primary causes of death during the immediate period following severe smoke inhalation.[3,4,17,19,21]

Thermal injury to the respiratory tract is frequently confined to the face, oral and nasal cavities, pharynx, and rarely into the trachea.[2,3,23] The lower respiratory tract is spared of thermal injury through the efficient cooling of hot gases by the upper airway and reflex laryngospasm and glottic closure.[3,5,6] Thermal injury to the upper airway results in blistering, edema, accumulation of thick saliva, and glottic closure in severe cases. These changes usually develop in the first 2 to 8 hours and can lead to partial or total airway obstruction. The presence of a large skin burn can intensify edema formation in the airways as a result of vascular leakage and resuscitation with large amounts of fluids.[11,13] Ventilatory failure can occur as a result of upper airway obstruction but may be delayed for some hours as the edema formation proceeds.

Chemical injury to the respiratory tract, brought about by inhalation of the toxic gases and irritant-laden soot particles, extends the injuries further into the lung causing acute tracheobronchitis, bronchospasm, bronchorrhea, and pulmonary edema[11,14,16,18,24] in severe cases. These changes are accompanied by an increase in bronchial blood flow, which can intensify the airway and alveolar edema.[2,13] Chemical exposure decreases mucosal ciliary transport, which may lead to mucus retention and infection.[4] In addition, the following abnormalities have been documented: surfactant dysfunction, increased lung water, decreased lung compliance, increased airway resistance, and increased pulmonary vascular resistance.[2-4,6,25,26] These changes will result in ventilation-perfusion ($\dot{V}/\dot{Q}$) mismatching and in increased physiologic dead space (V_D/V_T), which decreases Pao_2, increases the $P(A-a)o_2$, and increases the necessary minute ventilation to normalize the $Paco_2$ (Table 9–2).

Table 9–2 Changes in Blood Gases, Oxygen Consumption, and Acid-base Balance After Severe Burns*

	Period		
	Early	**Intermediate**	**Late**
Pao_2	−20%	+7%	−60%
Sao_2	−5%	−3%	−40%
Hematocrit	+3%	−30%	−30%
Oxygen transport	−15%	+25%	−60%
Oxygen consumption	+35%	+70%	−40%
$Paco_2$	−40%	−30%	+18%
pH	Normal	7.39–7.30	7.35–7.25

*From six patients (35–60% third-degree burns). The early period was the first 25% of their course, the late period was the last 25% of their course, and the intermediate period was the time between early and late periods. Values are expressed as percent change from data taken from 17 healthy control subjects.

Source: Adapted from Shoemaker, WC, et al: Burn pathophysiology in man. I. Sequential hemodynamic alterations. J Surg Res 14:64, 1973.

Table 9–3 Changes in Systemic Hemodynamics and Blood Volume After Severe Burns*

	Period		
	Early	**Intermediate**	**Late**
Heart rate	+50%	+75%	+25%
Blood pressure (mean)	Normal	+10%	−30%
Cardiac index	−15%	+65%	−15%
Left ventricular stroke work	−50%	Normal	−55%
Vascular resistance	+30%	−30%	−20%
Blood volume	−20%	+15%	−30%

*From six patients (35–60% third-degree burns). The early period was the first 25% of their course, the late period was the last 25% of their course, and the intermediate period was the time between early and late periods. Values are expressed as percent change from data taken from 17 healthy control subjects.

Source: Adapted from Shoemaker, WC, et al: Burn pathophysiology in man. I. Sequential hemodynamic alterations. J Surg Res 14:64, 1973.

Early systemic changes are associated with the degree of the decrease in oxygen transport and the area and depth of the skin burn. Hypovolemic shock is one of the primary systemic insults in the early period following a major full-thickness skin burn.[13,27] The early hypovolemia is secondary to massive fluid shifts out of the vascular compartment as a result of a leaky microvasculature. Although the exact mechanisms of the microvascular injury are not known, it is felt to be the result of various vasoactive mediators (e.g., histamine, prostaglandins, and oxygen radicals) being released from the burn site.[13] These mediators affect all organs of the body and result in edema in tissues some distance from the burn site.[13] This massive fluid shift results in a generalized edema that peaks within 8 to 24 hours and is dependent on the magnitude of the burn and the adequacy of the fluid resuscitation. Burned skin also loses its elasticity and becomes less compliant with the edema formation. In circumferential burns of the extremities and trunk, the tightening skin can further impair circulation and cause increased edema, distal tissue necrosis, and reduced chest wall compliance.[3,12,13] This reduction in chest wall compliance results in increased work of breathing that can lead to ventilatory compromise.

Cardiovascular and hematologic instability occurs from a loss of fluid volume that can exceed 4 mL/kg of body weight per hour in major burns[13,28] (Table 9–3). Cardiac output is decreased as a result of hypovolemia, myocardial hypoxia, the presence of myocardial depressant factors, and increased systemic vascular resistance.[27–29] Blood pressure may be normal or low, and heart rate is usually increased.[27] Immune suppression and alterations in leukocyte and macrophage function have been noted.[13] Hemolysis and the development of disseminated intravascular coagulation (DIC) may further compromise the microcirculation.[12]

The metabolic rate is often initially depressed as a result of the severe hypoxia and abnormal circulation. Stress stimulates a massive release of catecholamines and increases metabolism. The elevated metabolic rate, vasoconstriction, anxiety, pain, and muscle shivering result in an imbalance between oxygen demand and delivery. Anaerobic metabolism and metabolic acidosis may result.

Intermediate Pulmonary and Systemic Changes: 2 to 5 Days Postburn

Victims often demonstrate more obvious signs of respiratory distress during this period. Severely burned victims (more than 30 percent of total body surface area) without inhalation injury may have stable lung function unless fluid resuscitation has induced pulmonary edema. Increased capillary permeability may also induce pulmonary edema (e.g., ARDS) during this period, especially if shock has occurred. Pulmonary vascular resistance often returns to normal levels during this period, but a hypermetabolic state may develop and increase CO_2 production and O_2 consumption and increase the risk of respiratory failure (Table 9–2).

Patients with thermal injury usually begin to improve between days 2 and 4. Chemical injuries often persist, however, and result in increased mucus production and decreased mucus clearance. Injuries of the smaller airways usually peak on day 2 or 3. With more severe mucosal injuries, the mucosal tissue often becomes necrotic and sloughs, usually on day 3 or 4. The necrotic debris and mucus retention result in airway plugging and atelectasis. Atelectasis is further promoted by the victim's inability to take deep breaths and cough as a result of lowered chest and lung compliance, increased airway resistance, pain, use of narcotics, immobility, and inadequate airway care. The impaired secretion clearance, atelectasis, and burn-induced immune suppression set the stage for bacterial colonization, infectious bronchitis, and pneumonia.

Thirty percent of patients who develop major pulmonary complications may develop ARDS within a week after the injury.[10,30,31] The cause of ARDS in these patients is not known but is thought to include reduced surfactant production and microvascular hyperpermeability induced by mediator release from activated leukocytes that migrate to the lung and release free radicals[10,12,13,30–32] (see Chapter 11).

Hemodynamic changes are characterized by increased cardiac output during this period along with a persistent tachycardia secondary to the elevated catecholamines released from the sympathetic nervous system (Table 9–3). Systemic vascular resistance begins to drop and cardiac failure develops if the heart cannot support these added requirements. Cardiac failure causes 10 percent of the deaths during this period.[10] Erythrocyte damage secondary to cutaneous thermal injury is usually seen during this intermediate period as a decline in the hematocrit that levels off by day 4 or 5 (Table 9–2).

The metabolic rate during the intermediate phase is characterized by a catabolic hypermetabolism.[13] A negative nitrogen balance is often seen and signifies the catabolism of blood and muscle proteins. Stress-induced diabetes can result in hyperglycemia that frequently resolves during this period.[13] The use of Sulfamylon, a potent topical antibiotic, may complicate the patient's cardiorespiratory and metabolic status through its carbonic anhydrase inhibition, which causes metabolic acidosis.[33] If respiratory compensation for the metabolic acidosis is not possible because of pulmonary complications, an alternative topical antibiotic such as Silvedene is acceptable.

Late Pulmonary and Systemic Changes: Beyond 5 Days Postburn

The burn wound is a frequent site of infection and is the primary cause of death as a result of sepsis-induced multiorgan failure during the late period.[10] Sepsis compounds the pulmonary injuries and increases the metabolic rate. This may lead to a hyperdynamic circulatory status. The vascular hyperpermeability may persist for several weeks.

The hypermetabolic state seen during the intermediate phase often persists for 1 to 3 weeks. Resting CO_2 production frequently exceeds 400 mL/minute, as the metabolic rate may be twice the normal resting rate.[13] This added load on the respiratory system increases the work of breathing and, compounded by a possible muscle catabolism (breakdown of the muscle tissue), can result in respiratory muscle fatigue and ventilatory failure.

Pneumonia continues to be a major complication in the late stage of burn patients, both with and without inhalation injury. The control of burn wound sepsis through topical antibiotics and skin grafting has decreased the overall mortality rate. However, the incidence of pneumonia is approximately 35 percent and can be a cause of death.[2,10,12,13]

Pulmonary embolism usually develops within 2 weeks of the burn in 5 to 30 percent of burned patients.[34] Tachypnea, increasing minute ventilation, dyspnea, and a marked increase in $P(A-a)O_2$ suggest embolization. A $\dot{V}/\dot{Q}$ scan or pulmonary angiography may be needed to confirm the diagnosis of pulmonary embolism. Pulmonary emboli in this setting arise from deep venous thrombosis secondary to a hypercoaguable state and prolonged immobility[12,13,34] (see Chapter 7).

The long-term effects of severe inhalation injury can be the development of mixed restrictive and obstructive lung disease. This is thought to be due to the formation of alveolar fibrosis, squamous metaplasia of the respiratory mucosa, bronchial stenosis, bronchiectasis, and chronic lobar atelectasis.[35]

CLINICAL FEATURES

The increased morbidity and mortality associated with inhalation injury in the burn victim necessitate early recognition and treatment. There are a few important details that can help in the initial care of the smoke inhalation victim. The history of exposure to a smoke-filled enclosed environment, despite the absence of clinical findings, should suggest a high index of suspicion for potential injury.

Unconsciousness indicates a high risk for exposure to asphyxiating conditions and/or CO and HCN poisoning. Tables 9–4 and 9–5 list the major signs and symptoms associated with various levels of CO and HCN poisoning. The classic description of cherry-red skin during CO poisoning is an unreliable sign. CO oximetry is important to diagnose CO poisoning; however, low levels of Hbco do not rule out significant pulmonary injury in the intermediate or later postburn periods. Electrocardiograms (ECGs) often show tachycardia and may show signs of ischemic heart disease.

Pulse oximetry is rapidly becoming the *fifth* vital sign in monitoring acutely ill patients. However, SpO_2 does not accurately reflect HbO_2 concentration in patients poisoned by CO because oxyhemoglobin and Hbco have similar light absorption spectra. Thus, the reported SpO_2 reading will be falsely elevated in patients with CO.[36] Pulse oximetry will be useful only in burn victims with a Hbco that is near normal.

Facial burns, singed nasal hair, oral and laryngeal edema, and carbonaceous deposits in the airway and sputum suggest inhalation injury, but their absence does not rule it out.[6,9,10] Carbonaceous sputum, although considered a very sensitive sign

Table 9–4 Clinical Manifestations of CO Poisoning

Blood Hbco Concentration (%)	Signs and Symptoms
0–10	None, angina in those with coronary artery disease
10–20	Mild headache, exercise-induced angina, and dyspnea
20–40	Headache, dyspnea, vomiting, muscular weakness, dizziness, visual disturbance, impaired judgment
40–60	Syncope, increasing tachypnea and tachycardia, coma, convulsions, irregular breathing pattern
>60	Coma, shock, apnea, death

Table 9–5 Clinical Manifestations of Cyanide Poisoning

Blood Cyanide Concentrations (mg/L)	Signs and Symptoms
0.2–0.3	Tachycardia
	Tachypnea
	Dizziness
	Stupor
0.3–1.0	Progressive stupor
	Cardiac arrhythmias
	Apnea
	Seizures
>1.0	Death

for smoke inhalation, may not be seen for 8 to 24 hours and may only occur in about 40 percent of victims with pulmonary injury.[37] Stridor, hoarseness, difficulty speaking, and chest retractions suggest upper airway injury and the need for careful evaluation. Fiberoptic laryngoscopy and bronchoscopy have been found to be very useful in both evaluating the presence of upper airway injury and moving excessive saliva and debris.[4,38,39] Appearance of cough, dyspnea, tachypnea, cyanosis, wheezing, crackles, or rhonchi indicate more severe inhalation injury.

Chest radiographs frequently do not show the signs of inhalation injury. Scintiphotography for xenon-133, following the isotope's venous injection, will indicate small airway injury if it fails to clear from the lung after 90 seconds.[38] Unfortunately, the xenon-133 scan is often impractical in the initial treatment period.

Spirometry has been found to be useful in detecting small and upper airway injury. Peak expiratory flow and forced expiratory flow rates at 50 percent of the forced vital capacity are both markedly decreased.[39] The utility of spirometry, however, is limited to victims who can follow commands and make a good forced vital capacity effort.

ABG analysis is useful in evaluating the severity and progress of the patient's pulmonary insult. Reduced Pao_2 and an increased $P(A\text{-}a)o_2$ (greater than 300) or reduced Pao_2/Fio_2 (less than 350) are practical and sensitive signs of respiratory impairment.[3,40,41] Respiratory alkalosis is common in the early postburn period and often continues with the hypermetabolic phase. Respiratory acidosis is evidence of ventilatory failure and usually is associated with severe hypoxemia. Asphyxiation, elevated $Hbco$ (more than 40 percent), HCN poisoning, and poor cardiac output are all potential causes of severe metabolic acidosis.

ECG and hemodynamic monitoring are essential in patients with third-degree burns greater than 10 percent of their body surface area with or without inhalation injury. In large burns, especially those complicated by inhalation injury, pulmonary artery pressure, cardiac output, and other hemodynamic variables may be monitored to optimize fluid resuscitation and avoid hypotension, renal failure, and fluid overload.

The combination of physical assessment, fiberoptic bronchoscopy, chest radiography, ABG analysis, ECG, and hemodynamic monitoring form the core of diagnostic studies. Repeated evaluation of victims with these techniques will indicate appropriate and early intervention.

Assessment of cutaneous injury is carried out by physical examination, determination of body weight (for trending fluid balance), and total body surface area burned. The *rule of nines* can be used to estimate the total size of the injured area by determining the amount of injury to the head, the anterior and posterior trunk, and to each extremity. Each of these anatomic areas represents approximately 9

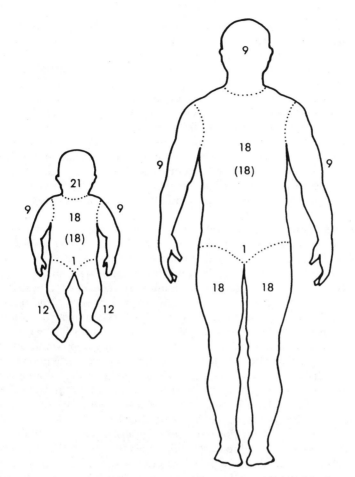

FIGURE 9–2 The percentage of surface area covered by skin in various body regions of the infant and adult.

percent to 18 percent of the body surface area (see Fig. 9–2). The burn depth is determined by its clinical appearance:

First degree: A burn to the epithelium that is manifested by erythema and pain
Second degree: A burn of the epithelium and dermis that is manifested by erythema, blisters, and pain
Third degree: A burn that destroys the skin through or into the hypodermis that is manifested by the pale or gray-brown leathery skin; pain not found in this area owing to the complete destruction of all sensory organs in the skin

TREATMENT

The goals of respiratory care for the burn patient are a patent airway, effective ventilation, adequate oxygenation, acid-base balance, cardiovascular stability, maintenance of lung volume, and suppression of infection.

Clinicians must closely monitor burn victims with minor upper airway injury for signs of airway closure or other signs of pulmonary involvement. The patient should be given supplementary oxygen via nasal cannula, and placed in high Fowler's position to reduce the work of breathing. Bronchospasm should be treated with aerosolized β-agonists (e.g., Alupent or albuterol).

Airway maintenance with an endotracheal tube of appropriate size is needed if upper airway obstruction is anticipated. Early tracheostomy is usually not recommended for burn patients because of its higher mortality and infection rates but may become necessary for long-term ventilatory support.[10,12,13] Early intubation has been found to precipitate transient pulmonary edema in some patients in the early stages following inhalation injury.[40] The addition of 5 to 10 cm H_2O of continuous positive airway pressure (CPAP) can help minimize the early pulmonary edema, maintain lung volume, support the edematous airways, optimize $\dot{V}/\dot{Q}$ matching, and decrease the early mortality rates.[10] The use of systemic corticosteroids to treat edema formation is not recommended because of increased risk of infections.[6,41-44]

Comatose victims must be treated for severe asphyxia and CO poisoning. Oxygen therapy is the cornerstone for the treatment of hypoxia and CO poisoning. Carboxyhemoglobin dissociation and elimination are accelerated when supplemental O_2 is employed (Table 9–6). Smoke inhalation victims with mildly elevated Hbco (less than 30 percent) and stable cardiopulmonary function are best treated with 100 percent O_2 therapy delivered by a tight-fitting nonrebreathing mask using 15 liters/minute of O_2 to maintain a full reservoir bag. Oxygen therapy should continue until the Hbco is reduced to levels below 10 percent. Mask CPAP with 100 percent O_2 may be adequate therapy for patients with increasing hypoxemia and who have minimal or no thermal injuries to the face and upper airway. Patients with refractory hypoxemia or inhalation injury associated with coma or cardiopulmonary instability need intubation and ventilatory support with 100 percent O_2 and rapid referral for hyperbaric O_2 therapy.[4] Hyperbaric oxygen therapy rapidly improves oxygen transport and increases the rate at which CO is removed from the blood (Table 9–6).

Ventilatory support with positive end-expiratory pressure (PEEP) will often be needed in those that develop early pulmonary edema, ARDS, and pneumonia. Ventilatory support is needed when the patient's ABGs indicate respiratory failure (Pao_2 less than 60 mm Hg, and/or $Paco_2$ greater than 50 mm Hg that results in a pH less than 7.25). The use of PEEP is indicated when the patient's Pao_2 falls below 60 and the patient's Fio_2 requirement climbs above 0.60. Ventilatory support is often prolonged because burn victims often have a high metabolic rate that requires an increased minute volume to maintain homeostasis. The ventilator should be capable of delivering a high minute ventilation (to 50 liters/minute), high peak airway pressures (to 100 cm H_2O), and stable inspiratory-expiratory (I:E) ratios with increasing pressure requirements. Refractory hypoxemia may respond to pressure-controlled inverse-ratio ventilation.

Good pulmonary hygiene is required to clear retained sputum. Chest physical therapy is helpful to mobilize secretions and prevent airway plugging and atelectasis. Recent skin grafts do not tolerate chest percussion and vibration. Therapeutic fiberoptic bronchoscopy may be needed to clear plugged airways.

Table 9–6 Half-life of Carboxyhemoglobin at Different Oxygen Exposures

Hbco Half-life	Inhaled O_2 Partial Pressure
280–320 min	Air (21% at 1 atm)
80–90 min	100% at 1 atm
20–30 min	100% at 3 atm

Careful maintenance of fluid balance is necessary to minimize the risk of shock, renal failure, and pulmonary edema. Resuscitation of the patient's fluid balance with the Parkland formula (4 mL isotonic crystalloids/kg per percentage burn per 24 hours) with a standard urine output target (30 to 50 mL/hour) and central venous pressure target (2 to 6 mm Hg) will usually result in hemodynamic stability.[44] In patients with inhalation injury, capillary permeability is higher and monitoring pulmonary artery pressures in addition to urine output is useful to guide fluid replacement therapy. Frequent analysis of the electrolyte panel and acid-base status is required.

The burned patient's hypermetabolic state requires careful nutritional analysis to avoid catabolic wasting of muscle tissue. Predictive formulas (e.g., Harris-Benedict and Curreri) have been used to estimate the metabolic rate of the burn patient. Commercially developed portable analyzers for serial measurements of indirect calorimetry have been found to produce more accurate estimates of the nutritional requirement.[45,46] Patients with large burns (greater than 50 percent of surface area) are often given diets with caloric contents that are 150 percent of their resting energy expenditure to facilitate wound healing and avoid catabolism. As the wounds heal, the nutritional support is tapered back to 130 percent of patient's resting energy expenditure.

Scar tissue may restrict chest wall movement if circumferential burns of the thorax have occurred. Escharotomy (cutting the burned skin) is done by making lateral incisions in the anterior axillary line extending from 2 cm below the clavicle to the 9th or 10th rib and transverse incisions across the chest at the top and bottom to form a square. Escharotomy of the chest should improve the elasticity of the chest wall and relieve the compressive effect of retracting scar tissue.

Treatment of the burn includes surgical debridement of the dead skin, application of topical antibiotic dressings (Silvedene and Sulfamylon), wound closure with temporary skin substitutes, and grafting of skin from unburned sites and cloned samples to the burn site. These methods reduce fluid loss and risk of infection.

Infections are most often coagulase-positive *Staphylococcus aureus* and gram-negative organisms such as *Klebsiella, Enterobacter, Escherichia coli,* and *Pseudomonas.* Isolation technique, room pressurization, air filtration, and wound covering form the front lines of infection defense. Antibiotic selection is based on serial wound, blood, urine, and sputum cultures. Prophylactic antibiotics should not be used in these patients because resistant bacterial strains quickly develop and produce resistant infections.[3,6,12,13] Prophylactic heparin therapy may be helpful to reduce the risk of pulmonary embolism in patients who remain immobile for a long time.

Case Study

HISTORY

Mr. A, a 33-year-old man, was in good health before his accident. While he was working above a vat of molten nickel in a foundry, a large tool was accidently dropped into the vat and broke through the semisolid surface crust and opened it. Upon contact with the air a tremendous amount of heat was released from the molten nickel, causing spontaneous combustion of Mr. A's clothes. He jumped down off the scaffolding and ran some distance, completely engulfed in flames, before the fire was put out by his fellow workers. His clothes were completely burned off and the only sites that were unburned appeared to be his head and feet, which were protected by his helmet and work boots. He was initially taken to a nearby community hospital.

Questions

1. What signs and symptoms will need to be evaluated immediately on his arrival?
2. What information can be acquired to help determine the severity of his injuries?
3. What therapeutic techniques should be available for use at the time of his arrival?

Answers

1. The patient should be evaluated for signs of a patent airway, spontaneous breathing, quality of breath sounds and their symmetry, pulse rate, blood pressure, and level of consciousness (Glasgow coma scale). Symptoms of respiratory distress, shock, and mental impairment are important to identify. Inspection of the nose and mouth should be performed to identify evidence of soot or upper airway burn.
2. The severity of the patient's injuries can be evaluated by determining if he was burned in an enclosed space, if there is evidence of inhalation injury, how long he was exposed to flame and smoke, the percentage of his body surface area that was burned and the degree or thickness of the burn, the length of time since his injury, his age, and any underlying medical conditions that may complicate his injuries.
3. Oxygen therapy (cannula or nonrebreathing mask); intubation equipment; manual resuscitation bag with proper mask, oxygen reservoir, and a PEEP capability; venous and arterial line placement equipment; crystalloid fluids for vascular support; appropriate resuscitation drugs; and medications for pain and agitation should be kept available for use on the patient.

PHYSICAL EXAMINATION

General *Mr. A is an average-sized man of approximately 80 kg who is burned over approximately 80 percent of his body. He is lying on an emergency room bed, restless, moaning, poorly responsive to questions, has a hoarse voice, and is in apparent respiratory distress. He is breathing with the aid of supplementary oxygen from a nonrebreathing mask. His Glasgow coma score is 13.*

Vital Signs *Temperature 38.6° C; respiratory rate 39/minute; blood pressure 121/76 mm Hg; pulse 147/minute*

HEENT *Most of head unburned; pupils equal and reactive to light; nasal flaring, nasal hairs singed; some sign of first- and second-degree burns on face and erythema in the oral cavity*

Neck *Third-degree burns starting at base of neck; trachea midline; mild inspiratory stridor; carotid pulses +++ bilaterally without bruit; no signs of lymphadenopathy, thyroidomegaly, or jugular vein distension; obvious tensing of sternocleidomastoid and scalene muscles during inspiration*

Chest *Circumferential third-degree burn; breath sounds revealing some scattered expiratory wheezes, otherwise clear bilaterally; some thoracoabdominal paradoxic motion noted*

Heart	*Regular rhythm at 145 to 150/minute; normal S_1 and S_2 sounds without murmurs, gallops, or rubs*
Abdomen	*Circumferential third-degree burn with exception of band around waist, possibly because of protection from belt; bowel sounds not heard clearly, no masses or organomegaly noted*
Extremities	*Able to move all extremities; circumferential third-degree burns on all extremities except feet, right elbow, and axillary areas; no clubbing, no obvious cyanosis; some generalized swelling*

Questions

4. What signs and symptoms indicate inhalation injury?
5. How are the circumferential burns of his thorax likely to influence respiratory function?
6. What are the possible causes of his accessory muscle usage and respiratory distress?
7. What diagnostic techniques should be used to evaluate his respiratory distress?
8. What laboratory test and other determinations are now needed to make a more complete evaluation?
9. What techniques are needed for monitoring cardiovascular status?

Answers

4. Inhalation injury is indicated by the presence of tachypnea, stridor, voice changes, use of accessory muscles of breathing, erythema about the face and in the mouth, nasal flaring, singed nasal hair, wheezing, and thoracoabdominal wall paradoxic motion.
5. Circumferential burns of the thorax are likely to result in decreased thoracic compliance, which would increase the work of breathing.
6. His respiratory distress is probably due to inhalation of hot gas and smoke. Upper airway edema, bronchospasm, and chemically induced acute tracheobronchitis are most common effects of smoke and hot air inhalation. Widespread burns may have caused generalized capillary permeability and resulted in pulmonary edema.
7. Bedside spirometry may be useful to evaluate further his respiratory distress if he can follow commands. Fiberoptic laryngoscopy and bronchoscopy would provide evaluation of the upper airway. A chest radiograph is indicated but may only serve as a baseline. A xenon-133 lung scan would be helpful in making the diagnosis of lung injury but may not be practical at this time.
8. Laboratory assessment of complete blood count (CBC), electrolytes, ABG, Hbco, standard blood chemistry, and screening for alcohol and illegal drugs are indicated. A more precise estimation of the burn size can be determined with careful physical examination and the use of a Lund-Browder burn chart to help guide therapy.
9. Monitoring ECG and placement of peripheral venous, central venous, and arterial lines will be needed to guide the maintenance of hemodynamic stability.

BEDSIDE AND LABORATORY EVALUATION

BURN SIZE

85% of total body surface area

ECG

Sinus tachycardia of 148/minute without any other abnormalities

ARTERIAL AND CENTRAL VENOUS LINE BLOOD PRESSURES

Blood pressure 130/81 mm Hg; central venous pressure (CVP) 3 mm Hg

BRONCHOSCOPY

Patchy erythema and some soot deposits on the mucosa of the nasal pharynx; epiglottic and laryngeal erythema and edema with some soot-streaked mucous membranes, scope not advanced beyond the vocal cords

CHEST RADIOGRAPH

(Fig. 9–3)

ABGs

pH 7.33, $Paco_2$ 32 mm Hg, Pao_2 94 mm Hg, Sao_2 91 percent, $Hbco$ 8 percent, Hco_3 18 mEq/liter while breathing 100 percent O_2 from a nonrebreathing mask

HEMATOLOGY

Hematocrit (Hct) 45 percent, red blood cells (RBC) $4.7 \times 10^6/mm^3$, white blood cells (WBC) 9.2×10^3, platelets 270×10^3

CHEMISTRY AND TOXICOLOGY

Results pending

Questions

10. How would you evaluate the ECG and hemodynamic findings?
11. What do the bronchoscopy results indicate?
12. How would you interpret the ABG data?
13. How do you interpret the chest radiograph?
14. What respiratory care is indicated at this time, and how should it be evaluated?
15. What hemodynamic support is indicated at this time, and how should it be evaluated?
16. What complications may occur in the next 24 to 48 hours?

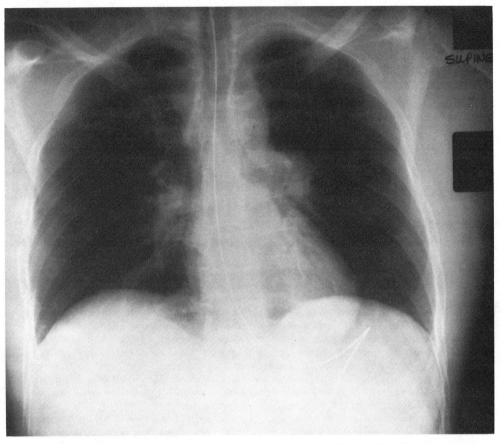

FIGURE 9–3 Chest radiograph taken approximately 5 hours after the burn and shortly after admission to the burn unit.

Answers

10. The ECG and hemodynamic measurements are consistent with the extent of injuries. A pulmonary artery catheter will be helpful to guide fluid replacement and use of vasoactive agents.

11. The bronchoscopy demonstrates thermal injury to the upper airway and suggests smoke inhalation. Bronchoscopy was limited to the supraglottic area to avoid upper airway obstruction.

12. The ABG analysis shows compensated metabolic acidosis with hyperventilation, hypoxemia, and minor CO poisoning. A $P(\text{A-a})\text{O}_2$ of 585 mm Hg and a $P\text{a}\text{O}_2/F\text{IO}_2$ of 94 indicate $\dot{V}/\dot{Q}$ abnormality, and venous-to-arterial intrapulmonary shunting.

13. The chest radiograph is essentially normal.

14. The patient will need to be intubated. An 8.5-mm internal diameter cuffed endotracheal tube is a good choice, and bronchoscopy assistance will make an otherwise potentially difficult intubation much easier. Following intubation, visual inspection of chest motion and breath sounds will help ensure proper tube placement. The patient will most likely need mechanical ventilatory support because of the high shunt fraction. Initial ventilator settings should be assist-control mode, set tidal volume (V_T) at 900 mL, rate set at 18/minute, adequate inspiratory flow to main-

tain an I:E greater than 1:3, PEEP of 5, and an F_{IO_2} of 1.0. The primary goal of oxygen therapy is adequate tissue oxygenation rather than treatment of the minor CO poisoning. In-line aerosolized bronchodilator treatment would be helpful for treatment of the bronchospasm.

15. Fluid resuscitation with crystalloid intravenous (IV) infusion according to the burn formula (e.g., 4 mL/kg per percentage of burn over 24 hours) should be started. Evaluation of CVP, pulmonary wedge pressure, cardiac output, and renal output will help avoid hypotension or fluid overload.

16. Intensive care in a burn unit will be required for the continued fluid resuscitation, ventilatory support, wound management, and monitoring of cardiovascular, pulmonary, and renal function. The patient is at risk for respiratory failure from ARDS, circulatory failure, renal failure, pulmonary edema, acid-base and electrolyte imbalance, DIC, and sepsis.

Mr. A was orally intubated in the emergency department and given mechanical ventilation with 100 percent O_2; IV and arterial lines were started, and fluid resuscitation was begun. A nasal gastric tube was placed and a urinary catheter inserted and attached to a closed collection system. He was stabilized at the community hospital and then transferred by air ambulance to a metropolitan burn center for intensive burn care. He was evaluated in the burn center 3 hours after the accident and found to have full-thickness burns over 88 percent of his body. His initial treatment concentrated on fluid resuscitation, escharotomies of the chest and extremities, and wound care with Silvedene cream and dressings. Ventilator support with 100 percent O_2 was continued with 5 cm H_2O of PEEP. Placement of a pulmonary artery catheter was done for fluid administration, monitoring of right atrial pressure, pulmonary artery wedge pressure, and cardiac output.

Over the next 2 days his fluid resuscitation continued and F_{IO_2} was successfully adjusted down to 0.70. During the second day his oxygenation began to deteriorate and he required higher F_{IO_2} and PEEP levels. At approximately 40 hours following the injury, his bedside findings, vital signs, chest radiograph, ventilator settings, and laboratory data were as follows.

BEDSIDE AND LABORATORY EVALUATION

Mr. A was lying in supine position with Silvedene cream and bandages covering all burned areas. He was developing generalized edema throughout the burned areas. He was responsive and followed commands. He was spontaneously initiating each breath from the Siemens Servo 900c ventilator through an 8.5-mm internal diameter oral endotracheal tube. The airway had 25 cm H_2O pressure in the cuff, and no gas leakage was heard over the cuff site. The airway was secured to the upper lip with waterproof tape and the 24-cm mark was seen at the lip. His breath sounds revealed scattered inspiratory crackles and expiratory wheezes and rhonchi with symmetrically diminished air movement. Suctioning of his airway removed small amounts of mucoid sputum flecked with soot. In-line ventilator circuit delivery of 2.5 mg of albuterol diluted in 3 mL of saline is being given every 4 hours. He was also receiving morphine sulfate and Versed for analgesia and sedation. His total fluid intake since the accident was 61.3 liters, with a total urine output of 4.2 liters. A large amount of fluid has leaked from the burn surfaces.

VITAL SIGNS, HEMODYNAMICS, AND URINE OUTPUT

Temperature 37.6° C; respiratory rate 30/minute; pulse 100/minute; systemic arterial blood pressure 110/53 mm Hg; CVP 9 mm Hg; pulmonary artery blood pressure 34/19 mm Hg; wedge pressure 18 mm Hg; cardiac output 7.7 liters/minute; urine output has averaged 55 to 65 mL/hour since admission

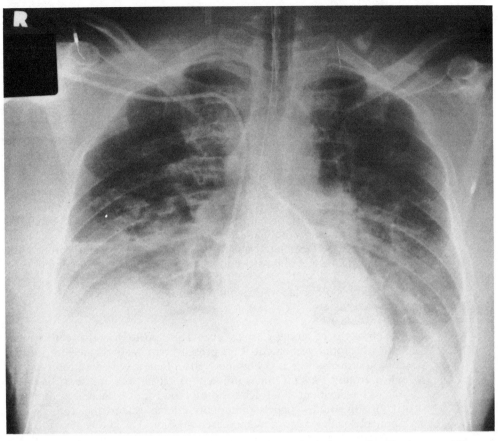

FIGURE 9–4 Chest radiograph taken approximately 40 hours after the burn and its treatment.

CHEST RADIOGRAPH

(Fig. 9–4)

VENTILATOR SETTINGS AND FINDINGS

Assist-control mode; V_T set at 1.0 liter; rate set at 12/minute; total rate 30/minute; FIO_2 0.85; inspiratory flow 80 liter/minute; $\dot{V}_E$ 30.4 liters/minute; peak pressure 55 cm H_2O; plateau pressure 38 cm H_2O; PEEP set at 10 cm H_2O; auto PEEP 15 cm H_2O; static compliance 40 mL/cm H_2O; airway resistance 13 cm H_2O/liter per second

LABORATORY FINDINGS

ABGs

pH 7.43, $Paco_2$ 34 mm Hg, Pao_2 65 mm Hg, HCO_3 22 mEq/liter, $P(A-a)o_2$ 498 mm Hg, Pao_2/FIO_2 76, Sao_2 92 percent (co-oximeter), Spo_2 91 percent (pulse oximeter)

Hematology

Hct 43 percent, RBC 4.7×10^6/mm³, WBC 11.1×10^3, platelets 253×10^3

Electrolytes and Chemistry
Na+ 139 mEq/L, K+ 3.5 mEq/L, Cl− 101 mEq/L, glucose 153 mg/dL, blood urea nitrogen (BUN) 20 mg/dL, creatinine 1.0 mg/dL
Microbiology
Blood, sputum, and wound smear and cultures pending

Questions

17. What do his airway care and breath sounds indicate? What treatment would you recommend at this time?
18. How would you interpret his hemodynamic parameters? What potential effects would you expect these hemodynamics to have on lung function?
19. How would you interpret the radiographic changes since the initial film taken shortly after admission to the burn center?
20. How would you evaluate the ventilator settings, breathing pattern, pulmonary mechanics, and ABG findings? What should be recommended at this time?
21. What do his other laboratory findings indicate?

Answers

17. His airway is of an appropriate size. Tube position and breath sounds indicate proper placement. Cuff pressure is effectively sealing the trachea at a pressure that is high enough to help avoid silent aspiration of saliva around the cuff but is unlikely to cause pressure necrosis of the mucosa. Placement of a tracheostomy tube is not indicated at this time. His breath sounds suggest pulmonary edema, retained secretions, continuing bronchospasm, and decreased aeration. The in-line aerosolization of albuterol is appropriate; however, its dosage should be doubled. Use of an in-line metered-dose inhaler with 10 to 20 "puffs" may be more effective. The sputum removed from the airway indicates inhalation injury. Special attention to the airway, its maintenance, and sterile technique will be necessary to help avoid infectious complications.
18. The hemodynamics are consistent with a moderate hyperdynamic state that is often seen following fluid resuscitation of a large burn complicated by inhalation injury. The filling pressures (central venous and pulmonary artery wedge pressures) indicate that the patient is adequately hydrated and may no longer need a rapid infusion rate. His moderately high cardiac output is typical of the response of a burn victim who is responding to stress. The possible pulmonary consequences of high pulmonary artery and wedge pressures is pulmonary edema and hypoxemia. However, if fluids are tapered too much, renal function and other organ function could be jeopardized as a result of hypovolemic shock.
19. The portable anteroposterior (AP) chest radiograph taken approximately 40 hours after injury (Fig. 9–4) shows the endotracheal tube in the same position, a nasogastric tube that extends into the stomach, and a pulmonary artery catheter that ends in the right pulmonary outflow tract. Pleural effusion, pulmonary edema, atelectasis, and air bronchograms are seen in the right middle and lower lobes. Some atelectasis is noted in the right upper lobe. Atelectasis and pulmonary edema are also seen in the left lung base. Overall lung volume has diminished. No signs of pneumothorax are present.

20. The ventilator settings indicate that he is requiring a high level of support. The tidal volume setting (10 mL/kg) is appropriate. He is receiving an increased FIO_2 and is triggering all breaths beyond the set rate of 12/minute with a high minute ventilation. He is generating occult or auto PEEP as a result of gas trapping. His respiratory pattern combined with the increased airway resistance is producing the air trapping. Tracking the auto PEEP is important to evaluate its effects on lung distension, lung mechanics, and hemodynamics. The auto PEEP can be reduced by lowering the respiratory rate, increasing the inspiratory flow, continuing the bronchodilator treatments and airway care, and sedating the patient. The compliance and resistance measurements are consistent with the chest radiographic and bedside findings of pulmonary edema, atelectasis, and increased airway resistance. His oxygenation is adequate but the FIO_2 is potentially toxic and needs reevaluation and adjustment to prevent oxygen toxicity. The very high minute ventilation and moderate respiratory alkalosis indicate increased dead space ventilation, increased metabolic rate, or combinations of the two. At this point it would be appropriate to control the patient's respiratory pattern through sedation and paralysis, perform an optimal PEEP study, reduce the respiratory rate, decrease fluid administration, and continue monitoring.

21. The hematologic data are acceptable. The mildly elevated WBC and increased band cell counts are consistent with this type of trauma but could also indicate early sepsis. The electrolytes, hemodynamics, and renal function are remarkably normal considering the amount of fluid that the patient has received. A slight hyperglycemia is noted, which may be a result of glucocorticoid and catecholamine release secondary to the trauma or of the IV fluids being given, or both.

Following assessment of Mr. A's cardiopulmonary status, he was paralyzed with IV Pavulon and his fluid administration was tapered down. An optimal PEEP study was then done.

$S\bar{v}O_2$ %	SpO_2 %	Blood Pressure mm Hg	Cs mL/cm H_2O	PEEP (cm H_2O)
66	90	108/53	42	5
64	90	111/54	41	8
62	89	109/53	41	10
64	90	109/52	42	12
65	91	106/54	44	14
61	88	99/48	37	16

Question

22. What is Mr. A's optimal PEEP level, and why is this the optimal level?

Answer

22. Mr. A's optimal PEEP level is 14 cm H_2O. At this level of PEEP the static lung compliance, mixed venous O_2 saturation, and pulse oximetry are best.

The PEEP of 14 cm H_2O was selected and an ABG measurement taken, with the ventilator on the same settings as noted earlier: pH 7.40, $Paco_2$ 38 mm Hg, Pao_2 92 mm Hg, HCO_3 24 mEq/liter while being ventilated with an FIO_2 of 0.85. Improved oxygenation is noted by the increase in the Pao_2, which continued through the next day. The patient's chest radiograph began to improve with signs of reduced atelectasis and reduction in pulmonary infiltrates. The Pavulon was discontinued and he was switched to synchronized intermittent mandatory ventilation plus pressure support (SIMV + PS), which was tolerated well despite a persistent tachypnea of 20 to 25 breaths/minute.

Mr. A's pulmonary status continued to improve over the next 5 days and he tolerated reductions in FIO_2, PEEP, and SIMV rate. His minute ventilation remained elevated in the range of 18 to 25 liters/minute. During this period, the first of many surgical excisions of burned tissue and grafting occurred. Following these procedures, his ventilation requirements would increase and necessitate increasing his SIMV and FIO_2 settings. Breath sounds were found to be coarse expiratory rhonchi in both lung fields and large amounts of tan sputum suctioned from his airway. His cultures revealed **Escherichia coli** *in areas of the wound,* **Streptococcus pneumoniae** *and yeast in his sputum, and negative blood cultures. He was started on appropriate antibiotics with repeat cultures planned.*

Nine days following his burn, weaning studies were found to be acceptable with a Pao_2/FIO_2 of 332 while breathing an FIO_2 of 0.40. He was placed on PS ventilation of 10 cm H_2O, PEEP of 5 cm H_2O, and 40 percent O_2. He tolerated this for 2 days and then became increasingly tachypneic to rates of 40/minute with large amounts of foul-smelling tan sputum suctioned from his airway. He was returned to SIMV + PS, and the decision was made to perform a tracheotomy for better airway clearance. Sputum cultures from this period showed **Staphylococcus aureus,** *and his antibiotic coverage was adjusted. His clinical picture and chest radiograph did not indicate the presence of pneumonia.*

Thirteen days postburn, his minute ventilation increased to 38 liters/minute while being supported in the SIMV + PS. His CO_2 production rate was found to be 505 mL/minute with a resting energy expenditure of 3813 kcal. This excessive minute ventilation was being driven by a very high metabolic rate and he was paralyzed to reduce both his metabolic rate and his required ventilatory support. He remained paralyzed for the next 10 days, continued to have weekly metabolic rate determinations, and had additional burn excisions and grafting. During this period his chest radiograph remained relatively clear despite suctioning tan sputum from his airway and sputum cultures, occasionally showing gram-positive cocci.

On the 24th day postburn the Pavulon was discontinued and he was gradually weaned to T tube with an FIO_2 of 0.40 during the next 10 days. His metabolic rate decreased 20 percent and his feedings were tapered. A fenestrated tracheostomy tube was placed to facilitate communication.

Sixty-five days following his admission to the burn unit, he continued to require the tracheostomy tube for secretion management. Effective wound size had been reduced to approximately 35 percent of his total body surface area. Extubation was planned when he was able to clear secretions effectively.

REFERENCES

1. Statistical Abstracts of the United States, National Data Book, ed 110. US Department of Commerce, 1990.

2. Herndon, DN, et al: Incidence, mortality, pathogenesis and treatment of pulmonary injury. J Burn Care Rehabil 7:184, 1986.

3. Trunkey, DD: Inhalation injury. Surg Clin North Am 56:1133, 1978.

4. Cohen, MA and Guzzardi, LJ: Inhalation of products of combustion. Ann Emerg Med 12:628, 1983.

5. Coleman, DL: Smoke inhalation. West J Med 135:300, 1981.

6. Moylan, JA and Alexander, LG: Diagnosis and treatment of inhalation injury. World J Surg 2:185, 1978.

7. Moylan, JA: Inhalation injury. J Trauma 21 (Suppl):720, 1981.

8. Nishimura, N and Hiranuma, N: Respiratory changes after major burn injury. Crit Care Med 10:25, 1982.

9. Cahalane, M and Demling, RF: Early respiratory abnormalities from smoke inhalation. JAMA 251:771, 1984.

10. Venus, B, et al: Prophylactic intubation and continuous positive airway pressure in the management of inhalation injury in burn victims. Crit Care Med 9:519, 1981.

11. Zawacki, B, Jung, R, and Joyce, J: Smoke, burns and the natural history of inhalation injury in fire victims. Ann Surg 185:100, 1977.

12. Burns and respiratory function. In Hedley-White, J, et al: Applied Physiology of Respiratory Care. Little, Brown, Boston, 1976.

13. Demling, RH: Management of the burn patient. In Shoemaker, WC, et al (eds): Textbook of Critical Care, ed 2. WB Saunders, Philadelphia, 1989.

14. Terrill, JB, Montgomery, RR, and Reinhardt, CF: Toxic gases from fires. Science 200:1343, 1978.

15. Crapo, RO: Smoke-inhalation injuries. JAMA 246:1694, 1981.

16. Dyer, RF and Esch, VH: Polyvinyl chloride toxicity in fires. JAMA 235:393, 1975.

17. Symington, IS, et al: Cyanide exposure in fires. Lancet 1:91, 1978.

18. Stone, JP, Hazlett, RN, and Johnson, JE: The transport of hydrogen chloride by soot from burning polyvinyl chloride. J Fire Flammability 4:42, 1973.

19. Okeda, R, et al: The pathogenesis of carbon monoxide encephalopathy in the acute phase—physiological and morphological condition. Acta Neuropathol 54:1, 1981.

20. Myers, RAM, Snyder, SK, and Emhoff, TA: Subacute sequela of carbon monoxide poisoning. Ann Emerg Med 14:1163, 1985.

21. Silverman, SH, et al: Cyanide toxicity in burned patients. J Trauma 28:171, 1988.

22. Halebein, P, et al: Whole body oxygen utilization during acute carbon monoxide poisoning and isocapneic nitrogen hypoxia. J Trauma 26:110, 1986.

23. Pruitt, BA, et al: Pulmonary complications in burn patients. J Thorac Cardiovasc Surg 59:7, 1970.

24. Chu, C: New concepts of pulmonary burn injury. J Trauma 21:958, 1981.

25. Robinson, NB, et al: Ventilation and perfusion alterations after smoke inhalation injury. Surgery 90:352, 1980.

26. Loke, J, et al: Acute and chronic effects of fire fighting on pulmonary function. Chest 77:369, 1980.

27. Shoemaker, WC, et al: Burn pathophysiology in man. I. Sequential hemodynamic alterations. J Surg Res 14:64, 1973.

28. Mason, AD, Pruitt, BA, and Moncrief, JA: Hemodynamic changes in the early postburn period: The influence of fluid administration and a vasodilator. J Trauma 11:36, 1971.

29. Petroff, P and Pruitt, BA: Pulmonary disease in the burn patient. In Artz, C, Moncreif, W, and Pruitt, B (eds): Burns: A Team Approach. WB Saunders, Philadelphia, 1979.

30. McArdle, CS and Finlay, WEI: Pulmonary complications following smoke inhalation. Br J Anaesth 47:618, 1975.

31. Pruitt, BA, Erickson, DR, and Norris, A: Progressive pulmonary insufficiency and other pulmonary complications of thermal injury. J Trauma 15:369, 1975.

32. Clark, WR and Nieman, GF: Smoke inhalation. Burns 14:473, 1988.

33. Asch, MJ, White, MG, and Pruitt, BA: Acid base changes associated with topical sulfamylon therapy. Retrospective study of 100 burn patients. Ann Surg 172:946, 1970.

34. Coleman, JB and Chang, FC: Pulmonary embolism: An unrecognized event in severely burned patients. Am J Surg 130:697, 1975.

35. Chu, C: Early and late pathological changes in severe chemical burns to the respiratory tract complicated with acute respiratory failure. Burns 8:387, 1982.

36. Craig, KC: Clinical application of pulse oximetry. In Hicks, GH (ed): Problems in Respiratory Care—Applied Noninvasive Respiratory Monitoring. 2:255, JB Lippincott, Philadelphia, 1989.

37. DiVencenti, FC, Pruitt, BA, and Reckler, JM: Inhalation injuries. J Trauma 11:109, 1971.

38. Hunt, JL, Agee, RN, and Pruitt, BA: Fiberoptic bronchoscopy in acute inhalation injury. J Trauma 15:641, 1975.

39. Petroff, PA, et al: Pulmonary function studies after smoke inhalation. Am J Surg 132:346, 1976.

40. Mathru, M, Venus, B, Tadikonda, LK, and Matsuda, T: Noncardiac pulmonary edema precipitated by tracheal intubation in patients with inhalation injury. Crit Care Med 11:804, 1983.

41. Skornik, WA and Dressler, DP: The effects of short-term steroid therapy on lung clearance and survival in rats. Ann Surg 719:415, 1974.

42. Welch, GW, Lull, RJ, and Petroff, PA: The use of steroids in inhalation injury. Surg Gynecol Obstet 145:539, 1977.

43. Robinson, NB, et al: Steroid therapy following isolated smoke inhalation injury. J Trauma 22:876, 1982.

44. Scheulenm, JJ and Munster, AM: The Parkland formula in patients with burns and inhalation injury. J Trauma 22:869, 1982.

45. Turner, WW, et al: Predicting energy expenditures in burned patients. J Trauma 25:11, 1985.

46. Saffle, JR, et al: Use of indirect calorimetry in the nutritional management of burned patients. J Trauma 25:32, 1985.

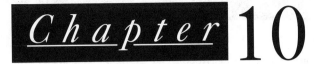

Chapter 10

David M. Stanton, MS, RRT, CPFT, RCP

NEAR DROWNING

INTRODUCTION

Drowning is defined as death by suffocation resulting from submersion.[1-6] Submersion under water, whether it be fresh, brackish, or salt water, is most frequent, but other fluids may also cause drowning. Approximately 10 to 15 percent of drowning victims do not aspirate fluid into their lungs. Death results from acute asphyxia, thought to be brought about by laryngospasm or prolonged breath holding. Laryngospasm may result from a small amount of fluid entering the region of the larynx as the victim gasps for air, while fully or partially submerged.

The majority (85 to 90 percent) of drowning victims aspirate fluid into their lungs. The volume aspirated is usually small (less than 22 mL/kg) and often includes vomit and other debris present in the fluid. Victims may swallow large amounts of liquid in their struggle to remain afloat, and vomiting with aspiration frequently occurs.

Near drowning is a term applied to those who are successfully resuscitated and survive at least 24 hours.[1-3,5] If death occurs within the first 24 hours, drowning is listed as the primary cause. Should the victim survive the initial 24 hours but die later from complications, the primary cause of death will be attributed to the complications (brain death, renal failure, sepsis, adult respiratory distress syndrome [ARDS]) with the near-drowning incident listed as the secondary cause. Wet or dry near-drowning terminology is applied to near-drowning victims based on whether or not the patient aspirated.

Other pertinent nomenclature includes immersion syndrome,[3-6] the development of asystole or ventricular fibrillation resulting from sudden immersion in very cold water; postimmersion syndrome[3,5-6] (secondary drowning), the development of ARDS following a near-drowning incident; and hyperventilation-submersion syndrome[3,4] (shallow water blackout), which is unconsciousness brought about by brain hypoxia that occurs after hyperventilation prior to diving or swimming underwater. In hyperventilation-submersion syndrome unconsciousness may occur before blood carbon dioxide levels increase sufficiently to stimulate respiration.

Drownings are responsible for 150,000 deaths worldwide[3,7] each year, with between 6000 and 8000[1,3-5,7] occurring in the United States. An estimated 80,000 near-drowning incidents occur annually in the United States. A high incidence occurs in men between 10 and 19 years of age,[1,6] and in children under 5 years of age.[3,5] Drowning is the third most common cause of mortality in children[1,5,7] and the fourth most common cause of accidental death overall.[5,7] Alcohol is a related feature in 40 to 50 percent of the teenage drownings.[1,3,6] Poor judgment and lack of supervision are also major contributing factors in drownings.[2]

PATHOLOGY AND PATHOPHYSIOLOGY

Neurologic Insult

Hypoxia and ischemia are important concepts which require clarification. Hypoxia is insufficient oxygen supply to a particular tissue of the body. Ischemia results when blood flow to a tissue or organ system is diminished or when the blood oxygen content is markedly diminished. In near-drowning incidents the brain may become hypoxic before cardiac arrest occurs. Blood flow may continue under anaerobic conditions for a period even after the oxygen supply has been depleted. Most people lose consciousness after 2 minutes of anoxia and brain damage may occur after 4 to 6 minutes.

Submersion times as long as 40 minutes have been reported with full recovery.[8] These unique incidents are more common in cold water. An intact diving reflex[3,4] (breath holding, bradycardia, and peripheral vasoconstriction when the face is immersed in cold water) is a possible explanation. The brain-protective effects of a rapidly induced hypothermia by reducing metabolic demand, especially to the brain, is likely to contribute to recovery.

Energy in the form of adenosine triphosphate (ATP) is produced by metabolic pathways which include glycolysis, the tricarboxylic acid (TCA) cycle, and oxidative phosphorylation[9] under aerobic conditions (Fig. 10–1). Glycolysis occurs in the cell cytoplasm, whereas the TCA cycle and oxidative phosphorylation take place in the mitochondria of the cell. Under anaerobic conditions the TCA cycle and oxidative phosphorylation no longer function, leaving glycolysis as the major ATP producer.[9] Glycolysis, under anaerobic conditions, is rapid but tissue perfusion must continue in order to provide a new supply of glucose. The anaerobic metabolism of each glucose molecule produces a net of 2 ATP compared with 36 ATP produced when aerobic conditions exist. ATP provides energy for many active transport mechanisms (sodium-potassium pumps, calcium pumps, and so on) found in cellular membranes that maintain homeostasis.[10]

Brain cells are strictly aerobic and during hypoxic conditions, injury can rapidly occur as oxygen and energy supplies diminish. Active transport mechanisms begin to slow down or quit working altogether owing to the diminished supply of energy. Cellular integrity becomes jeopardized as potassium is lost from within the cell and sodium and calcium flood into it.

Mitochondria and the endoplasmic reticulum (ER) are cellular organelles that assist in intracellular calcium regulation by absorbing it when it is in excess.[10] During hypoxic events, as the cellular integrity becomes compromised, calcium absorption may ultimately cause the uncoupling of oxidative phosphorylation, which greatly reduces energy production and further compromises cellular metabolism. Water follows sodium and calcium into the cell, causing swelling.[11,12]

The end point of the glycolytic pathway under aerobic conditions is pyruvate, but when anaerobic conditions exist lactate (lactic acid) is produced. Accumulation of lactate decreases pH and may alter enzyme function, leading to cell death if oxygenation and perfusion are not restored.

Pulmonary Insult

Aspiration occurs in 85 to 90 percent of near-drowning patients. Pulmonary injury is more frequent in this group than in those who do not aspirate. The volume, type of fluid aspirated, and components found in the aspirated fluid determine the extent of pulmonary injury.

Fresh water is hypotonic compared to the blood and when aspirated is rapidly absorbed into the bloodstream. It destroys surfactant, thereby increasing surface tension of the alveoli, and inducing alveolar collapse.[13–17] Sea water is hypertonic

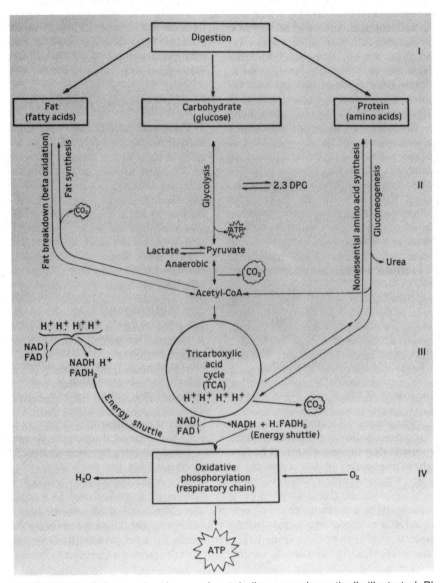

FIGURE 10–1 Four major phases of metabolism are schematically illustrated. Phase I: Digestion and nutrient absorption of fat, carbohydrate, and protein. Phase II: Breakdown of fatty acids, glucose, and amino acids to acetylcoenzyme A (acetyl = CoA), which can either go on to synthesize, directly or indirectly, fat, carbohydrate, or amino acids, as need may be, or go on to have more energy extracted from it in phases III and IV. Phase III: Tricarboxylic acid cycle, where most of the body's carbon dioxide (CO_2) is produced, as well as where most of the molecular energy shuttles (nicotinamide-adenine dinucleotide [NAD], flavin adenine dinucleotide [FAD]) receive their energy supply (in form of hydrogen atoms). Shuttles transport energy to respiratory chain. Phase IV: Inner mitochondrial membrane where oxidative phosphorylation occurs (production of adenosine triphosphate [ATP] in presence of oxygen), and oxygen is final acceptor of the now energy-depleted electrons and hydrogen ions. (From Wilkins, R, Sheldon, R, and Krider, S: Clinical Assessment in Respiratory Care. ed. 2, CV Mosby, St Louis, 1990, with permission.)

compared to the blood (approximately 3 percent saline) and causes fluid from the blood to flood into the alveoli when aspirated. Alveolar collapse occurs as surfactant is washed out and surface tension forces increase.

Atelectasis results in ventilation-perfusion ($\dot{V}/\dot{Q}$) mismatching, intrapulmonary shunting ($\dot{Q}_S/\dot{Q}_T$), a decrease in functional residual capacity, and a decrease in lung compliance. These abnormalities often lead to refractory hypoxemia.[18]

Aspirated substances may include mud, sand, bacteria, and gastric contents, which create inflammatory processes throughout the respiratory tract, resulting in alveolitis, bronchitis, and pneumonitis.

ARDS is a common complication of near drowning and probably results from microvascular injury associated with aspiration and/or an inflammatory response. Activated granulocytes can cause alveolar-capillary membrane injury by release of lysosomal enzymes and oxygen free radicals. As the alveolar-capillary membrane is damaged, protein-rich fluid floods the interstitial space. This protein-rich fluid is not easily removed from the interstitial space. Protein attachment to the alveolar walls can form hyaline membranes, producing the white-out appearance on chest radiograph, consistent with ARDS (see Chapter 11). Once ARDS occurs, it resolves slowly.

Hemodynamic and Electrolyte Effects

Animal studies have not demonstrated a difference between hypoxic animals and animals made to aspirate hypotonic, isotonic, or hypertonic saline.[19] The pulmonary vascular resistance, central venous pressure, and pulmonary capillary wedge pressure increased in all animals, whereas cardiac output and effective dynamic lung compliance decreased. An equally important finding was that there were no significant cardiovascular or hemodynamic differences between solution aspiration and the hypoxic control subjects. Initial changes in cardiovascular and hemodynamic function are more likely to result from hypoxia rather than aspiration of fluids.[19]

Evaluations of near-drowning patients have not demonstrated severe electrolyte or hemoglobin abnormalities with either saltwater or freshwater drowning. This means that hemoglobin and hematocrit changes cannot be used to determine whether fresh water or salt water has been aspirated.[20]

Renal Function

Most near-drowning patients do not develop renal dysfunction; however, acute tubular necrosis may result from myoglobinuria, diminished renal blood flow secondary to the hypoxic event, hypotension, lactic acid production, or trauma. Maintenance of adequate cardiac output will usually prevent development of renal insufficiency.

CLINICAL FEATURES

The initial assessment of drowning victims should be rapid and directed toward the victim's level of consciousness, pulse, and breathing rate. Information from onlookers can also be very helpful in determining the extent of injury.

If possible, the history should include information regarding the approximate length of time the patient was submerged; the type of fluid or water in which the victim was submerged; whether vital signs were present upon removal of the victim from the water; the approximate length of time that transpired between submersion and the initiation of cardiopulmonary resuscitation (CPR); whether CPR was performed immediately after removal of the victim from the water; how long CPR was performed before the return of vital signs; the approximate temperature of the water; the individual's age; and any other circumstances related to the near-drowning incident (e.g., diving or other accident, alcohol ingestion, and so on).

Vital signs may be highly variable in near-drowning victims. Patients may be in a full arrest state or have a pulse and respirations within normal limits. The body temperature is variable, depending on the water temperature in which they were submerged, the patient's body surface area, and the duration of exposure. Hypothermia is common when the patient is recovered from cold water and it may improve survival. Careful rewarming of the patient is required. The cardiac effects of near drowning are usually bradycardia, possibly followed by asystole.[21]

Neurologic impairment from hypoxia and medication used during resuscitation results in dilated pupils that respond slowly or not at all to light.

The head and neck should be carefully inspected for trauma. Near-drowning victims may incur injuries resulting from diving into shallow waters. Suspected spinal cord injuries require immobilization before transport.

Auscultation over the chest may reveal wheezing as a result of bronchospasm or foreign body aspiration and/or late inspiratory crackles associated with atelectasis or pulmonary edema.[18] The presence of adventitious lung sounds (e.g., coarse crackles) suggests that the patient has aspirated and is at risk for pneumonia and ARDS.

The extremities of the near-drowning patient are often cool to the touch owing to hypothermia and peripheral vasoconstriction. A slow capillary refill is present when peripheral circulation is reduced.

Arterial blood gas (ABG) studies often reveal hypoxemia, especially when aspiration has occurred, and metabolic acidosis. The severity of the metabolic acidosis is usually related to the severity of the tissue hypoxia. Hemoglobin, hematocrit, and electrolyte concentrations may decrease when large volumes of fresh water are swallowed or aspirated. This is the result of the dilution effects of the water when it enters the circulating blood volume.

INITIAL ASSESSMENT AND PROGNOSIS

Several scoring systems have been devised for assessment of near-drowning victims. No system can predict outcome with 100 percent accuracy. Three commonly used systems are the Glasgow coma scale (GCS), the Orlowski score,[1,22-24] and the postsubmersion neurologic classification system from Modell and Conn.[25,26]

The Glasgow coma scale[1,22-24] has three categories with the best response from each category determined and given the numeric value assigned to that response (Table 10-1). Scores from each category are then added for a total score. A score of 3 is the lowest possible, a score of 7 or less indicates coma, and a score of 14 indicates full consciousness. Prognosis should be based on the initial GCS examination.

Near-drowning patients with an initial GCS of less than or equal to 4 have an 80 percent chance of dying or of having permanent neurologic sequelae.[22] Patients with a GCS greater than or equal to 6 have a very low risk for permanent neurologic sequelae or mortality.[27]

The Orlowski score[1,22-24] is based on evidence of unfavorable factors related to the patient's recovery (Table 10-2). Patients with two or less unfavorable prognostic factors have a 90 percent chance for good recovery, whereas those with 3 or more unfavorable factors have less than a 5 percent chance for good recovery.

In 1980, Conn[26] and Modell[25] and their associates independently published a postresuscitation neurologic classification system based on the near-drowning patient's initial level of consciousness (Table 10-3). Conn and colleagues subcategorized the coma group, whereas Modell did not.

All patients in one retrospective study with an admission assessment of cate-

Table 10–1 Glascow Coma Scale*

Eye opening
  1. None
  2. To pain
  3. To speech
  4. Spontaneous
Best verbal response
  1. None
  2. Incomprehensible
  3. Inappropriate
  4. Confused
  5. Oriented
Best motor response
  1. None
  2. Extension (decerebrate)
  3. Flexion (decorticate)
  4. Localizing pain
  5. Obeying commands

*The Glascow coma score is determined by assessment of the patient's best response from each category. The numeric value to the left of each chosen response is then added together for all three categories for a total value. A total score less than 7 indicates presence of coma, whereas 14 signifies full consciousness.

Source: From Orlowski, J: Drowning, near-drowning, and ice-water submersions. Pediatr Clin North Am 34(1):75, 1987, with permission.

Table 10–2 Orlowski Score*

Unfavorable Prognostic Factors
1. Age ≤3 years
2. Estimated submersion time longer than 5 minutes
3. No resuscitative measures attempted for at least 10 minutes
4. Patient comatose upon arrival at the emergency room
5. Arterial blood gas pH ≤7.10

*The Orlowski score is determined by the number of unfavorable factors listed that apply to the near-drowning victim. Lower scores are prognostic of a more favorable outcome.

Source: From Orlowski, J: Drowning, near-drowning, and ice-water submersions. Pediatr Clin North Am 34(1):75, 1987, with permission.

Table 10–3 Postsubmersion Neurologic Classification System*

Category	Description
A. Awake	Alert, fully conscious and oriented
B. Blunted	Blunted consciousness, lethargic but rousable, purposeful response to pain
	Not arousable, abnormal response to pain
C. Comatose	
C_1	Decorticate flexion in response to pain
C_2	Decerebrate extension in response to pain
C_3	Flaccid or no pain response

*By Modell and Conn. Prognosis is determined by category, with those in categories A and B having excellent prognosis. Prognosis worsens in category C with the depth of coma.

Source: From Conn A, et al: Cerebral salvage in near-drowning following neurological classification by triage. Can Anaesth Soc J 27(3):201, 1980, with permission.

gory A (Table 10–3) survived without complications.[25] Ninety percent of category B patients survived with complete recovery, but 10 percent died. Fifty-five percent of category C patients completely recovered, but 34 percent died and 10 percent had permanent neurologic sequelae.

TREATMENT

Basic life support[28] and activation of the Emergency Medical Services (EMS) system should begin as soon as possible. The rescuer should carefully open the victim's airway and, if there is no breathing, begin mouth-to-mouth resuscitation until the victim resumes spontaneous breathing. Assessment for a heartbeat should be done when the victim is either brought to shore or placed on a flotation device large enough for both the rescuer and the victim. Chest compressions performed in the water cannot be effective enough to restore brain perfusion. If the victim is recovered from cold water, the recommended pulse check may take up to 1 minute[1,29] in order to rule out bradycardia or a faint heartbeat. Chest compressions started in haste might result in ventricular fibrillation and actually decrease cerebral perfusion. As soon as possible, the victim should be transported to a hospital.

The Heimlich maneuver should *not* be performed unless an airway obstruction is present.[2,30] Drowning victims may swallow a large amount of water and the Heimlich maneuver may result in vomiting and aspiration of the stomach contents.

Health care practitioners at the hospital should prepare appropriate equipment for intubation including laryngoscope, an assortment of blades, various tube sizes, stylettes, Magill forceps, syringe to check cuff patency and for cuff inflation, equipment for suctioning, tape to secure the endotracheal tube, and an appropriate bag-valve-mask device. An ABG kit should be available as well as appropriate gowning provisions for universal precautions.

Treatment for near-drowning patients is based on initial assessment and categorization. The following summary is based on the postsubmersion neurologic classification system.

Category A (Awake)

The neurologic status of these patients is alert and awake with a GCS of 14, indicating minimal hypoxic injury. These patients should be hospitalized and placed under continuous observation for 12 to 24 hours to allow early intervention should pulmonary or neurologic deterioration occur. Laboratory evaluation should include a complete blood count (CBC), serum electrolytes, chest radiograph, ABGs, sputum cultures, blood glucose levels, and clotting times.[21,26] A drug toxicologic screen may also be necessary. The cervical spine should be radiographed if there is a possibility of neck injury.

Treatment for this group is primarily symptomatic. Oxygen may be delivered via cannula or mask to maintain a Pao_2 above 60 mm Hg. An incentive spirometry device (volume type) may be helpful. Foreign body aspiration may be evaluated by chest radiograph. Bronchospasm can be treated with aerosolized β_2-adrenergic agents. Intravenous (IV) access is important for fluid and electrolyte management and allows rapid intervention should deterioration occur.

Neurologic deterioration may result from:

1. Hypoxemia due to worsening pulmonary condition
2. An increase in intracranial pressure (ICP) due to hypoxic injury
3. Drug ingestion before the event

If the patient is stable and no neurologic or pulmonary deterioration has occurred within 12 to 24 hours, the patient may be discharged. Physician follow-up within

2 to 3 days after discharge is strongly recommended and may detect a developing pulmonary infection.

Category B (Blunted)

The neurologic status of these patients is obtunded, or semiconscious but rousable. GCS is usually 10 to 13, indicating a more serious and prolonged episode of asphyxia. They have purposeful pain responses, normal respirations, and normal pupillary reactions. They may be irritable and combative. Following resuscitation and initial evaluation in the emergency department, these patients should be placed in the intensive care unit (ICU) with close attention paid to any neurologic, pulmonary, and/or cardiovascular changes. Their hospital stay is usually longer than with category A patients. All testing and treatment mentioned above in category A should be implemented. Blood, sputum, and possibly urine cultures should be performed daily. Vitamin K administration may improve clotting times. Antibiotics should be implemented only when culture specimens show evidence of bacterial growth other than normal flora. Changes in the patient's neurologic status can rapidly occur and a normal routine for head injury should be followed. Pulmonary edema, intractable metabolic acidosis, and a prolonged resuscitation period (with the exception of victims found in cold waters) generally indicate severe hypoxia. Hypoxemia may become refractory to increased inspired oxygen concentrations. Continuous positive airway pressure (CPAP) delivered via mask or mechanical ventilator may be necessary to maintain a Pao_2 greater than 60 mm Hg. Fluid restriction may be necessary but serum osmolality should not exceed 320 mOsm/liter.

Category C (Comatose)

The neurologic status of these severely ill patients is unarousable. The GCS is less than 7. Treatment should ultimately be directed toward maintaining normal oxygenation, ventilation, perfusion, blood pressure, and blood sugar and electrolyte levels.

Limited animal studies on brain resuscitation have brought new hope for salvaging comatose patients who have suffered severe anoxic episodes.[31–44] The goals of brain resuscitation are to prevent increases in ICP and to preserve brain cells that are viable but nonfunctional. Treatment might include use of hypothermia, hyperventilation, calcium blockers, barbiturates, muscle relaxation or paralysis, etomidate, and fluorocarbon infusions. Unfortunately the results of brain resuscitation have been mixed and the therapies remain controversial.[4,48] A serious ethical issue is whether brain resuscitation improves postresuscitation quality of life or merely prolongs the dying process by creating a greater population of patients in a persistent vegetative state.

The following sections are based on Conn's brain resuscitation recommendations. He uses the term "HYPER" because seriously brain-injured patients are frequently hyperhydrated, hyperventilating, hyperpyrexic, hyperexcitable, and hyper-rigid.

HYPERHYDRATION The hyperhydrated state may contribute to an increase both in ICP and in pulmonary edema. In an attempt to limit these problems, diuretics are usually implemented. Hemodynamic monitoring is used to avoid excessive fluid restriction that may lead to renal insufficiency and failure. Small doses of dopamine (less than 5 µg/kg per minute) will act on dopaminergic receptors in the kidneys to increase renal perfusion and possibly urine output. Attempts at diuresis should not drive the serum osmolality above 320 mOsm/liter. Invasive hemodynamic monitoring requires use of a pulmonary artery catheter for monitoring central venous pressure and pulmonary artery and wedge pressures. Arterial lines may also be necessary if blood pressure is unstable or frequent ABG measurements are needed.

ICP monitoring was widely used during the 1980s to control or prevent increases in ICP. It is now most commonly used for patients in category A or B who show signs of mental and neurologic deterioration. It is hoped that hyperventilation, osmotic diuretics, and thiopental will reverse the cerebral edema resulting from ischemia. Unfortunately, successful control of ICP does not ensure intact survival.[45−48]

HYPERVENTILATION   Patients requiring mechanical ventilation should be hyperventilated and their $Paco_2$ kept between 25 and 30 mm Hg. Cerebral vascular resistance is controlled by the arterioles, which respond to changes in pH. Because pH is affected by $Paco_2$ changes, hyperventilation causes cerebral vasoconstriction and a lower ICP. Patient tidal volumes can be set in the range of 10 to 15 mL/kg at a rate necessary to achieve the appropriate reduction in $Paco_2$.

Oxygen delivery to the tissues is an important goal in patients with more extensive lung involvement. Maintaining an arterial oxygen percent saturation (Sao_2) near 96 percent (Pao_2 of 100 mm Hg) is ideal but not always possible. The use of positive end-expiratory pressure (PEEP) is a valuable adjunct to achieve adequate oxygenation (Pao_2 greater than 60 mm Hg). In adults and older pediatric patients, PEEP levels should be increased in increments of 5 cm H_2O until acceptable oxygenation is achieved. Smaller increases in PEEP should be made in younger patients.

HYPERPYREXIA   Hypothermia (body temperature 30 ± 1°C or less) has been advocated for brain-injured comatose patients, as it may decrease cerebral oxygen requirements and ICP.[26] Hypothermia is known to protect the brain when induced before cerebral hypoxia. However, it has not improved neurologic outcome in patients who have already suffered cerebral hypoxia, and it can induce other complications such as suppression of the normal immune response, a left shift in the oxyhemoglobin dissociation curve, and cardiac dysrhythmias. Normothermia should be maintained via antipyretics and a cooling mattress when fever is present since fever increases oxygen consumption.

HYPEREXCITABILITY   Barbiturates are thought to bring about reduction of ICP via cerebral vasoconstriction, suppression of seizure activity, and reduction of cerebral metabolic rate. Thiopental is probably the only barbiturate that may remove oxygen free radicals. Induction of a barbiturate coma has not been shown to improve survival or neurologic outcome in near-drowning patients with severe deficit and may enhance cardiovascular instability. Barbiturate coma is no longer a part of the recommended treatment because of these problems.[47−49] Barbiturates are used, however, to control seizure activity. Steroid use was also advocated in near-drowning treatment in the hope of controlling ICP. Subsequent studies have shown steroids to be ineffective in the postanoxic near-drowning patients. Steroid use may also mask normal immune responses to bacterial infection, resulting in a higher incidence of sepsis.[4,49]

HYPERRIGIDITY   Decerebrate and decorticate rigid posturing are signs of raised ICP. ICP may be elevated because of brain swelling from hypoxia, mechanical ventilation and PEEP, coughing, and Trendelenburg's positioning. Suctioning procedures may elevate ICP for as long as 30 minutes. ICP might be reduced in patients requiring mechanical ventilation with sedation and use of paralytic agents.

Case Study No. 1

HISTORY

JR is a 1-year-old white male infant who was found floating face down in his grandparents' swimming pool after having been missed for approximately 5 minutes. The patient's mother immediately began mouth-to-mouth resuscitation, and he *responded after four to five breaths. He began breathing spontaneously, cried, and vomited a large amount of water. He was taken to the local emergency medical services facility, where he was alert, active, and crying. His initial ABG analysis on room air was pH 7.34, Paco$_2$ 34 mm Hg, Pao$_2$ 51 mm Hg, Sao$_2$ 84 percent, HCO$_3^-$ 19 mEq/liter, and base excess (BE) −5.6 mEq/liter. His temperature at that time was 38.8°C (rectally) and auscultation revealed bilateral coarse crackles.*

Questions

1. Interpret the acid-base and oxygenation status of this patient's initial ABG. What accounts for the acid-base abnormality?
2. What could be the cause of the coarse crackles?

Answers

1. His acid-base status is consistent with a partially compensated metabolic acidemia. The metabolic acidosis is probably the result of lactic acidosis from anaerobic metabolism. He is moderately hypoxemic on room air.
2. The coarse crackles are most likely due to aspiration.

The patient was given oxygen by cannula and was warmed with blankets.

PHYSICAL EXAMINATION

General *Upon physical examination, he was alert, oriented, and in no acute respiratory distress.*

Vital Signs *Temperature 35.8°C (rectally), pulse 156/minute, respirations 46/minute, blood pressure 98/58 mm Hg, arterial mean pressure 72 mm Hg, weight 10.87 kg, height 88 cm.*

HEENT *Normocephalic; atraumatic; pupils equal, round, reactive to light, and accommodation (PERRLA); sclera and conjunctiva nonicteric; nasopharynx showing nasal crusting, no nasal flaring; oropharynx clear; tympanic membranes showing erythema on left with a decreased light reflex on the right with some cerumen; head circumference is 47.4 cm*

Neck *Supple, full range of motion without rigidity or tenderness*

Lungs *Auscultation of the lower lung fields revealed coarse crackles anteriorly and posteriorly*

Heart *Regular rhythm and normal S$_1$ and S$_2$, no murmurs, gallops, or rubs.*

Back *Straight, without presacral edema or gross abnormalities*

Extremities *Full range of motion with ++ pulses, and normal reflexes*

Skin *Warm and pink*

Neurologic *Patient is alert and oriented; cranial nerves II through XII fully intact; motor and sensory examination within normal limits*

Questions

3. Based on his initial evaluation, how would you rate JR on the Glasgow coma scale? What Orlowski score would he have? Under what category would he be placed by the Conn-Modell Postsubmersion Neurologic Classification System?
4. Based on these evaluation methods what is his prognosis?

Answers

3. His GCS score is 14; his Orlowski score shows only one unfavorable prognostic factor; his postsubmersion neurologic classification is category A.
4. His prognosis is 100 percent full recovery without neurologic deficit.

LABORATORY EXAMINATION

CBC shows white blood cells (WBC) 14.9 $\times$ 10³/µL, red blood cells (RBC) 4.41 $\times$ 10⁶/µL, hemoglobin (Hb) 12.0 g/dL, hematocrit (Hct) 34.7 percent, platelets 480 $\times$ 10³/µL with differential segs 33 percent, bands 47 percent, lymphocytes 19 percent, monocytes 1 percent. Electrolytes show sodium 133 mEq/liter, potassium 3.6 mEq/liter, chloride 106 mEq/liter, total CO_2 18 mM/liter, blood urea nitrogen (BUN) 6 mg/dL, creatinine 0.4 mg/dL. ABGs on 2L/min pH 7.37, $Paco_2$ 33 mm Hg, Pao_2 73 mm Hg, Sao_2 94 percent, oxygen concentration (Cao_2) 13.7 vol%, HCO_3^- 19 mEq/liter, BE −5 mEq/liter, Hb 10.7 g/dL. Chest radiograph reveals patchy opacifications in both lower lobes with the left clearer than the right, consistent with bibasalar subsegmental atelectasis. There is mild central pulmonary congestion and interstitial edema consistent with noncardiogenic interstitial pulmonary edema (Fig. 10–2).

Questions

5. Interpret the ABG analysis.
6. Electrolytes show a diminished sodium. What might be the cause?
7. What pathophysiology might account for hypoxemia in this patient?
8. How soon could the child return home and what follow-up is necessary?

Answers

5. The acid-base status is consistent with a completely compensated metabolic acidosis. There is mild hypoxemia on 2 L/min.
6. The drop in sodium is most likely due to dilutional hypervolemia resulting from swallowing large amounts of water. Dilution may also occur from aspiration and absorption of water through the lungs.
7. The $Paco_2$ is low, ruling out hypoventilation as a source of hypoxemia. The Pao_2 response to supplemental oxygen helps determine whether the hypoxemia was due to $\dot{V}/\dot{Q}$ mismatching (which is associated with an improved Pao_2 as in this case) or shunt (which would not be associated with an improved Pao_2).
8. The patient is stable and can be discharged after 24–48 hours of observation. He should be reevaluated after 2 to 3 days in the outpatient clinic.

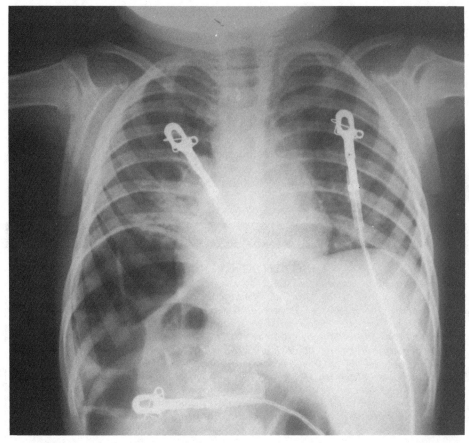

FIGURE 10–2 This radiograph is consistent with mild noncardiogenic interstitial pulmonary edema. Note the elevation of the left hemidiaphragm resulting from subsegmental atelectasis.

Case Study No. 2

HISTORY

JM is a 2-year-old Hispanic boy who had been missing for 10 to 15 minutes and was found floating face down under the solar cover of the family's backyard swimming pool. He was unresponsive upon removal from the pool.

Questions

1. What treatment is indicated and when should it be implemented?
2. Should the Heimlich maneuver be implemented? Why or why not?

Answers

1. The ABCs of CPR should immediately be started. Determine unresponsiveness by shaking and shouting. Call for help! Open the *Airway*. Evaluate whether *Breathing* is present by looking, listening, and feeling for breathing. Give two breaths if the victim is apneic. Assess if *Circulation* is present

by establishing pulselessness for 5 to 10 seconds. Begin chest compressions if there is no pulse. Continue CPR at a ratio of chest compressions to ventilations of 5:1. If this had been an adult victim, the ratio of chest compressions to ventilations would have been 15:2 in one-rescuer CPR and 5:1 for two-rescuer CPR. Activate the EMS system as soon as possible!

2. The Heimlich maneuver should not be implemented at this time. It is used only when complete airway obstruction is present. Near-drowning patients frequently swallow large quantities of water and the likelihood for vomiting and aspiration is increased when the Heimlich maneuver is performed.

One family member started CPR while another activated the EMS system. The paramedics arrived shortly thereafter and took over CPR performance. The patient was transported to the nearest EMS facility, arriving there within 20 minutes from the time of initial discovery.

Question

3. What airway preparations should be made in the emergency room before the patient arrives?

Answer

3. Ensure that the appropriate intubation equipment is present—laryngoscope with various blade sizes (straight and curved), endotracheal tubes (cuffed and uncuffed), batteries, replacement bulbs for the blades, stylet, tape, Magill forceps, syringe for cuff, inflation, nonpetroleum-base lubricating gel—and is in good working condition. Once the tube size is determined, if there is a cuff, check for cuff patency by inflation and then remove the air, insert stylet, and lubricate the distal end of the tube.

Ensure that appropriate suctioning equipment is present (wall or portable suction device, reservoir, tubing, suction catheters, Yankauer's suctioning device) and is in good working condition.

Ensure that an appropriate bag-valve-mask device with a face mask assortment and an adequate 100 percent oxygen source is available and working.

Ensure that appropriate equipment is available for drawing blood for ABG analysis.

Gown as appropriate for universal precautions.

The patient remained in a full arrest state upon arrival to the EMS facility. The initial ABG with CPR in progress and the patient on 100 percent oxygen by bag-valve device showed pH 6.69, $Paco_2$ 55 mm Hg, Pao_2 70 mm Hg, BE −30 mEq/liter, and plasma bicarbonate (HCO_3^-) 7 mEq/liter. He was orally intubated with a 4.5-mm endotracheal tube, given one dose (0.2 mg IV) of epinephrine and 2 mg of sodium bicarbonate. CPR continued and after 10 minutes a second round of drug therapy was administered.

Questions

4. Interpret the initial ABG analysis.
5. What treatment is indicated by the ABG results?
6. Following intubation, what should be done to determine endotracheal tube placement?

Answers

4. The acid-base status is consistent with a severe combined respiratory and metabolic acidemia. The oxygenation status is consistent with a mild hypoxemia in spite of manual ventilation with 100 percent oxygen.
5. The extreme acidemia indicates the need for bicarbonate administration. The elevation of the Pa_{CO_2} indicates the need to increase alveolar ventilation.
6. Assessment of endotracheal tube position can be done by auscultating the lungs for equal, bilateral breath sounds; by checking the linear measurement of the tube at the lip to determine how far it was inserted; and by reviewing the chest radiograph to assess proper tube placement. The right main stem bronchus is shorter, wider, and straighter than the left so that the endotracheal tube will usually enter the right side if it is inserted too far. Intubation of the right main stem bronchus usually leaves the left lung without ventilation and breath sounds.

The patient remained asystolic in the emergency room for about 1 hour. He required several dosages of epinephrine, sodium bicarbonate, and atropine. A nasogastric tube was inserted and 15 mL of clear fluid removed. The advanced cardiac life support measures restored the patient's heartbeat. An ABG analysis was performed while the patient was receiving 100 percent oxygen via manual resuscitator. Results were pH 7.02, Pa_{CO_2} 11 mm Hg, Pa_{O_2} 464 mm Hg, BE −26 mEq/liter, and HCO_3^- 3 mEq/liter.

After resuscitation, the patient's initial temperature was 34.4°C rectally, respirations were sporadic requiring assistance, pulses ranged from 80 to 130/minute, blood pressure varied from 99/25 to 134/69 mm Hg, and pupils were 4 mm and reacted sluggishly to light. The patient was unresponsive to stimuli (without eye opening, without verbal response) and exhibited decorticate posturing. His initial glucose level was 744 mg/dL. Initial electrolytes revealed sodium 118 mEq/liter, potassium 3.6 mEq/liter, chloride 92 mEq/liter, total CO_2 less than 5 mmol/liter, BUN 18 mg/dL, and creatinine 0.9 mg/dL. His initial CBC revealed a WBC 7.2 × 10³/µL, RBC 4.5 × 10⁶/µL, Hb 12.2 g/dL, Hct 35.6 percent, and differential morphology showed segs 22 percent and lymphocytes 78 percent. Warming measures were started and the patient was transported to a tertiary care facility. The initial chest radiograph showed proper endotracheal tube placement; bilateral fluffy infiltrates, more extensive on the left, consistent with noncardiogenic pulmonary edema; and a right-sided pleural effusion. The heart was normal in size, and a nasogastric tube was present with the tip in the fundus of the stomach (Fig. 10–3).

Questions

7. What GCS score would you give the patient? What category would you place him based on the Conn-Modell postsubmersion neurologic classification system? What Orlowski score would he have?
8. What is his prognosis?

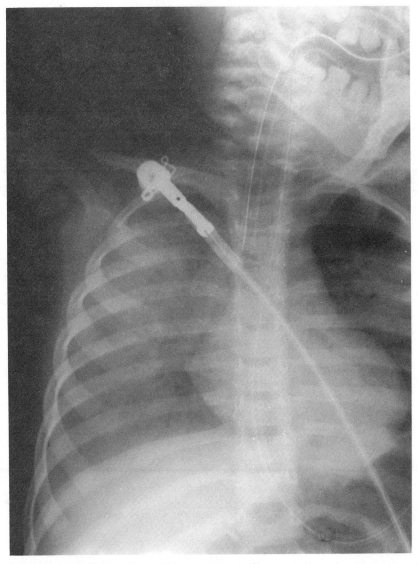

FIGURE 10–3 This radiograph is consistent with noncardiogenic pulmonary edema with probable right-sided pleural effusion.

9. What do his initial electrolytes and CBC reveal, and what is the most likely cause for these results?
10. What is indicated by the bilateral fluffy infiltrates and normal heart size on his chest radiograph?
11. Should life support efforts be continued?

Answers

7. His GCS is 5; his postsubmersion neurologic classification category is C_1; and his Orlowski score shows four unfavorable prognostic factors.
8. Orlowski would give him a 5 percent chance of a good recovery. His GCS predicts 80 percent mortality or permanent neurologic sequelae. Modell and Conn would predict approximately 33 percent mortality, 10

to 23 percent permanent neurologic sequelae, and a 44 to 55 percent chance of full recovery.

9. His electrolytes reveal hyponatremia and hypochloremia, which are likely the result of hypervolemia resulting from swallowing and aspirating water. The diminished total CO_2 is consistent with marked acidemia. His CBC reveals mild anemia, again consistent with hypervolemia.

10. The radiography results are consistent with aspiration or noncardiogenic pulmonary edema.

11. Yes, resuscitation should continue because there is a chance of full recovery.

Upon arrival to the tertiary care facility, his initial physical examination revealed the following:

PHYSICAL EXAMINATION

General	*Patient responsive to deep pain only; difficult to assess secondary to decorticate movements involving all extremities, head, and trunk*
Vital Signs	*Temperature 36.7°C, pulse rate 169/minute, respiratory rate 28/minute by manual resuscitator, blood pressure 140/90 mm Hg, and weight 35 lb*
HEENT	*Head normocephalic, atraumatic; patient unable to focus; pupils sluggishly reactive, 4 mm, sclerae not icteric or injected; ears showing normally shaped pinna, auditory canals patent, tympanic membranes clear, without sign of infection; nose without nasal discharge; patient intubated*
Neck	*No adenopathy or thyromegaly*
Heart	*Regular rate and rhythm, normal S_1 and S_2, without gallop*
Lungs	*Coarse crackles heard throughout chest*
Abdomen	*Soft, nondistended; no spleen tip or other masses palpated*
Back	*Intact, no spina bifida, hair tuft, or sacral dimple*
Extremities	*Pulses barely palpable in axillae, carotids, and femoral; nail beds dusky*
Skin	*Very poor perfusion, cool to the touch, no rashes, no signs of trauma*
Neurologic	*Responds to deep pain only; deep tendon reflexes are hyper-reflexic; has decorticate posturing*

Questions

12. What is the significance of the sluggish pupils?
13. What is the significance of the dusky nailbeds?

Answers

12. The sluggish pupils indicate an impaired neurologic function that may be due to the hypoxic event. Atropine, that was given during the resuscitation, may contribute to the sluggish pupils.

13. The dusky nailbeds indicate poor cardiac output, poor peripheral perfusion, or hypothermia. Shock and poor cardiac output are the most likely causes of the dusky nailbeds in this situation.

Ventilator settings were intermittent mandatory ventilation (IMV) 20/minute, inspired fraction of oxygen (FIO_2) 0.70, tidal volume (V$_T$) 170 mL, PEEP 5 cm H$_2$O. ABG analysis on these parameters revealed pH 7.42, PaCO_2 30 mm Hg, PaO_2 75 mm Hg, BE −4 mEq/liter, HCO$_3^-$ 19 mEq/liter.

During the first 8 hours the patient's intake was 282 mL and output 497 mL. After 12 hours his neurologic status improved with some purposeful movements, pupils 4 mm bilaterally and reactive, purposeful response to pain, and occasional back arching. Breath sounds were improved. Electrocardiogram (ECG) showed a regular rate and rhythm. There was a smelly, bloody discharge from his rectum. This was thought to be consistent with a compromised gastrointestinal track caused by severe ischemia.

LABORATORY EVALUATION

Electrolyte evaluation showed sodium 133 mEq/liter, potassium 3.3 mEq/liter, chloride 105 mEq/liter, total CO$_2$ 19 mM/liter, BUN 20 mg/dL, creatinine 0.5 mg/dL, and glucose 181 mg/dL. His serum osmolality was 273 mOsm/liter. CBC showed the WBC 5.6 × 10^3/μL and RBC within normal limits, hemoglobin 14.7 g/dL, and hematocrit 42.8 percent. His platelet count was 368 × 10^3/μL, prothrombin time (PT) was 13.3 seconds and his partial thromboplastin time (PTT) was 32 seconds.

Questions

14. List data that indicate the presence of a persistent metabolic acidosis?
15. Interpret the ABGs.
16. Why is the serum sodium rising?
17. What changes in ventilator parameters would you make, if any?

Answers

14. The parameters that indicate persistent metabolic acidosis include BE −4 mEq/liter, HCO$_3^-$ 19 mEq/liter, and total CO$_2$ 19 mM/liter.
15. The acid-base status is consistent with a completely compensated metabolic acidosis. There is mild hypoxemia on an FIO_2 of 0.70 and PEEP 5 cm H$_2$O. The calculated CaO_2 is 18.5 vol %, which is within normal limits.
16. The hyponatremia is resolving as diuresis occurs, ridding the body of excess fluids.
17. If tolerated, a PEEP increase might improve his PaO_2 and allow the FIO_2 to be diminished below 0.50. This would reduce the risk for onset of oxygen toxicity.

On the 14th hour of hospitalization, there was a sudden drop in the pulse oximeter saturation accompanied by an increase in both pulse and respiratory rate. The patient began fighting the ventilator and was paralyzed. Auscultation revealed his breath sounds to be markedly dimished on the left side.

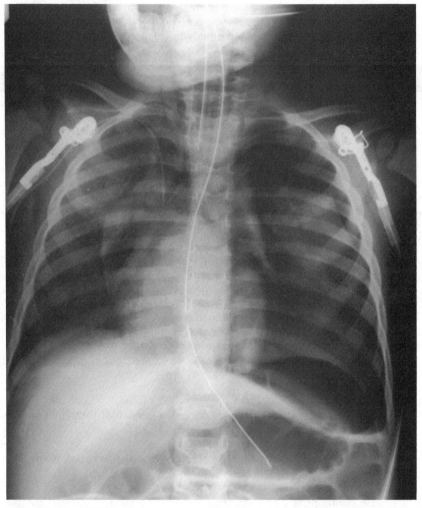

FIGURE 10–4 This radiograph is consistent with pneumomediastinum and a fairly large left pneumothorax. Also, there is persistent bilateral diffuse pulmonary edema and subcutaneous emphysema extends into the soft tissues of the neck.

Questions

18. What are possible causes of the sudden fall in the pulse oximeter saturation, increase in pulse and respiratory rate, and decreased breath sounds on the left side?
19. How can the cause be confirmed and treated?

Answers

18. Causes of the sudden deterioration might include advancement of the endotracheal tube into the right main stem bronchus, pneumothorax, or mucus and debris obstructing the left main stem bronchus.
19. Check the position of the endotracheal tube to determine if it has slipped. If so, reposition it and auscultate for equal bilateral breath sounds. Obtain a chest radiograph immediately to confirm endotracheal tube position and rule out pneumothorax and atelectasis. Pneumothorax may be corrected by chest tube placement. Mucus plugging can usually

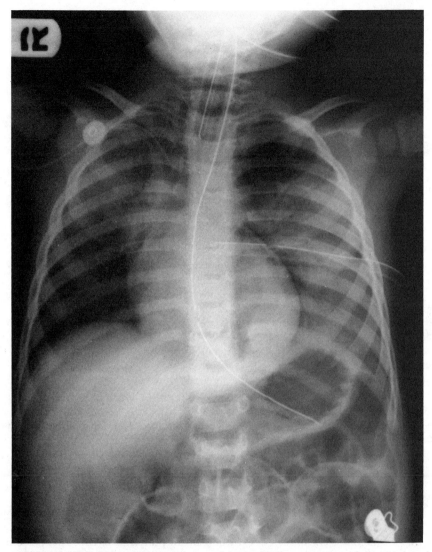

FIGURE 10–5 This radiograph is consistent with the presence of chest tube placement on the left with reinflation of the left lung. Pneumomediastinum is present and the bilateral pulmonary edema is worsening. Also, left lower lobe subsegmental atelectasis is present.

be corrected by postural drainage and vibration of the chest wall. Bronchoscopy may be used as a last resort.

His chest radiograph revealed a moderate-sized pneumothorax on the left side with pneumomediastinum. The bilateral diffuse pulmonary edema was essentially unchanged from the previous chest radiograph. Also, the endotracheal tube had been retracted to the level of the thoracic inlet, a central venous line was present with the tip in the right atrium and the nasogastric tube tip remained in the fundus of the stomach (see Fig. 10–4). A chest tube was placed on the left side and the follow-up radiograph showed marked decreases of the pneumomediastinum and left pneumothorax. The left hemidiaphragm was elevated, associated with atelectasis in the *left lower lobe. The bilateral pulmonary edema appeared to be worsening as evident by increased hazy opacification of the lungs (see Fig. 10–5). The ventilator parameters were changed to FIO_2 1.00, PEEP 12 cm H_2O, and resulted in a Pao_2 of 77 mm Hg.*

The patient never regained consciousness and expired after 6 weeks from respiratory complications.

REFERENCES

1. Orlowski, J: Drowning, near-drowning, and ice-water submersions. Pediatr Clin North Am 34(1):75, 1987.

2. Ornato, J: The resuscitation of near-drowning victims. JAMA 256(1):75, 1986.

3. Neal, J: Near-drowning. J Emerg Med 3(1):41, 1985.

4. Gonzalez-Rothi, R: Near drowning: Consensus and controversies in pulmonary and cerebral resuscitation. Heart Lung 16(5):474, 1987.

5. Martin, T: Neardrowning and cold water immersion. Ann Emerg Med 13:263, 1984.

6. Spyker, D: Submersion injury: Epidemiology, prevention, and management. Pediatr Clin North Am 32(1):113, 1985.

7. Shepherd, S: Immersion injury: Drowning and near drowning. Postgrad Med 85:183, 1989.

8. Siebke, H, et al: Survival after 40 minutes' submersion without cerebral sequelae. Lancet 1:1275, 1975.

9. Stryer, L: Biochemistry, ed 3. WH Freeman, New York, 1988.

10. Darnell, J, Lodish, H, and Baltimore, D: Molecular Cell Biology. Scientific American Books, New York, 1986.

11. Brierley, J, Meldrum, B, and Brown, A: The threshold and neuropathology of cerebral anoxic-ischemic cell change. Arch Neurol 29:367, 1973.

12. Brown, A and Brierley, J: The earliest alterations in rat neurones and astrocytes after anoxia-ischemia. Acta Neuropathol (Berlin) 23:9, 1973.

13. Modell, J, et al: Serum electrolyte concentrations after fresh-water aspiration. Anesthesiology 30(4):421, 1969.

14. Modell, J, et al: The effects of fluid volume in seawater drowning. Ann Intern Med 67(1):68, 1967.

15. Giammona, S and Modell, J: Drowning by total immersion: Effects on pulmonary surfactant of distilled water, isotonic saline, and sea water. Am J Dis Child 114:612, 1067.

16. Halmagyi, D: Lung changes and incidence of respiratory arrest in rats after aspiration of sea and fresh water. J Appl Physiol 16:41, 1961.

17. Reidbord, H and Spitz, W: Ultrastructural alterations in rat lungs: Changes after intratracheal perfusion with freshwater and seawater. Arch Pathol 81:103, 1966.

18. Nichols, D and Rogers, M: Adult respiratory distress syndrome. In Rogers, M: Textbook of Pediatric Intensive Care. Williams & Wilkins, Baltimore, 1987.

19. Orlowski, J, et al: The hemodynamic and cardiovascular effects of near-drowning in hypotonic, isotonic, or hypertonic solutions. Ann Emerg Med 18:1044, 1989.

20. Modell, J, Graves, S, and Ketover, A: Clinical course of 91 consecutive near-drowning victims. Chest 70:231, 1976.

21. Gilbert, J, Puckett, J, and Smith, R: Near drowning: Current concepts of management. Respir Care 30(2):108, 1985.

22. Dean, J and Kaufman, N: Prognostic indicators in pediatric near-drowning: The Glasgow coma scale. Crit Care Med 9(7):536, 1981.

23. Frewen, T, et al: Cerebral resuscitation therapy in pediatric near-drowning. J Pediatr 106(4):615, 1985.

24. Allman, F, et al: Outcome following cardiopulmonary resuscitation in severe pediatric near-drowning. AJDC 140:571, 1986.

25. Modell, J, Graves, S, and Kuck, E: Near-drowning: Correlation of level of consciousness and survival. Can Anaesth Soc J 27(3):211, 1980.

26. Conn, A, et al: Cerebral salvage in near-drowning following neurological classification by triage. Can Anaesth Soc J 27(3):201, 1980.

27. Jacobsen, W, et al: Correlation of spontaneous respiration and neurologic damage in near-drowning. Crit Care Med 11(7):487, 1983.

28. Health care provider's manual for basic life support. American Heart Association, Dallas, 1990.

29. Steinman, A: Cardiopulmonary resuscitation and hypothermia. Circulation 74(Suppl IV):29, 1986.

30. Modell, J: Near drowning. Circulation 74(Suppl IV):27, 1986.

31. Steen, P and Michenfelder, J: Barbiturate protection in tolerant and non-tolerant hypoxic mice: Comparison with hypothermic protection. Anesthesiology 50:404, 1979.

32. Carlsson, C, Hagerdal, M, and Siesjo, B: Protective effect of hypothermia in cerebral oxygen deficiency caused by arterial hypoxia. Anesthesiology 44:27, 1976.

33. Hagerdal, M, et al: Protective effects of combination of hypothermia and barbiturates in cerebral hypoxia in the rat. Anesthesiology 49:165, 1978.

34. Bleyaert, A, et al: Thiopental amelioration of brain damage after global ischemia in monkeys. Anesthesiology 49:390, 1978.

35. Lafferty, J, et al: Cerebral hypometabolism obtained with deep pentobarbital anesthesia and hypothermia (30 C). Anesthesiology 49:159, 1978.

36. Michenfelder, J, Milde, J, and Sundt, T: Cerebral protection by barbiturate anesthesia. Use after middle cerebral artery occlusion in Java monkeys. Arch Neurol 33:345, 1976.

37. Hoff, J, et al: Barbiturate protection from cerebral infarction in primates. Stroke 6:28, 1975.

38. Hankinson, H, et al: Effect of thiopental on focal cerebral ischemia in dogs. Surg Forum 25:445, 1974.

39. Bleyaert, A, et al: Amelioration of post ischemic brain damage in the monkey by immobilization and controlled ventilation. Crit Care Med 6:112, 1978.

40. Soloway, M, et al: The effect of hyperventilation on subsequent cerebral infarction. Anesthesiology 29:975, 1968.

41. Safar, P, et al: Resuscitation after global brain ischemia-anoxia. Crit Care Med 6:215, 1978.

42. Pappius, H and McCann, W: Effects of steroids on cerebral edema in cats. Arch Neurol 20:207, 1969.

43. Rovit, R and Hagan, R: Steroids and cerebral edema: The effect of glucocorticoids on abnormal capillary permeability following cerebral injury in cats. J Neuropathol Exp Neurol 27:277, 1968.

44. Wilkinson, H, Wepsic, J, and Austen, G: Diuretic synergy in the treatment of acute experimental cerebral edema. J Neurosurg 34:203, 1971.

45. Sarnaik, A, et al: Intracranial pressure and cerebral perfusion pressure in near-drowning. Crit Care Med 13(4):224, 1985.

46. Nussbaum, E and Galant, S: Intracranial pressure monitoring as a guide to prognosis in the nearly-drowned, severely comatose child. J Pediatr 102:215, 1983.

47. Dean, J and McComb, J: Intracranial pressure monitoring in severe pediatric near-drowning. Neurosurgery 9:627, 1981.

48. Bohn, D, et al: Influence of hypothermia, barbiturate therapy, and intracranial pressure monitoring on morbidity and mortality after near-drowning. Crit Care Med 14(6):529, 1986.

49. Conn, A and Barker, G: Fresh water drowning and near-drowning: An update. Can Anaesth Soc J 31(3):S38, 1984.

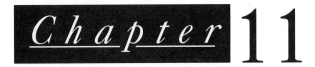
Kenneth D. McCarty, MS, RRT

ADULT RESPIRATORY DISTRESS SYNDROME

INTRODUCTION

Adult respiratory distress syndrome (ARDS) was first described by Ashbaugh et al in 1967.[1] It is characterized by hypoxemic respiratory failure from damage to the alveolar-capillary membrane, which increases pulmonary vascular permeability and leads to interstitial and alveolar edema. The syndrome may occur after injury or illness in previously healthy people at any age. Many synonyms have been used to describe ARDS including noncardiogenic pulmonary edema and shock lung (Table 11–1).

ARDS is often accompanied by multiple organ failure.[2,3] The most commonly affected organ systems include cardiovascular, renal, hepatic, central nervous, and bone marrow[4–6] (Table 11–2). When ARDS was first described its mortality rate was approximately 95 percent and the majority of deaths were due to respiratory failure.[7] More recently the mortality rate is between 50 and 70 percent and is due most often to nonpulmonary multiple organ system failure.[5]

ETIOLOGY

Many disorders are associated with ARDS (Table 11–3); however, shock (see Chapter 6), infection, and trauma (see Chapter 12) are most common. Although the potential causes of ARDS are varied, each disorder ultimately results in serious

Table 11–1 Synonyms for ARDS

Shock lung
Da Nang lung
Increased permeability pulmonary edema
Noncardiogenic pulmonary edema
White lung syndrome
Hemorrhagic atelectasis
Capillary leak syndrome
Post-traumatic pulmonary insufficiency
Wet lung syndrome

Table 11–2 Frequency of Nonpulmonary Organ Failure in ARDS

Cardiovascular	10–23%
Renal	40–55%
Hepatic	12–95%
Gastrointestinal	7–30%
Central nervous system	7–30%

Source: From Dorinsky, PM and Gadek, JE: Mechanisms of multiple nonpulmonary organ failure in ARDS. Chest 96:885, 1989, with permission.

Table 11–3 Disorders Associated with ARDS

Shock (any cause)
Infection (pneumonia, sepsis)
Trauma (thoracic and nonthoracic)
Aspiration (gastrointestinal fluid, near-drowning)
Drug toxicity (overdose or toxic effects)
Inhalation injury (oxygen toxicity, smoke inhalation, caustic chemicals)
Hematologic disorders (disseminated intravascular coagulation, multiple transfusions)
Metabolic disorders (pancreatitis, uremia)
Neurologic disorders (head trauma, brain tumor)

---

damage to the alveolar-capillary membrane. Exactly how this damage to the lung parenchyma occurs is not known. Numerous humoral and cellular agents are probably involved. Chemical mediators may be released by neutrophils, which are known to accumulate in the pulmonary capillary bed of the patient with acute lung injury.[8-10] Pulmonary edema is generally evident within approximately 24 hours after the precipitating event. Fluid flow through the damaged capillary membranes results in the accumulation of protein-rich fluid in the interstitium and alveolar spaces.

PATHOLOGY

The predominant pathologic abnormalities of ARDS change as the syndrome progresses and are often described as the exudative, proliferative, and fibrotic phases. The exudative phase begins after the precipitating event and lasts for up to 1 week. This phase is characterized by endothelial cell swelling, widening of the intercellular junctions, and widespread type I pneumocyte damage.[11,12] As a result, interstitial and alveolar edema occur, and dense eosinophilic hyaline membranes are formed.[13] Lungs from patients who die of ARDS during this stage are edematous, hemorrhagic, heavy, and relatively airless. The proliferative phase is characterized by regeneration of alveolar epithelial cells. The fibrotic phase occurs 3 to 4 weeks after the onset of the syndrome and is characterized by widespread formation of collagenous tissue by fibroblasts causing thickened alveolar septa.[14]

Alterations and remodeling of the pulmonary vasculature also occur in addition to pulmonary alveolar changes associated with ARDS. The exudative phase is associated with hypoxemia-induced pulmonary vasoconstriction, thrombi formation, and interstitial edema, which all contribute to a reversible increase in pulmonary artery pressure (PAP). The fibrotic phase is associated with fibrous obliteration of the pulmonary microvasculature and increased arteriolar muscularization and may produce prolonged pulmonary hypertension.[15]

PATHOPHYSIOLOGY

ARDS affects lung mechanics, gas exchange, and the pulmonary vasculature.[16] Intravascular fluid leaks from the pulmonary capillaries and floods the alveoli diluting surfactant. Injury of type II pneumocytes decreases their production of surfactant. As a result, microatelectasis occurs and lung compliance decreases.[17,18] These changes in lung mechanics increase the patient's work of breathing.

Alveolar flooding and atelectasis produce areas of perfusion without ventilation (shunt). Uneven pathologic changes in the pulmonary parenchyma and capillaries produce local areas of ventilation-perfusion ($\dot{V}/\dot{Q}$) mismatching.[19,20] These abnormalities cause hypoxemia that responds poorly to supplemental oxygen administration (refractory hypoxemia).

Hypoxemia, microemboli, and capillary compression increase the pulmonary vascular resistance (PVR). This alters the distribution of blood flow through the lungs, contributes to the $\dot{V}/\dot{Q}$ mismatch, and produces pulmonary hypertension.[21,22] Right ventricular pressure, size, and work increase in order to maintain cardiac output.[23] Right ventricular failure develops when these demands can no longer be met.

CLINICAL FEATURES

Regardless of the etiology, the clinical course of ARDS usually follows a specific pattern[24]:

1. Initial injury
2. Apparent respiratory stability
3. Respiratory deterioration and insufficiency
4. Terminal stage

After the initial insult, a period of time occurs in which patients do not appear to have any pulmonary abnormalities. This lasts from a few hours to about 1 day after injury. Respiratory deterioration is accompanied by dyspnea, an apparent increase in the work of breathing, tachypnea, tachycardia, and cough. Chest radiographs and auscultation are often normal at this stage. Arterial blood gases (ABGs) reveal an uncompensated respiratory alkalosis with moderate hypoxemia with an increased alveolar-arterial difference in partial pressure of oxygen $P(A\text{-}a)O_2$.[25]

As intravascular fluid leaks into the interstitial and alveolar spaces, respiratory dysfunction becomes increasingly severe. Physical examination of the ARDS patient in this stage often reveals tachypnea, labored breathing, and cyanosis. Auscultation typically reveals inspiratory crackles due to pulmonary edema and atelectasis. Severe hypoxemia is usually present at this point.

Respiratory acidosis commonly occurs late in the course of ARDS as the patient's work of breathing causes respiratory muscle fatigue. Severe hypoxemia and high metabolic rate, combined with a poor cardiac output, can result in metabolic acidosis from anaerobic metabolism and lactic acid production. Results of other diagnostic tests including electrocardiogram (ECG), complete blood count (CBC), and chemistry profile are usually abnormal in response to the stress associated with the patient's illness, but these results rarely provide information leading to a diagnosis of the cause for the ARDS.

The chest radiographic findings, which may lag behind the pathology and symptoms of ARDS, can be divided into three stages according to the extent of lung injury.[26] In stage I (radiographically latent), pathophysiologic changes are occurring but the radiograph shows minimal abnormalities.[27] Stage II (acute) usually develops about 24 hours after the initial injury and is characterized by bilateral, diffuse, "fluffy" interstitial and alveolar infiltrates that are the hallmark of ARDS.[27,28] In contrast to "cardiogenic" pulmonary edema, the heart size is normal in patients with ARDS.[28] Fluid in the lung tissue highlights air in the airways and produces "air bronchograms." The third stage (chronic) begins late in the first week after lung injury. Alveolar fluid begins to clear, leaving interstitial edema. Pulmonary interstitial emphysema may also occur.[27] Most patients who survive ARDS eventually return to nearly normal gas exchange and chest radiograph findings.

Pulmonary capillary wedge pressure (PCWP) measured with a pulmonary artery catheter is usually normal or low in patients with ARDS. This contrasts sharply with the patient with cardiogenic pulmonary edema who has markedly elevated PCWP measurements.

TREATMENT

The treatment of ARDS is primarily supportive. Care for the patient with ARDS includes[29]:

1. Treatment of the precipitating problem.
2. Ensuring adequate tissue oxygenation (ventilation plus cardiovascular support)
3. Nutritional support

ARDS is a syndrome in which one of many different precipitating factors results in similar pulmonary damage. Some causes of ARDS are not amenable to intervention, but when treatment is available, such as in shock and sepsis, early treatment of the precipitating problem is crucial in limiting the severity of the ARDS.

Pharmacologic treatment of ARDS is aimed at correcting the underlying disorder and providing cardiovascular support. An example of this would include antibiotics for treatment of infection and vasopressors for treatment of hypotension.

Tissue oxygenation depends on adequate oxygen delivery (O_{2del}) which is a function of arterial oxygen content and cardiac output. This means that both ventilation and cardiac function are vital to the patient's survival. Mechanical ventilation with positive end-expiratory pressure (PEEP) is vital to ensure adequate oxygenation of the arterial blood in patients with ARDS. Positive pressure ventilation, however, may decrease cardiac output while improving arterial blood oxygenation (see farther on). Increases in arterial oxygenation from positive pressure ventilation are of little or no value if the cardiac output is correspondingly reduced by the increased intrathoracic pressure. As a result, the maximum level of PEEP tolerated by the patient is usually determined by cardiac function. Severe ARDS may cause death from tissue hypoxia when maximum fluid and vasopressor support for the heart do not provide adequate cardiac output with the level of PEEP required for adequate gas exchange in the lung.

Malnutrition often occurs in patients who are severely ill and particularly in patients receiving mechanical ventilation.[30-31] The effects of malnutrition on the pulmonary system include immunosuppression (decreased macrophage and T-lymphocyte activity), decreased hypoxic and hypercapneic drive, abnormal surfactant function, decreased intercostal and diaphragmatic muscle mass, and decreased strength owing to catabolism of respiratory muscles.[32] Malnourishment, therefore, can affect many factors critical not only to patient maintenance and supportive care but also to weaning from the mechanical ventilator. Enteral alimentation (food supplement via the nasogastric tube) is preferable whenever possible; but if the bowel is not functional, parenteral (intravenous) feeding is mandatory to provide adequate protein, fat, and carbohydrate along with minerals and vitamins.

Mechanical Ventilation in ARDS

Mechanical ventilation and PEEP neither prevent nor directly treat ARDS but rather keep the patient alive until the underlying problem resolves and the lungs heal enough to support the patient again. The mainstay of continuous mechanical ventilation (CMV) in ARDS is conventional volume-limited ventilation using tidal volumes of 10 to 15 mL/kg.[33-34] Full ventilatory support (usually with assist-control or intermittent mandatory ventilation [IMV]) is administered during the acute stages of the disease. Partial support usually is reserved for the recovery phase or ventilatory weaning.[33] Atelectatic regions may be reopened by PEEP, thereby converting areas of shunt to functional gas exchange units, resulting in increased arterial oxygenation at a lower fraction of inspired oxygen (F_{IO_2}). Recruitment of atelectatic alveoli also increases functional residual capacity (FRC) and pulmonary compliance.[35] Generally, the goal of CMV with PEEP is to obtain a PaO_2 greater than 60 mm Hg on an FIO_2 less than 0.60.

Although PEEP is an important part of maintaining adequate gas exchange in the lung of the ARDS patient, side effects are possible. Decreased pulmonary compliance from overdistended alveoli, decreased venous return and cardiac output, increased PVR, increased right ventricular afterload, and barotrauma may occur.[33,36,37] For these reasons, the use of "optimal" or "best" PEEP is suggested. Optimal or best PEEP is generally defined as that level of PEEP with the best O_{2del} at an FIO_2 less than 0.60.[33,35] PEEP levels that improve oxygenation but significantly reduce cardiac output are not optimal, as O_{2del} is reduced. In addition, the partial pressure of mixed venous oxygen ($P\overline{v}O_2$) provides information related to tissue oxygenation. A $P\overline{v}O_2$ less than 35 mm Hg indicates that tissue oxygenation is not optimal. Reductions in cardiac output (as may occur with the application of PEEP) typically result in a low $P\overline{v}O_2$. For this reason $P\overline{v}O_2$ can also be used to monitor optimal PEEP.

Failure of PEEP with conventional CMV is the most common reason for switching to ventilation with an inverse inspiratory-expiratory (I:E) ratio or high-frequency ventilation. Inverse I:E ratio ventilation is now more commonly used than high-frequency ventilation.[38-41] It works best when the patient is paralyzed and the ventilator is set (in a time-cycled mode) to a rate that allows each breath to start when exhalation from the previous breath has just reached the desired PEEP level. Respiratory rate can be lowered by adding inspiratory hold. This often results in lower average intrathoracic pressures in spite of higher PEEP and thus provides better O_{2del} as a result of improved cardiac output.

High-frequency positive-pressure ventilation (HFPPV), high-frequency oscillation (HFO), and high-frequency jet ventilation (HFJV) are methods that can sometimes provide adequate ventilation and oxygenation without the use of high lung volumes and high pressures. Only HFJV has been widely evaluated for the treatment of ARDS. No conclusive benefits have yet been shown for HFJV over those of conventional CMV with PEEP.[33]

Extracorporeal membrane oxygenation (ECMO) was studied during the 1970s as a method for providing adequate oxygenation without any mechanical ventilation so that the lung could heal without injury from positive pressure ventilation. Unfortunately, patients who were sick enough to fail conventional ventilation and qualify for ECMO had such severe lung injury that they developed pulmonary fibrosis and never regained pulmonary function.[33]

Weaning from Mechanical Ventilation in ARDS

Assurance of the patient's ability to survive without ventilator support is required before weaning the patient from the ventilator. The minimum criteria for these weaning parameters or "respiratory mechanics" are listed in Chapter 1.[34,42] Mechanical indices such as maximum inspiratory pressure (MIP), vital capacity (VC), and spontaneous tidal volume (VT) measure the patient's ability to move air in and out of the chest. None of these measurements, however, reflects the endurance capabilities of the respiratory muscles. Physiologic indices such as pH, dead space to tidal volume ratio (VD/VT), $P(A-a)O_2$, nutritional status, cardiovascular stability, and metabolic acid-base status reflect the patient's general reserve and ability to tolerate the stress of weaning.

Weaning from mechanical ventilation is done in a stepwise fashion to provide assurance that the patient has recovered to the point that weaning will be successful before the endotracheal tube can be removed. Weaning is usually initiated when the patient is medically stable, FIO_2 requirement is less than 0.40, PEEP requirement is 5 cm H_2O or less, and weaning parameters indicate a reasonable chance for spontaneous ventilation. IMV is popular as a weaning mode for patients recovering from ARDS because it allows the use of a small amount of PEEP until the patient is extubated and lets the patient gradually assume the work of breathing required for spontaneous ventilation.

Monitoring during weaning is an important adjunct for ensuring its success. Changes in blood pressure, increases in heart rate and respiratory rate, fall in pulse oximeter–measured arterial blood oxygen saturation, and decreased mental function indicate weaning failure. Gradual lengthening of the weaning periods can help prevent weaning failure caused by fatigue while the patient reacquires independent pulmonary function. The different methods of weaning from mechanical ventilation are described in more detail in Chapter 1.

Monitoring in ARDS

Pulmonary artery monitoring allows measurement of cardiac output, calculation of O_{2del}, and measurement of $P\bar{v}o_2$. These parameters are essential for the management of hemodynamic complications. Pulmonary artery monitoring also allows measurement of the filling pressures for the right (CVP) and left (PCWP) ventricles of the heart, which is useful in optimizing cardiac output (see Chapter 6).

A pulmonary artery catheter for hemodynamic monitoring becomes important when blood pressure is unstable enough to require vasoactive drugs (e.g., dopamine, norepinephrine [Levophed]) or when pulmonary function deteriorates to the point that PEEP greater than 10 cm H_2O is needed. Unstable blood pressure requiring large volumes of fluid in a patient with cardiac or pulmonary instability may also require placement of a pulmonary artery catheter and hemodynamic monitoring even before vasopressors are needed.

Positive-pressure ventilation may affect hemodynamic monitoring by falsely increasing the measured PCWP. Higher levels of PEEP may be transmitted to the monitoring catheter and falsely elevate CVP and PCWP.[43] This is more likely if the tip of the monitoring catheter is near the anterior chest (zone I) while the patient is lying supine. Zone I is the nondependent region of the lungs, where blood vessels are minimally distended with blood. If the catheter tip is located in one of these vessels, the pulmonary capillary pressure readings will be greatly affected by alveolar pressures, and therefore will be inaccurate. Zone III is the most dependent portion of the lung, where blood vessels are almost always distended with blood. If the catheter tip is located in zone III, the catheter measurement is minimally influenced by ventilation pressures.[43] The zone III location can be assessed by obtaining a lateral chest radiograph. When positioned in zone 3 the catheter tip will be positioned below the left atrium on the radiograph.

Static compliance (Cst) gives valuable information regarding stiffness of the lungs and chest wall, whereas dynamic compliance (Cdyn) provides information about airway resistance. Cst is calculated by dividing tidal volume (VT) by static (plateau) pressure (Pstat) less PEEP pressure (Cst = VT/Pstat − PEEP). Pstat is measured by obtaining a short inspiratory hold after a volume-limited breath. This hold can be achieved by using the pause control on the ventilator or by manual occlusion of the expiratory leg of the patient circuit. Pressure is monitored on the ventilator manometer during volume hold and should be less than the peak airway pressure (Ppk). Dynamic compliance is similarly calculated and measured, although Ppk is used instead of static pressure (Cdyn = VT/Ppk − PEEP).

Normal Cst is from 60 to 100 mL/cm H_2O and may be decreased to around 15 or 20 mL/cm H_2O by severe cases of pneumonia, pulmonary edema, atelectasis, fibrosis, and ARDS.[43] Because pressure is required to overcome airway resistance during ventilation, a portion of the peak airway pressure generated during the mechanical breath represents resistance to flow through the airways and ventilator circuit. Cdyn thus measures total impairment in airway flow resulting from both compliance and resistance. Normal Cdyn is 35 to 55 mL/cm H_2O. Cdyn can be adversely affected by all of the problems that decrease Cstat, plus factors that affect resistance (bronchoconstriction, airway edema, retained secretions, airway compression by tumor).[43]

Case Study

HISTORY

Ms. Y is a 23-year-old woman who was feeling fine until the morning of admission, when she began having severe chills, vomiting, diarrhea, headache, and a fever of 40°C. The symptoms persisted throughout the day and caused her to seek medical attention at the local emergency room about 6 PM. Ms. Y had an intrauterine device (IUD) inserted at a local family planning clinic 3 days before admission. At the time of admission she denied shortness of breath, wheezing, sputum production, cough, hemoptysis, orthopnea, chest pain, illicit drug use, or exposure to tuberculosis.

PHYSICAL EXAMINATION

General   *Patient is well-nourished, alert, and oriented to time, place, and person; she appears anxious but there is no evidence of respiratory distress.*

Vital Signs   *Temperature 40.3°C; respiratory rate 24/minute; pulse 104/minute; and blood pressure 126/75 mm Hg*

HEENT   *Sinuses not tender, throat not inflamed*

Neck   *Supple with full range of motion; trachea midline and mobile, carotid pulse ++ bilaterally with no bruits, no jugular venous distension; no cervical or supraclavicular lymphadenopathy*

Chest   *Normal configuration and normal expansion with breathing; normal resonance to percussion bilaterally*

Heart   *Regular rhythm with a rate of 104/minute; no murmurs, heaves, or rubs noted*

Lungs   *Clear breath sounds bilaterally*

Abdomen   *Lower abdominal tenderness to palpation; no masses or organomegaly; bowel sounds present*

Extremities   *No cyanosis, edema, or clubbing; pulses and reflexes are ++ and symmetric*

LABORATORY DATA

CHEST RADIOGRAPH

(Fig. 11–1).

CBC

White blood cells (WBC) 15,500 or 15.5×10^3 bands 16 percent, segs 65 percent, hemoglobin 10.2 g/100 mL.

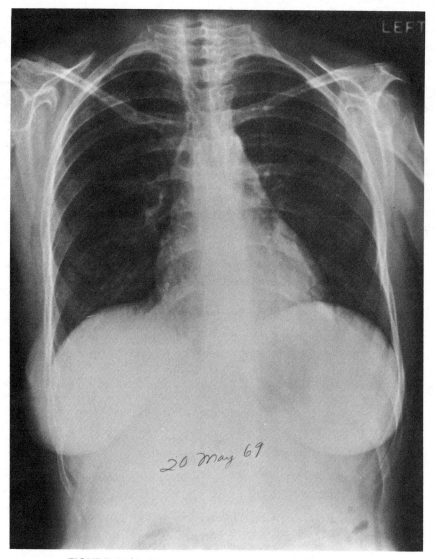

FIGURE 11–1 Chest radiograph taken upon admission.

ELECTROLYTES

Na$^+$ 135 mEq/liter, k$^+$ 4.5 mEq/liter, Cl$^-$ 105 mEq/liter, HCO$_3^-$ 15 mEq/liter

Questions

1. Does the patient appear to have a pulmonary problem at this time?
2. Does the patient's medical problem predispose her to the development of ARDS?
3. What signs and symptoms might suggest the onset of ARDS?
4. What is the significance of the lower abdominal tenderness?
5. What is the significance of the CBC and electrolyte findings?

Answers

1. No, the patient does not appear to have a pulmonary problem at this time.
2. Yes, the patient's problem does predispose her to the development of ARDS. Severe chills and fever suggest that an infection may be present and the most common cause of ARDS in medical intensive care units (ICUs) is infection.
3. Typical signs of ARDS include dyspnea, tachypnea, tachycardia, increased work of breathing, use of accessory muscles of ventilation, and cyanosis. On laboratory evaluation, ABGs may reveal hypoxemia in spite of a normal chest radiograph early in the course of the disorder.
4. Lower abdominal tenderness 2 to 4 days after placement of an IUD suggests infection in the lining of the uterus.
5. The elevated WBC count suggests infection. The increase in bands and segmented neutrophils also suggests acute infection. Bands are immature forms of neutrophils used in defense against infection only under severe conditions. Electrolytes show a decreased serum HCO_3^- which is consistent with metabolic acidosis or compensation for respiratory alkalosis.

Ms. Y has been started on intravenous (IV) antibiotic therapy. Results of a uterine swab show gram-negative diplococci, and a preliminary blood culture also shows gram-negative cocci. Twelve hours later, she begins complaining of increased shortness of breath. Respiratory rate is 34/minute, pulse 120/minute, and temperature 39.6°C. She is using her accessory muscles to breathe and chest auscultation now reveals fine, inspiratory crackles bilaterally.

An emergency ABG analysis shows pH 7.25, $Paco_2$ 21 mm Hg, Pao_2 62 mm Hg, HCO_3^- mEq/liter, base excess (BE) −17, and Sao_2 88 percent on room air. Based on these ABG results, the patient is placed on nasal cannula at 3 liter/minute.

Questions

6. What is the patient's acid-base and oxygenation status on the most recent ABG?
7. What is the most likely explanation for the sudden onset of dyspnea, tachypnea, and tachycardia?
8. Why is the chest radiograph normal just 4 hours before the onset of the respiratory problems?
9. What pathophysiology accounts for the adventitious lung sounds (fine, inspiratory crackles)?
10. What is the most likely cause of the accessory muscle usage?

Answers

6. The acid-base status of the patient suggests a metabolic acidosis, probably as a result of lactic acidosis. Moderate hypoxemia is present on room air. The hypoxemia would probably be worse if the patient was not hyperventilating.
7. The sudden onset of dyspnea, tachypnea, and tachycardia are most likely due to the acute onset of noncardiogenic pulmonary edema, also known as ARDS. The leakage of pulmonary edema into the lung causes the patient to experience hypoxemia and an increase in the work of breathing. These changes often occur suddenly and result in acute changes in

the clinical condition of the patient. Less likely causes for sudden onset of dyspnea would be pulmonary embolus and pneumothorax.

8. The chest radiograph is not sensitive to the early detection of damage to the alveolar capillary membrane. For this reason, it often lags behind the clinical findings in patients with ARDS.

9. Fine, inspiratory crackles are common in any disease that allows peripheral airways to stick shut during exhalation and pop open during inhalation. In ARDS patients, damage to the alveolar capillary membrane allows fluid to leak into the interstitial spaces and peripheral airways. The edema fluid sticks the small airways shut during exhalation and results in the presence of fine, inspiratory crackles over the entire chest.

10. The patient is using her accessory muscles to breathe because her lungs are much less compliant and more difficult to expand, as a result of the pulmonary edema and atelectasis associated with ARDS.

The patient continues to experience severe respiratory distress and is given an F_{IO_2} of 0.60 by entrainment device with the following ABG results: pH 7.26, P_{CO_2} 35 mm Hg, P_{O_2} 49 mm Hg, and HCO_3^- 16 mEq/liter. Her respiratory rate is now 38/minute and pulse 134/minute. A portable chest radiograph is obtained (Fig. 11–2).

Questions

11. Interpret the ABGs.
12. What treatment is needed at this point?
13. What does the chest radiograph demonstrate, and what are the findings typical for ARDS?

Answers

11. The ABGs show metabolic acidosis with moderate hypoxemia on 60 percent oxygen. Although the Pa_{CO_2} is not elevated, it is increased compared with the previous ABG results. This suggests relative hypoventilation that would accompany respiratory muscle fatigue.

12. Mechanical ventilation with PEEP is required because of the refractory nature of the hypoxemia. Refractory hypoxemia is most often caused by intrapulmonary shunting. PEEP holds the airways open and improves the distribution of ventilation thereby reducing shunt and increasing Pa_{O_2}. PEEP allows adequate oxygenation at a lower F_{IO_2} and reduces the chance for oxygen toxicity. Mechanical ventilation may not be required initially as the major problem is hypoxemia, but the patient with stiff lungs will soon tire and need ventilatory support.

13. The chest radiograph now shows bilateral alveolar infiltrates and air bronchograms with no cardiomegaly, which is typical for ARDS.

The patient is sedated, intubated, and placed on a volume ventilator.

Questions

14. What ventilator settings do you recommend?
15. How should the position of the endotracheal tube be assessed?

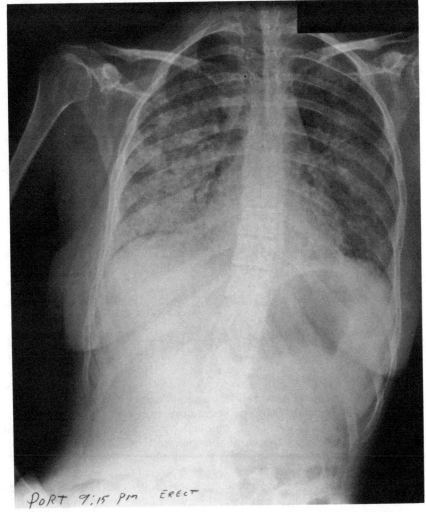

PoRT 9:15 PM ERECT

FIGURE 11–2 Portable chest radiograph taken approximately 14 hours after admission.

Answers

14. The patient should be placed on a volume ventilator with a tidal volume of 10 to 15 mL/kg of ideal body weight. Because she weighs 55 kg, an ideal tidal volume would be about 500 to 700 mL. The ventilator should be set in the assist-control or IMV mode with a backup rate of 10 to 14 breaths/minute. Initially a PEEP of 5 cm H_2O and an F_{IO_2} of 0.60 is reasonable.

15. The endotracheal tube position should be evaluated by listening to breath sounds bilaterally and by inspecting the chest radiograph.

After being mechanically ventilated, the patient's vital signs were pulse 150/minute, respiratory rate 22/minute, temperature 38.9°, and blood pressure 70/30 mm Hg. A pulmonary artery catheter was inserted because of the hypotension. An ABG analysis *showed pH 7.26, PCO_2 35 mm Hg, PO_2 55 mm Hg, HCO$_3^-$ 16 mEq/liter. Chest auscultation revealed bilateral inspiratory crackles. Chest radiograph showed diffuse bilateral fluffy infiltrates and normal heart size, consistent with noncardiogenic pulmonary edema. It also shows that the endotracheal tube is in good position. During a mechanical breath the peak pressure is 72 cm H$_2$O and static (plateau) pressure is 57 cm H$_2$O, with an exhaled tidal volume of 630 mL and a PEEP of 5 cm H$_2$O.*

Questions

16. What is the patient's static and dynamic compliance, and how do you interpret the measurements?
17. What pathophysiology accounts for the static compliance measurement?
18. What can be done therapeutically to increase the patient's static lung compliance?
19. What changes do you recommend for the mechanical ventilator settings?

Answers

16. Static compliance is calculated by dividing the static pressure minus the PEEP level into the exhaled tidal volume. In this case, the static compliance is 630 mL/57 − 5 cm H$_2$O = 12 mL/cm H$_2$O. The dynamic compliance is calculated by dividing the peak pressure minus the PEEP level into the tidal volume. In this case the dynamic compliance is 630 mL/72 − 5 cm H$_2$O = 9 mL/cm H$_2$O.

    Since normal static compliance is from 60 to 100 mL/cm H$_2$O and dynamic compliance is normally 35 to 55 mL/cm H$_2$O, the aforementioned values are well below normal. The measurements indicate that an increased pressure is required to inflate the lungs to a specific volume. This increases the work of breathing during spontaneous breathing and eventually will fatigue the respiratory muscles.

17. Pulmonary compliance is reduced when fluid moves from the injured pulmonary capillaries into the interstitial spaces, airways, and alveoli. Loss of surfactant, atelectasis, and fibrous tissue also reduce lung compliance.

18. Application of appropriate PEEP levels improves compliance by reducing alveolar opening pressures and increasing the distribution of ventilation.

19. Because the PaO_2 is still less than 60 mm Hg on an FIO_2 greater than 0.60, an increase in PEEP is indicated. No change in the tidal volume or rate is needed because the PaCO_2 is acceptable.

A PEEP study was performed, with the following results:

PEEP (cm H$_2$O)	PaO_2 (mm Hg)	P$\bar{v}O_2$ (mm Hg)	PAP (mm Hg)	PCWP (mm Hg)	Cardiac Output (l/min)	Cst (mL/ cmH$_2$O)
5	55	32	28/14	18	4.2	12
10	71	36	27/16	22	4.1	25
15	82	33	32/20	29	3.1	18

Questions

20. Based on these data, what is the best PEEP and why?
21. Are the PAP and PCWP readings believable when the PEEP level is at 15 cm H_2O? Why or why not?
22. Why did the $P\overline{v}O_2$ drop when the PEEP was increased from 10 to 15 cm H_2O?
23. Why did the static compliance fall when the PEEP was increased from 10 to 15 cm H_2O?
24. How can the zone position of the pulmonary artery catheter be assessed?

Answers

20. The best or optimal PEEP level at present is 10 cm H_2O. At a PEEP level of 10 cm H_2O, the cardiac output and PaO_2 are both at acceptable levels. The cardiac output dropped significantly when the PEEP was increased to 15 cm H_2O, suggesting that tissue oxygenation was not as good as it was when the PEEP was 10 cm H_2O.
21. No, the pulmonary artery measurements are not believable at a PEEP level of 15 cm H_2O. A PCWP that is almost equivalent to the systolic pulmonary artery pressure indicates that blood would be flowing backward through most of the cardiac cycle. This is probably impossible and certainly not consistent with life. Pressure from the airways is apparently being transmitted to the pulmonary artery catheter at higher levels of PEEP. The catheter may be in a zone I position.
22. The $P\overline{v}O_2$ dropped when the PEEP was increased from 10 to 15 cm H_2O because of the drop in cardiac output and oxygen delivery to the tissues. A lack of adequate tissue oxygenation causes severe desaturation of the blood in the tissues and venous blood returning to the heart thus has lower than normal levels of oxygen.
23. Initially PEEP increases pulmonary compliance by increasing alveolar recruitment; however, as PEEP is increased beyond optimal levels, over-distension of alveoli can occur, reducing lung compliance.
24. Because patent blood vessels are present in true zone III conditions, a wedged catheter in zone III shows an undamped waveform with distinct a and v waves. Location of the wedged pulmonary artery catheter can also be assessed via chest radiograph. A lateral chest radiograph will show the catheter tip below the left atrium when positioned in zone III.

A few hours later the patient suddenly developed labored breathing, a pulse rate of 140/minute, and a blood pressure of 70/40 mm Hg. A check of the ventilator revealed a significant increase in the peak inspiratory pressure with each mechanical breath and frequent sounding of the pressure limit alarm. The patient's level of consciousness deteriorated and peripheral cyanosis was present.

Questions

25. What may be causing the sudden deterioration of the patient?
26. What assessment procedures should be done to identify the cause of the sudden clinical deterioration?
27. What therapeutic procedures should be done in response to each of the most likely causes of the patient's problem?

25. The most likely causes of the sudden increases in peak pressure and clinical deterioration of the patient are pneumothorax or mucus plugging or kinking of the endotracheal tube.

26. Auscultation should be done to see if bilateral breath sounds are present. An immediate chest radiograph should be ordered. Attempts to pass a suction catheter should help determine whether the endotracheal tube is blocked.

27. The patient's F_{IO_2} should be increased to 1.0. If breath sounds are present on only one side and increased resonance to percussion is present on the side with absent breath sounds, a pneumothorax is probably present. A chest radiograph would confirm the pneumothorax; however, the patient may not survive the time needed to obtain and develop a chest radiograph. The attending physician should insert a large-bore needle between the ribs on the affected side if a pneumothorax is strongly suggested by the clinical findings and the patient is rapidly deteriorating. If the patient is stable, a chest radiograph can be ordered and a chest tube inserted if the film confirms the pneumothorax. If the endotracheal tube is blocked, it should be cleared or removed and replaced.

A portable emergency chest radiograph confirmed a right-sided pneumothorax. A chest tube was inserted, which resulted in immediate improvement in pulmonary and cardiovascular function. The patient was stabilized within a few hours.

Over the next 5 days the patient was maintained on mechanical ventilation with a PEEP of 10 to 12 cm H_2O and an F_{IO_2} of 0.40 to 0.45. Her vital signs remained stable and body temperature gradually decreased to near normal. Her hemodynamic status stabilized and on day 6 her cardiac output was 5.2 liters/minute with a PCWP of 14 mm Hg. Her static compliance was calculated to be 35 mL/cm H_2O and her chest radiograph demonstrated minimal improvement in the alveolar infiltrates. Auscultation revealed bilateral inspiratory crackles, especially in the dependent regions. Spontaneous respiratory mechanics demonstrated a vital capacity of 1100 mL, V_T of 420 mL, and MIP of −28 cm H_2O.

25. Is the patient ready to begin weaning from the mechanical ventilator? Why or why not?
26. What modes of ventilation can be used to wean the patient?
27. How should weaning proceed?

25. The patient appears to be ready for weaning because the values for respiratory mechanics (VC, V_T, and NIP) are acceptable; her static compliance is much improved; her cardiovascular parameters and vital signs (cardiac output, blood pressure, and PCWP) are stable; and the infection appears to be clearing.

26. Weaning can take place by using IMV and slowly decreasing the mechanical rate, by using pressure support, or by using continuous positive airway pressure (CPAP) for increasing periods of time as tolerated. The patient should be allowed to gradually resume her own work of breath-

ing without producing undue stress. The weaning can continue as long as the stress of weaning does not produce more than a 20 percent change in blood pressure, respiratory rate, or pulse rate.

27. After the F_{IO_2} is less than 0.45, the PEEP can be decreased in increments of 3 to 5 cm H_2O, as tolerated, to approximately 5 cm H_2O. Waiting at least 3 to 4 hours to assess the patient's response to each decrease in the PEEP before proceeding is desirable. Mechanical support can then be decreased until the patient is breathing on her own. After 12 to 24 hours of stability, the endotracheal tube can be removed.

Over the next 24 hours the patient was weaned from PEEP and mechanical ventilation. She was extubated and placed on a nasal cannula at 3 liters/minute. Over the next several days the chest radiograph continued to demonstrate improvement of the alveolar infiltrates with no residual fibrotic changes. Auscultation revealed improved breath sounds, although scattered inspiratory crackles remained. The patient was discharged on the 12th hospital day.

REFERENCES

1. Ashbaugh, DG, et al: Acute respiratory distress in adults. Lancet 2:319, 1967.

2. Murray, JF, et al: Mechanisms of acute respiratory failure. Am Rev Respir Dis 115:1071, 1977.

3. Dorinsky, PM and Gadek, JE: Mechanisms of multiple nonpulmonary organ failure in ARDS. Chest 96:885, 1989.

4. Bell, RC, et al: Multiple organ system failure and infection in adult respiratory distress syndrome. Ann Intern Med 99:293, 1983.

5. Montgomery, AB, et al: Causes of mortality in patients with the adult respiratory distress syndrome. Am Rev Respir Dis 132:485, 1985.

6. Matuschak, GM, et al: Effect of end stage liver failure on the incidence and resolution of the adult respiratory distress syndrome. J Crit Care 2:162, 1986.

7. Dorinsky, PM and Gadek, JE: Multiple organ failure in adult respiratory distress syndrome. Clin Chest Med 11(4):581, 1990.

8. Mizer, L, et al: Neutrophil accumulation and structural changes in nonpulmonary organs following phorbol myristate acetate-induced acute lung injury. Am Rev Respir Dis 139:1017, 1989.

9. Brigham, KL and Meyrick, B: Endotoxin and lung injury. Am Rev Respir Dis 133:913, 1987.

10. Goldblum, SE, et al: Interleukin-1-induced granulocytopenia and pulmonary leukostasis in rabbits. J Appl Physiol 62:1, 1987.

11. Albertine, KH: Ultrastructural abnormalities in increased-permeability pulmonary edema. Clin Chest Med 6:345, 1985.

12. Schnells, G, et al: Electron microscopic investigation of lung biopsies in patients with traumatic respiratory insufficiency. Acta Chir Scand (Suppl) 499:9, 1980.

13. Teplitz, C: The core pathobiology and integrated medical science of adult acute respiratory insufficiency. Surg Clin North Am 56:1091, 1976.

14. Tomashefski, JF: Pulmonary pathology of the adult respiratory distress syndrome. Clin Chest Med 11(4):593, 1990.

15. Tomashefski, JF: The pulmonary vascular lesions of the adult respiratory distress syndrome. Am J Pathol 112:112, 1983.

16. Snapper, JR: Lung mechanics in pulmonary edema. Clin Chest Med 6:393, 1985.

17. Petty, TL, et al: Abnormalities in lung elastic properties and surfactant function in adult respiratory distress syndrome. Chest 75:571, 1979.

18. Seeger, W, et al: Alteration of surfactant function due to protein leakage: Special interaction with fibrin monomer. J Appl Physiol 58:326, 1985.

19. Lamy, M, et al: Pathologic features and mechanisms of hypoxemia in adult respiratory distress syndrome. Am Rev Respir Dis 114:267, 1976.

20. Dantzker, DR, et al: Ventilation-perfusion distributions in the adult respiratory distress syndrome. Am Rev Respir Dis 120:1039, 1979.

21. Calvin, JE, Langlois, S, and Garneys, G: Ventricular interaction in a canine model of acute pulmonary hypertension and its modulation by vasoactive drugs. J Crit Care 3:43, 1988.

22. Zapol, WM and Snider, MT: Pulmonary hypertension in severe acute respiratory failure. N Engl J Med 296(9):476, 1977.

23. Stool, EW, et al: Dimensional changes of the left ventricle during acute pulmonary arterial hypertension in dogs. Am J Cardiol 33:868, 1974.

24. Bone, RC: The adult respiratory distress syndrome: Diagnosis and treatment. Proc Cardiol 5:49, 1979.

25. Flick, MR: Pulmonary edema and acute lung injury. In Murray, JF and Nadel, JA (eds): Textbook of Respiratory Medicine. WB Saunders, Philadelphia, 1988, pp 1359.

26. Aberle, DR and Brown, K: Radiologic considerations in the adult respiratory distress syndrome. Clin Chest Med 11(4):737, 1990.

27. Greene, R: Adult respiratory distress syndrome. Acute alveolar damage. Radiology 163:57, 1987.

28. Milne, EN, et al: The radiologic distinction of cardiogenic and noncardiogenic edema. AJR 144:879, 1985.

29. Taylor, RW: The adult respiratory distress syndrome. In Kirby, RR and Taylor, RW (eds): Respiratory Failure. Year Book Medical, Chicago, 1986.

30. Driver, AG and LeBrun, M: Iatrogenic malnutrition in patients receiving ventilator support. JAMA 244:2195, 1980.

31. Larca, L and Greenbaum, DM: Effectiveness of intensive nutritional regimens in patients who fail to wean from mechanical ventilation. Crit Care Med 10:297, 1982.

32. Procter, CD: Nutritional support. In Kirby, RR and Taylor, RW (eds): Respiratory Failure. Year Book Medical, Chicago, 1986.

33. Stoller, JK and Kacmarek, RM: Ventilatory strategies in the management of the adult respiratory distress syndrome. Clin Chest Med 11(4):755, 1990.

34. Balk, RA and Bone, RC: Mechanical ventilation. In Bone, RC, George, RB, and Hudson, LD (eds): Acute Respiratory Failure. Churchill Livingstone, New York, 1987, p 213.

35. Gong, H: Positive-pressure ventilation in the adult respiratory distress syndrome. Clin Chest Med 11(4):69–88, 1982.

36. Kuckelt, W, et al: Effect of PEEP on gas exchange, pulmonary mechanics, and hemodynamics in adult respiratory distress syndrome (ARDS). Intensive Care Med 7:177, 1981.

37. Suter, PM, et al: Optimum end-expiratory airway pressure in patients with acute pulmonary failure. N Engl J Med 292:284, 1975.

38. Gurevitch, MJ, et al: Improved oxygenation and lower peak airway pressure in severe adult respiratory distress syndrome. Treatment with inverse ratio ventilation. Chest 89(2):211, 1986.

39. Lain, DC, et al: Pressure control inverse ratio ventilation as a method to reduce peak inspiratory pressure and provide adequate ventilation and oxygenation. Chest 95:1081, 1989.

40. Tharratt, RS, et al: Pressure controlled inverse ratio ventilation in severe adult respiratory failure. Chest 94:755, 1988.

41. Abraham, E and Yoshihara, G: Cardiorespiratory effects of pressure-controlled inverse ratio ventilation in severe respiratory failure. Chest 96:1356, 1989.

42. Spence, TH: Acute respiratory failure in chronic obstructive lung disease. In Kirby, RR and Taylor, RW (eds): Respiratory Failure. Year Book Medical, Chicago, 1986, p 260.

43. Williams-Colon, S and Thalken, FR: Management and monitoring of the patient in respiratory failure. In Scanlan, CL, Spearman, CB, and Sheldon, RL (eds): Fundamentals of Respiratory Care. CV Mosby, St Louis, 1990, p 780.

Chapter 12

George H. Hicks, MS, RRT

CHEST TRAUMA

INTRODUCTION

Trauma is one of the more serious public health concerns in the United States today. Trauma continues to be responsible for approximately 130,000 deaths, 70 million injuries, and economic losses that exceed 80 billion dollars annually.[1-3] It is the leading cause of death in people less than 40 years of age and is the third leading cause of death in the general population, after heart disease and cancer.[1,2] Approximately one fourth of these injuries results in a bed-disabling condition that requires extended care and rehabilitation. Owing to the younger age of most of its victims, trauma causes more disability and loss of productivity than heart disease and cancer combined.[2]

Motor vehicle accidents, suicide, homicide, and accidental falls are the most common causes of trauma-related deaths.[1] The North American Major Trauma Outcome Study has found the chest to be the third most common anatomic site of injury (Table 12–1) and further found chest wall (e.g., rib fracture) and lung parenchymal injuries (e.g., lung contusion) to be the most common consequences of severe chest trauma (Fig. 12–1).[4] Approximately 25 percent of all trauma-related deaths per year are attributable to chest injuries.[3-5] In patients with multiple trauma injuries, the presence of major chest trauma (e.g., flail chest or lung contusion) increases the overall mortality rate from 27 to as high as 68 percent.[6] Those chest trauma victims who present with respiratory distress and require endotracheal intubation in the emergency department have a mortality rate of 58 percent and, if complicated by the presence of shock, their mortality rate increases to 73 percent.[7]

Table 12–1 Distribution of Various Injuries from Motor Vehicle Accidents

Location	Percent
Extremities	34
Head and neck	32
Chest	25
Abdomen	15

Source: Adapted from LoCicero, J and Mattox, KL: Epidemiology of chest trauma. Surg Clin North Am 69:15, 1989.

Distribution of Injuries Following Chest Trauma

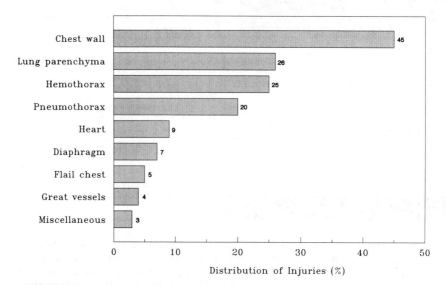

FIGURE 12–1 The distribution of specific types of injuries in 15,047 chest trauma patients from the North American Trauma Outcome Study. (Developed from data presented in LoCicero, J and Mattox, KL: Epidemiology of chest trauma. Surg Clin North Am 69:15–19, 1989.)

ETIOLOGY

Chest trauma injuries are classified as penetrating, blunt, or a combination of these two types of injuries (Table 12–2). Most penetrating injuries of the chest are caused during homicides, suicides, or the attempts to commit these acts. Penetrating wounds are produced by knives, bullets, and metal fragments from explosions. The injuries from high-speed missiles are proportional to the kinetic energy they impart to the tissues. The mass of the missile and its velocity determine the extent of the injury. For example, a rifle bullet traveling 1000 m/second may induce 36 times more damage than a pistol bullet of similar size that is traveling 170 m/second.[3]

Missiles traveling at high speeds and possessing high kinetic energy damage both the objects they pierce and the surrounding tissues. The explosive effect of high-speed bullets can cause not only massive tissue and blood vessel destruction

Table 12–2 Mechanisms of Injuries in Chest Trauma

Mechanism	Example
Blunt Trauma	
Acceleration or deceleration	Motor vehicle accident
Compression	Crushing, blasts, or falls
Penetration Trauma	
High-speed impact or penetration	Gunshot wound
Low-speed penetration	Stab wound

along their trajectory, but also cavitational effects which pull external debris deep into the tissue.[3] In contrast, slower bullets often cause minimal soft tissue injuries to surrounding tissues.[8] The extent of tissue damage is increased when softer bullets (e.g., unjacketed lead or hollow-point bullets) break up upon contact with bone and the fragments penetrate into more tissue or deform and impart all their kinetic energy to the surrounding tissue.

Wounds from close-range shotgun blasts often cause severe damage by producing one large entrance wound and extensive underlying tissue damage from numerous pellet penetrations. These wounds are further complicated by the wad, a plastic casing that separates the pellets and the gunpowder, which enters the tissue and can cause severe infections.[9] Long-range shotgun blast injuries are associated with multiple small-caliber pellet entrance wounds that cause less deep tissue destruction.[9] Low-speed penetrating knife wounds cause chest injuries that are largely localized to the tissues that have been pierced and the resulting hemorrhage.

Blunt trauma to the chest, which is much more frequently encountered, causes severe damage by crushing tissue, fracturing bones, and shearing tissue upon rapid acceleration or deceleration.[3,5,10] Sudden and severe deceleration causes violent motion or crushing of mobile structures. This violent motion and resultant shearing forces cause microscopic and macroscopic tears in the tissues, especially at junctions with more firmly supported tissues. In the United States, blunt chest trauma occurs most frequently during motor vehicle accidents.[4]

INJURY PATHOPHYSIOLOGY

Chest Wall Injuries

Cutaneous injuries are rarely fatal (with the exception of a burn injury; see Chapter 9), but they may be the source of considerable morbidity. Subcutaneous emphysema, a common manifestation of chest injuries, usually develops secondary to air leakage from a disrupted airway. Air migrates along the great vessels and fascial planes to the mediastinum and then into the soft tissues of the neck and chest. Subcutaneous emphysema is usually only a temporary cosmetic problem because of the skin's distensible behavior; however, it indicates underlying problems that could be life threatening.

Open or "sucking" chest wounds can act as oneway valves that allow air entry on inspiration and air trapping during exhalation. This can lead to a pneumothorax that can rapidly escalate to a fatal tension pneumothorax. An open chest wound that approaches or exceeds the diameter of the glottis can cause ventilatory failure as a result of the wound's better properties as an "airway" between the thorax and atmosphere. The loss of lung volume, compromised alveolar ventilation, and ventilation-perfusion ($\dot{V}/\dot{Q}$) mismatching that result from an open chest wound and pneumothorax may lead to respiratory failure and shock.

Clavicular fractures are rarely a clinical problem unless their sharp bony ends lacerate the underlying blood vessels, brachial plexus, or lung.

Rib fractures are more common in adults than in children because of the child's highly elastic costochondral cartilage. In contrast, the ribs of the older patient are more brittle and more likely to break on impact. Fractures to ribs 1 and 2 are rare because of the added protection and support provided by the bones and tissues of the shoulder. An impact great enough to fracture the first and second ribs is associated with severe injuries to the head, neck, lung, great vessels, and tracheobronchial tree.[3,11,–13] Ribs 5 through 9 are more often broken with fractures that occur along the posterior aspect and midaxillary line.[13,14] High-intensity impacts to local areas of the chest can cause the ribs to break and then force them through the pleural membranes and result in hemothorax, pneumothorax, or hemopneumothorax. Impacts that fracture ribs 9 through 11 can cause abdominal injuries and have a higher association with intra-abdominal bleeding and shock from liver or splenic laceration.[3,14] Rib fractures often cause pain, shallow breathing, guarded cough, and atelectasis. Fifty to 70 percent of patients with multiple rib fractures have associated complications including pneumothorax, hemopneumothorax, flail chest, pulmonary contusion, cardiac contusion, and abdominal injuries (Fig. 12–2).[13,14]

Sternal fractures and costochondral separations are often the product of a high-speed deceleration impact to the anterior chest during a motor vehicle accident. Sternal injuries are frequently associated with flail chest, cardiac contusion, great vessel rupture, or tracheobronchial rupture.[3] The most common site of sternal fractures is along the junction of the manubrium and sternal body or transversely through the sternal body.

Flail chest is characterized by an unstable chest wall that has an asymmetric paradoxic motion during the breathing cycle. It is caused by two fractures along the length of the same rib in three or more adjacent ribs (Fig. 12–3).[13–15] The two-point fracture results in an unsupported portion of the chest wall that can produce paradoxic or "flail" motion (Fig. 12–4). During the inspiratory phase, the unsupported region is pulled in while the rest of the chest is pulled out, and the reverse occurs during exhalation. Hypoxemia and CO_2 retention may occur as a result of both increased work of breathing and underlying pulmonary contusion.[3,14,15] The paradoxic motion associated with a flail chest becomes more apparent over the first 48 hours as lung compliance decreases and the respiratory effort increases. As the work of breathing increases and $\dot{V}/\dot{Q}$ mismatch intensifies, respiratory failure may eventually occur. Mortality has been reduced from approximately 50 percent to

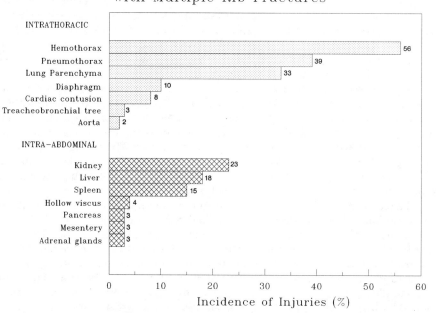

FIGURE 12–2 The incidence of intrathoracic and intra-abdominal injuries associated with multiple rib fractures in 542 chest injury cases. (Developed from data presented in Wilson, JM, et al: Severe chest trauma: Morbidity implication of first and second rib fracture in 120 patients. Arch Surg 113:846, 1978.)

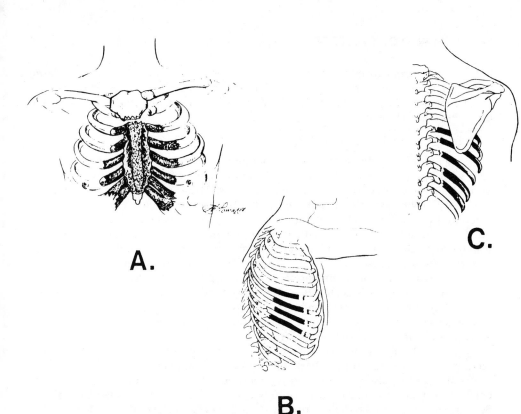

FIGURE 12–3 Areas of the thoracic cage involved in flail chests. *A*, Anterior sternal flail; *B*, lateral flail; *C*, posterior flail. (From Pate, JW: Chest wall injuries. Surg Clin North Am 69:59–70, 1989, with permission.)

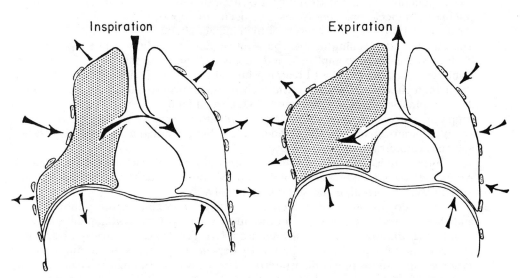

FIGURE 12–4 Paradoxic or flail motion of the chest following multiple rib fractures. The resulting motion produces a very inefficient movement of gas that can lead to respiratory muscle fatigue and respiratory failure. (From Wilkins, EW: Non-cardiovascular thoracic injuries: Chest wall, bronchus, lung, esophagus, and diaphragm. In Burke JF, Boyd, RJ, and McCabe, CJ (eds): Trauma Management. Year Book Medical, Chicago, 1988, with permission.)

less than 3 percent through the use of positive-pressure ventilation to "splint" the flail segment internally and support the patient's breathing.[15-17] In very severe cases, the use of surgically placed rib plates or wiring has been successful in stabilizing the chest wall.[14,18,19]

Lung Parenchymal Injuries

Pneumothorax, hemothorax, and hemopneumothorax are frequently associated with blunt chest trauma (see Fig. 12–1) and are characterized by air, blood, or air and blood collection in the pleural cavity. These conditions are commonly caused by broken ribs that penetrate the lungs or tear intercostal arteries or both. Bleeding from the lung's low-pressure pulmonary circulation is relatively slow and often self-limiting, compared with that from higher-pressure intercostal arteries, which can produce more brisk bleeding. Air and blood in the pleural cavity decrease lung volume and cause increased $\dot{V}/\dot{Q}$ mismatching. Pneumothorax is usually not associated with physiologic impairment until more than 30 percent of the lung has collapsed. The diagnosis is suggested by diminished breath sounds on the affected side and confirmed by chest radiographic findings of air or fluid or both in the pleural space. Placement of a chest tube is the treatment of choice to evacuate the air and blood and to reexpand the lung.

A bronchopleural fistula is characterized by a persistent leak of air into the pleural space despite proper chest tube placement and suction. Its occurrence is rare and is almost always associated with a severe lung laceration or tracheobronchial rupture and the use of positive-pressure ventilation. The leakage can exceed 50 percent of a delivered tidal breath during mechanical ventilation and can be further exacerbated by the application of positive end-expiratory pressure (PEEP). As the leakage increases, effective ventilation and oxygenation become more difficult. Use of multiple chest tubes, independent lung ventilation, high-frequency jet ventilation, and surgical repair or resection have been used successfully.[19,20]

Pulmonary contusion is associated with interstitial edema and hemorrhage that is generally localized to the area of lung underlying the impact site of blunt trauma.[3] On occasion, contusions can occur on opposite sides of the chest or throughout both lungs as a result of high-impact shock waves from a blast injury. The edema and bleeding in the contused region of the lung cause a progressive decline in local lung compliance and airway inflammation that lead to atelectasis. Hypoxemia and the work of breathing intensify during the first 48 to 72 hours as the pathologic changes evolve.[3] These changes can progress to the development of adult respiratory distress syndrome (ARDS). Small contusions can be managed with supplemental oxygen and monitoring. Ventilatory support with PEEP is needed when respiratory failure occurs. Independent lung ventilation may be necessary if severe asymmetric lung injury is present.[19]

Intrabronchial bleeding occurs in many chest trauma victims with penetrating wounds. Massive bleeding can rapidly lead to asphyxiation. Therapeutic efforts aim at reducing the bleeding and suctioning the airway.

Aspiration of stomach contents is relatively common in the trauma patient and should always be suspected in the unconscious patient with an elevated alveolar-arterial difference in partial pressure of oxygen $P(\text{A-a})o_2$. Airway obstruction and aspiration pneumonitis in the gravity-dependent portions of the lungs are the major complications of gastric aspiration. The signs of inflammatory changes in the lung are often delayed for 12 to 24 hours. The combination of chest trauma and aspiration increase the risk of ARDS.[21]

Airway Injuries

Impact injury to the larynx may produce sudden airway occlusion secondary to a crushed larynx or cricotracheal dislocation. A more common problem is progressive airway obstruction from edema. Most laryngeal injuries are caused by steering wheel or dashboard impacts in unrestrained drivers involved in motor vehicle accidents. Symptoms of laryngeal and tracheal injury include hoarseness, inability to lay supine, dysphagia, laryngeal tenderness, tracheal deviation, and subcutaneous emphysema.[22] These signs and symptoms produce important clues to tracheal injury. Inspiratory stridor may not be apparent until the airway is 70 to 80 percent occluded.[3] Lateral neck radiographs may be deceptively negative, whereas the computed tomography (CT) scan can produce a more accurate noninvasive evaluation of the laryngeal anatomy. Initial laryngoscopy should be done cautiously in the operating room in case sudden airway obstruction occurs and emergent tracheostomy is required. Placement of an endotracheal tube with the aid of a bronchoscope or emergent tracheostomy if emergent bronchoscopy is impossible is the treatment of choice for severe laryngeal trauma and airway obstruction.[3,22]

Blunt and penetrating chest injuries can lead to tracheal and bronchial injuries. Sudden compression of the thorax can cause deceleration shearing of the trachea or bronchus.[23] Most of these injuries occur within 2 cm of the carina and result in pneumothorax and subcutaneous emphysema.[23] Almost all victims of transection of the trachea are dead upon arrival to the emergency department and frequently have two or more other major injuries.[24] Tracheal and bronchial laceration or rupture requires rapid evaluation by bronchoscopy and direct repair by thoracotomy. Surgical repair of a lacerated trachea or bronchus is the treatment of choice. Diagnostic and therapeutic bronchoscopy is an important tool in managing the patient with tracheobronchial injuries.

Heart and Great Vessel Injuries

Chest trauma can lead to a variety of cardiac injuries, which include penetration, rupture, tamponade, coronary artery lacerations and occlusion, myocardial contusion, pericardial effusion, septal defects, valvular injuries, and great vessel rupture.[3] These injuries are often rapidly fatal.

Cardiac penetrating injuries are more frequently caused by knife and gunshot wounds to the chest and have a mortality rate of 50 to 85 percent.[21] Blunt trauma is more often associated with cardiac rupture injuries (right ventricle more common than left) and has been found to have a survival rate of approximately 50 percent for those patients who present to the emergency department with vital signs.[26] Following rupture of a cardiac chamber or lacerations of the coronary or great vessels, blood will rapidly fill the pericardial sac and result in tamponade. As little as 60 to 100 mL of blood can produce cardiac tamponade and cardiogenic shock as a result of reduced diastolic filling.[25] Puncture wounds through the pericardial sac and cardiac chamber cause brisk bleeding, which will dominate the clinical picture. Interestingly, the presence of tamponade following a cardiac gunshot wound is actually associated with a higher survival rate owing to its effects of reducing the blood loss and associated hypotension.[27] Cardiac tamponade is often associated with clinical signs of Beck's triad—distended neck veins, hypotension, and diminished heart tone.[3] However, Beck's triad may not be seen in those patients who are hypovolemic following hemorrhage. A widened mediastinum on the chest radiograph may suggest mediastinal bleeding and/or tamponade. Echocardiography is more helpful in establishing the diagnosis of tamponade. Emergency exploratory thoracotomy with heart-lung bypass, surgical repair, and adequate transfusion are the corrective measures of choice.

Myocardial contusion following blunt chest trauma is not easily identified, but in carefully monitored patients the incidence probably approaches 25 percent.[3] The pathologic changes in the contused heart include intramyocardial hemorrhage, myocardial edema, coronary artery occlusion, myofibril degeneration, and myocardial cell necrosis.[28] These changes lead to arrhythmias and hemodynamic instability that are very similar to those found following a myocardial infarction. Electrocardiographic findings often show tachycardia, ST-segment elevation, T-wave changes, and occasional premature ventricular contractions.[3,25,29] Plasma enzyme levels (e.g., serum glutamic-oxaloacetic transaminase [SGOT], lactate dehydrogenase [LDH], and creatine phosphokinase [CPK]) are almost always elevated following blunt chest trauma and are therefore of little diagnostic value. Plasma CPK-MB isoenzyme elevation appears to be more discriminatory and contributes to the diagnosis of myocardial contusion.[25,29] Pulmonary artery catheterization is often useful in monitoring hemodynamic performance and for treating signs of failure. Echocardiography, radionuclide angiography, and serial electrocardiography, hemodynamics, and CPK-MB monitoring form the diagnostic array for detecting myocardial contusion. Patients are treated in the same fashion as if they had a myocardial infarction. In those patients with cardiac failure, use of an intra-aortic balloon pump has been found useful in supporting cardiac output.[30] Often there is complete clinical recovery with minimal scarring of the myocardium. The overall mortality in patients with myocardial contusion is approximately 10 percent.[31]

Aortic rupture and exsanguination following blunt chest trauma in a motor vehicle accident leads to rapid death. Approximately 8000 people have aortic ruptures in this country each year and about 80 to 90 percent die in the first few minutes following the event.[29,32] The upper descending thoracic aorta is the most common site of rupture in those who are admitted to the emergency department with vital signs.[29] The patient frequently presents in profound hypotension and often with chest radiographic findings showing a widened mediastinum. Aortic angiography is the diagnostic method of choice for detecting a ruptured or lacerated aorta. If the patient presents in shock and with an obviously widened mediastinum, emergent thoracotomy, surgical repair, and transfusion are needed.

Diaphragmatic Injuries

Penetrating trauma is the most frequent cause of diaphragmatic injury. Blunt trauma causes diaphragmatic rupture in only 5 percent of blunt abdominal injuries, with the left diaphragm injured 90 percent of the time.[18,33] Rupture of the diaphragm is associated with splenic rupture, hemothorax, impaired diaphragmatic motion, shock, ventilatory failure, CO_2 retention, coma, and bowel herniation up into the thorax, resulting in bowel strangulation and reduced lung volume.[3,18,33] The mortality rate is reported at 29 percent, but it is certainly associated with other injuries rather than the diaphragmatic lesion alone.[33] The diagnosis is usually made by evaluation of the chest and abdominal radiographs, CT scans, or during exploratory laparotomy. Diaphragmatic rupture requires surgical evaluation and closure. Diaphragmatic contusion and weakness are much less frequently diagnosed and are probably associated with ventilatory fatigue and impaired cough.

Delayed Complications of Chest Wall Trauma

Chronic pain, recurring atelectasis, and pneumonia are the most common delayed and prolonged chest wall problems following chest injuries.[34] In most patients the cause remains unclear and is usually managed with analgesics and reassurance. Occasionally, surgery may be necessary to repair painfully persistent fractures of the ribs and sternum. Pleural infection can arise from retained hemothorax or foreign body and result in empyema, pleurisy, and fibrothorax.[34] Thoracotomy, pleural drainage, antibiotics, and pleural decortication are frequently used to correct poorly responding pleural infections and avert the formation of a fibrothorax.

Penetrating and blunt chest injuries can lead to pulmonary artery-to-vein fistula, aortic aneurysm, cardiac valvular insufficiency, constrictive pericarditis, diaphragmatic herniation, and esophageal stricture or fistula.[35] Retained foreign bodies have been found to migrate or erode into other areas many years following the initial injury. Foreign body migration can result in embolic events. Erosion of a sharp body can result in hemoptysis, pneumonia, and lung abscess. Acute and rehabilitative care coupled with surgical repairs is often needed for these long-term complications.

CLINICAL FEATURES

Gathering a proper history about the events of the trauma is vital to understanding the extent of injuries. Information about the nature of the motor vehicle accident (e.g., whether seat restraints were used, whether the victim was ejected, size of vehicle, and so on), the caliber or type of gun used, and how long the victim went untreated or was in shock are useful pieces of information. Preexisting heart, lung, vascular, and renal disease and a history of substance abuse are important because they often complicate the response to trauma.

A rapid and careful physical examination should include evaluation of the patient's airway, breathing efforts, blood pressure, signs of flail chest, presence of subcutaneous emphysema, and symmetry and quality of breath sounds. A rapid and systematic method of initial evaluation of the nervous, circulatory, and respiratory systems is found in the trauma score.[36] This scoring system is a simple method for evaluating trauma patients and determining the severity of their injuries (Table 12–3). In a recent study of 2166 patients, the revised trauma score was able to identify survivors and the fatally injured (e.g., trauma scores equal to 12 and 6 were associated with 99.5 percent and 63 percent survival, respectively) for better triaging to trauma centers.[37] The findings from these examinations then dictate which additional tests and care should be performed.

A variety of studies and laboratory procedures are frequently used to better define the nature and extent of chest injuries. The portable anteroposterior (AP) chest radiograph is virtually necessary in all cases to evaluate the patient further and help guide emergent care. Complete blood count (CBC), electrolytes, arterial blood gases (ABGs), and electrocardiogram (ECG) are done on admission and then serially. More specialized studies such as CT, magnetic resonance imaging (MRI), and angiography are done to determine more precisely the extent of injuries.

Table 12–3 Revised Trauma Score

Glasgow Coma Scale	Systolic Blood Pressure	Respiratory Rate	Points
13–15	>89	10–29	4
9–12	76–89	>29	3
6–8	50–75	6–9	2
4–5	1–49	1–5	1
3	0	0	0

Example: Glasgow coma scale* = 14; blood pressure = 80; respiratory rate = 35
   Points   4
Trauma score = 10

*Glasgow coma scale is a simple neurologic examination system that awards points according to the patient's best eye movement, verbal response, and motor response to various stimuli (see Chapter 10 for a more detailed explanation of the Glasgow coma scale).

Source: Adapted from Champion, HR, et al: A revision of the trauma score. J Trauma 29:623, 1989.

TREATMENT

Approximately 80 percent of all trauma-related deaths occur in the first few hours following injury (Fig. 12–5).[38] Victim survival improves with rapid access to advanced life support and to trauma center care. Acute care for chest trauma includes maintenance of a patent airway, supplementary oxygen with an FIO_2 of 1.0 (e.g., nonrebreathing mask, resuscitation bag with reservoir, or high-flow oxygen delivery system), mechanical ventilation, placement of peripheral and central intravenous (IV) lines for fluid or blood administration, chest tube placement, and possible direct admission to the operating room (OR) for emergency thoracotomy. Placement of a pulmonary artery catheter is useful when managing a patient who is hemodynamically unstable or who requires large amounts of fluids to maintain fluid balance or both. Pain management is also important. Use of patient-controlled analgesia (PCA) devices for the infusion of pain medication (e.g., systemic infusion or thoracic epidural analgesia) improves the patient's pain toleration, cooperation in deep breathing, improvement in pulmonary function, and avoidance of ventilatory support.[39,40]

Airway Management

Airway obstruction following trauma is felt to be the leading cause of preventable death.[38] Airway obstruction is most commonly caused by the tongue slipping back into the oropharynx. Aspiration of vomitus, blood, excessive saliva, dentures, and oral-laryngeal injuries with swelling are also causes of airway obstruction. Manual reposition of the victim's head and placement of an oral-pharyngeal airway facilitates a patent airway and bag-mask ventilation with 100 percent oxygen.

A proper-sized cuffed oral endotracheal tube is the artificial airway of choice for most emergency airway maintenance procedures. It permits positive-pressure ventilation, facilitates endotracheal suctioning, and helps protect the lungs from aspirating gastric contents. If the patient has a suspected cervical fracture, bronchoscopic-assisted placement of a nasotracheal tube is recommended because this method requires less extension of the head for placement. Inadequate preoxygenation, mainstem intubation, esophageal intubation, respiratory alkalosis secondary to excessive ventilation, and/or vasovagal reflex bradycardia may result in cardiac arrest during attempted endotracheal tube placement.

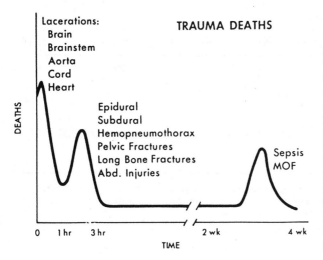

FIGURE 12–5 The trimodal distribution and principal causes of death following trauma. The initial 50 percent die almost immediately, another 30 percent within hours of admission to the hospital, and the remaining 20 percent later from complications (multiple organ failure [MOF]). (From Trunkey, DD: Organization of trauma care. In Burke, JF, Boyd, RJ, and McCabe, CJ (eds): Trauma Management. Year Book Medical, Chicago, 1988, with permission.)

Careful examination of the endotracheal tube placement should be done to ensure bilateral ventilation. Right mainstem bronchial intubation occurs in approximately 30 percent of victims who require resuscitation.[41] A chest radiograph and fiberoptic bronchoscopy are indicated to evaluate excessive blood being suctioned from the airway. Diagnostic and therapeutic fiberoptic bronchoscopy is often very useful in patients with persistent or recurring atelectasis. A double-lumen endotracheal tube may be required in cases of severe asymmetric lung contusion or tracheobronchial rupture, which necessitates independent lung ventilation. In situations when endotracheal intubation and tracheostomy tube placement are difficult or not possible, cricothyrotomy can be performed until it is possible to place a tracheostomy tube. In situations when no other airway access is available, the insertion of a 12-gauge cricothyroid needle can provide short-term percutaneous transtracheal oxygenation and ventilation until a tracheostomy tube can be placed.[42]

Ventilatory Support

Patients who present in apnea, who are in impending respiratory failure (respiratory rate greater than 35/minute), or who are in frank respiratory failure (Pao_2 less than 60 mm Hg, $Paco_2$ greater than 50, and pH less than 7.20) will require ventilatory support. Initial ventilator settings for a patient with an unknown degree of chest injury should be directed toward complete support with assist-control volume-limited ventilation with a tidal volume setting of 10 mL/kg, set rate of 15/minute, flow setting to provide an inspiratory-expiratory rate (I:E) of 1:3, and an Fio_2 of 1.0. Adjustments can then be made after further clinical examination and ABG results are available. PEEP of 5 to 15 cm H_2O is frequently necessary to improve lung volume and oxygenation. However, caution is always necessary when using positive-pressure ventilation and PEEP in chest trauma victims because of their higher risk for hypotension and barotrauma. As the patient can spontaneously breathe more effectively, synchronized intermittent mandatory ventilation (SIMV) combined with pressure support (PS) is useful in weaning these patients from ventilatory support. A final step before extubation is trial spontaneous ventilation in the continuous positive airway pressure (CPAP) mode with 5 cm H_2O to maintain oxygenation and improve lung mechanics.

A variety of more complicated modes of ventilation and gas exchange support exist as potential solutions for complicated injuries. In severe cases of ARDS the use of pressure-controlled inverse-ratio ventilation may improve oxygenation and ventilation and reduce high-peak airway pressure.[43-46] Those patients who present with severe asymmetric lung injury and who develop poor oxygenation, despite the application of 100 percent oxygen and PEEP during conventional mechanical ventilation, may improve with independent lung ventilation through a double-lumen endotracheal tube.[47-50] High-frequency jet ventilation or independent lung ventilation may support the ventilatory needs of patients who develop bronchopleural fistula.[51,52] Extracorporeal membrane oxygenation (ECMO) is apparently not any more beneficial than conventional mechanical ventilation in the adult.[53] The use of ECMO in the pediatric population appears to be more beneficial. When the treatment of multiple organ failure secondary to trauma is improved in the adult, the use of ECMO may be more beneficial.[19]

Other Techniques of Respiratory Care

The patient with chest trauma often requires additional forms of respiratory care. Heated and/or cool humidity therapy are frequently used for the management of secretions. Airway clearance is very important for those who have prosthetic airways and secretion retention. Chest physical therapy is often effective in mobilizing retained airway secretions and may help reexpand atelectatic areas. Aerosolized bronchodilator therapy is frequently employed to reduce airway resistance, facilitate lung expansion and reduce the work of breathing. These "low-tech" forms of respiratory care are important in the management of the patient following chest trauma.

Case Study

HISTORY

Ms. M, a 20-year-old woman, was in good health when she accidently drove off the roadway at high speed and struck a tree head-on as an unrestrained driver. She was conscious when discovered a short while later, resuscitated in the field, and had a reported trauma score of 10. She was initially taken to a community hospital where she was assessed and trauma life support begun.

Questions

1. What signs and symptoms need to be evaluated immediately upon her arrival?
2. What diagnostic techniques can be used to help determine the severity of her injuries?
3. What therapeutic support should be available upon her arrival?

Answers

1. Signs of a patent airway, spontaneous breathing, quality of breath sounds and their symmetry, pulse rate, blood pressure, and level of consciousness should be evaluated.
2. The nature and severity of her injuries can be better understood by determining the nature of the motor vehicle accident. A careful and rapid physical evaluation, followed by radiographs of her spine, chest, abdomen, and extremities, will be needed as indicated. Other important features include the degree and duration of shock, signs of gastric aspiration, signs of hypothermia, and any underlying medical conditions or history of substance abuse that may complicate her injuries.
3. Oxygen therapy (via cannula or nonrebreathing mask); intubation equipment; bag-valve device with proper mask, oxygen reservoir, and a PEEP capability; venous and arterial line placement equipment; fluids for vascular support; resuscitation drugs; chest tube placement equipment; and medications for pain and agitation should all be available. The capability to admit directly to the operating room upon arrival is important for those patients in shock from internal bleeding.

PHYSICAL EXAMINATION

General   *Ms. M is a tall woman with an approximate weight of 55 kg, awake, with a cervical collar on, combative, and moving all extremities while breathing air. Her Glasgow coma score is 13 (see Table 12–3).*

Vital Signs   *Temperature 35.5°C; respiratory rate 32/minute; blood pressure is 91/61 mm Hg; pulse 138/minute; nailbed refill 5 seconds*

HEENT   *Pupils equal and reactive to light; no obvious nasal flaring; no signs of blood or vomit in mouth*

Neck	*Trachea shifted to the left of midline; no signs of inspiratory stridor or contusion to the larynx; carotid pulses are + + bilaterally without bruit; no signs of lymphadenopathy or thyroidomegaly; some jugular vein distension noted with patient head elevated; some tensing of sternocleidomastoid and scalene muscles noted during inspiration*
Chest	*Abrasions over the right chest; obvious flail motion of the right lateral and anterior chest with 1- to 2-cm depression on inspiration; subcutaneous air felt over the anterior and lateral right chest; breath sounds diminished in the right lung compared with left lung; some thoracoabdominal paradoxic motion noted*
Heart	*Regular rhythm at a rate of 135 to 145/minute; distant S_1 and S_2 sounds without murmurs, gallops, or rubs*
Abdomen	*Abrasions over the right upper quadrant; slightly distended and tender; bowel sounds hypoactive*
Extremities	*Moving all extremities; no signs of fracture or dislocations; no clubbing and no obvious cyanosis*

Questions

4. What signs and symptoms indicate chest injuries?
5. How will the chest injuries influence respiratory function?
6. What are the possible causes of her respiratory distress?
7. In addition to the physical examination, how should the patient's cardiorespiratory status be further evaluated?
8. What other laboratory tests would be helpful?

Answers

4. Chest injuries are indicated by the presence of chest wall abrasions, flail motion, tachypnea, accessory muscle tensing, tracheal deviation, subcutaneous emphysema, diminished breath sounds in the right lung, and thoracoabdominal wall paradoxic motion.
5. Flail chest will result in increased work of breathing and decreased efficiency of gas exchange. ABGs are almost always abnormal as a result of this type of injury.
6. Her respiratory distress is probably due in part to the flail chest and pain from broken ribs. Other possible causes include pneumothorax and/or hemopneumothorax, lung contusion, tracheobronchial rupture, cardiac contusion, great vessel fracture, diaphragmatic herniation, and intra-abdominal injuries. These changes may be inducing increased airway resistance; decreased pulmonary compliance; and causing $\dot{V}/\dot{Q}$ mismatching, hypoxemia, and ventilatory failure.
7. To evaluate further her cardiorespiratory distress, ABG analysis, ECG monitoring, and a chest radiograph are needed. Placement of peripheral venous, central venous, and arterial lines will be needed to guide and maintain hemodynamic stability.
8. Laboratory assessment of CBC, electrolytes, standard blood chemistry, and screening for alcohol and illegal drugs is indicated. Her hypothermia secondary to exposure following the accident may be contributing to her hypotension and altered mental status and will require care and continued monitoring. Abdominal injuries should be evaluated by peritoneal lavage

for the presence of blood. Blood in the peritoneum signifies ruptured abdominal organs and requires explorative and corrective surgery.

BEDSIDE AND LABORATORY EVALUATIONS ─────────

ECG

Sinus tachycardia of 137/minute without any other abnormalities

CHEST RADIOGRAPH

Shows subcutaneous air over the right hemithorax, ribs 3 through 8 fractured on the right, hemopneumothorax in the right pleural space, mediastinal shift to the left indicating tension pneumothorax, signs of hazy infiltrate in the right consistent with pulmonary contusion, normal mediastinal width and no signs of pneumomediastinum; no foreign bodies are seen (film taken at community hospital)

ABGs

pH 7.07, $Paco_2$ 61 mm Hg, Pao_2 31 mm Hg, HCO_3 = 18 mEq/liter while breathing room air

Hematology

Hematocrit (Hct) 21 percent, hemoglobin (Hb) 7 g/dL, red blood cells (RBC) 2.3 × 10^6/mm³, white blood cells (WBC) 9.2 × 10^3, platelets 210 × 10^3

CHEMISTRY AND TOXICOLOGY

Results pending

Questions

10. How would you interpret the ECG?
11. What does the chest radiograph indicate and what should be done based on these findings?
12. How would you interpret the ABG data?
13. What do the hematologic data indicate?
14. What respiratory care is indicated at this time and how should it be evaluated?
15. What hemodynamic support is indicated at this time and how should it be evaluated?
16. What complications may occur in the next 24 to 48 hours?

Answers

10. The ECG findings indicate a compensatory tachycardia in response to blood loss, hypoxemia, hypotension, and stress.
11. The chest radiographic findings reveal the magnitude of injuries following a severe blunt impact injury to the right chest. The tension hemo-

pneumothorax indicates the need for rapid chest tube placement to drain both blood and air.

12. The ABG data show severe respiratory and metabolic acidosis, hypoventilation, and hypoxemia. These findings are consistent with shock, $\dot{V}/\dot{Q}$ abnormality, diffusion defect, and/or venous-to-arterial intrapulmonary shunting following severe blunt chest injuries.

13. The hematologic data indicate anemia secondary to severe blood loss, requiring immediate fluid replacement and transfusion. Peritoneal lavage revealed substantial blood in the peritoneal cavity and the need for emergent exploratory laparotomy.

14. The patient will need to be fully supported. Following intubation, visual inspection of chest motion and auscultation of breath sounds will need to be done for initial determination of proper tube placement. Her initial ventilator support should be: assist-control mode, set VT 800 mL, set rate 16/minute, adequate inspiratory flow to maintain an I:E 1:3, PEEP 0, and an FIO$_2$ of 1.0 to help correct the hypoxemia and acidosis. Placement of chest tubes in the right hemithorax. Physical examination, vital signs, ABG analysis, and chest radiograph should be repeated to determine the patient's initial response to therapy.

15. Fluid resuscitation with crystalloid IV infusion should be started. Blood should be given as soon as available. Evaluation of central venous pressure, systemic blood pressure, and renal output should be monitored to avoid hypotension or fluid overload. If hemodynamic instability persists, placement of a pulmonary artery balloon catheter for monitoring preload pressures, cardiac output, and afterload may be needed.

16. The severity of her blunt impact injuries and shock provides multiple risk factors for the development of ARDS and multiple organ failure. She will require intensive care for continued ventilatory support, IV fluid administration, and monitoring of neurologic, cardiovascular, pulmonary, and renal function.

In the operating room Ms. M was anesthetized, orally intubated with a 7.5-mm cuffed tube, and provided with mechanical ventilation with 100 percent O$_2$. Peripheral venous and arterial lines were placed, and fluid resuscitation was begun. Two 36-F chest tubes were placed in the right pleural space and 25 cm H$_2$O of suction applied by underwater seal drainage systems. Air and 600 mL of blood were immediately removed. Exploratory laparotomy resulted in discovery and removal of a large amount of free blood, a ruptured spleen, and a lacerated right lobe of the liver. The peritoneal cavity was then lavaged with warm saline and betadine. During surgery and over the next 12 hours, she received 35 units of packed RBCs and 3.5 liters of Ringer's lactate. A CT scan of her head was done after admission to the intensive care unit (ICU) and no signs of closed head injury were found despite the persistent reduction in the level of consciousness. After 24 hours of care and stabilization at the community hospital she was transferred to the regional trauma center.

On admission to the trauma center her problem list included the following:

1. *Status after shock and respiratory failure from blunt trauma to chest and abdomen*
2. *Multiple rib fractures, flail chest, lung contusion, and subcutaneous emphysema on the right side with chest tubes*
3. *Midline abdominal incision following repair of multiple abdominal injuries*
4. *Possible closed head injury or hypoxic brain injury*
5. *Rule out spinal injuries and pelvic fractures*
6. *Status after hypothermia*
7. *Positive disseminated intravascular coagulation (DIC) screen*

The goals of her initial treatment at the trauma center concentrated on improving cardiovascular stability and respiratory function. A central venous catheter was placed and the administration of fluids, fresh frozen plasma, and blood continued along with full ventilatory support.

Shortly after her arrival at the trauma center, her bedside findings, vital signs, chest radiograph, ventilator settings, and laboratory data were as follows.

BEDSIDE FINDINGS

Ms. M is lying in semi-Fowler's position, orally intubated, two chest tubes exit her right thorax, and bandages cover a distended abdomen that has a bandaged midline incision. A small amount of blood (less than 20 mL/hour) continues to be drained from the chest tubes and no air leaks are crossing the water seal. She is moving all four extremities and periodically becomes combative, requiring reassurance and analgesics for sedation. She is spontaneously initiating approximately every other breath from the Siemens Servo 900C ventilator through a 7.5-mm internal diameter endotracheal tube. The endotracheal tube has 25 cm H_2O pressure in the cuff, and no gas leakage is heard over the cuff site. The airway is secured to the upper lip with waterproof tape and is showing the 23-cm mark at the lip. The right hemithorax is noted to have a flail motion when she becomes agitated and makes spontaneous efforts to breathe. Her breath sounds are generally diminished over the right lung with better aeration noted in the left lung with occasional expiratory rhonchi heard. On suctioning her airway, small amounts of mucoid sputum are removed. In-line ventilator circuit delivery of 2.5 mg of albuterol diluted in 3 mL of saline is being given every 4 hours and prn.

VITAL SIGNS, HEMODYNAMICS, AND URINE OUTPUT

Rectal temperature 37.2°C; respiratory rate 20/minute; pulse 100/minute; systemic arterial blood pressure is 123/78 mm Hg; central venous pressure (CVP) 6 mm Hg; urine output averaging 65 to 80 mL/hour since admission.

CHEST RADIOGRAPH

(Fig. 12–6)

VENTILATOR SETTINGS AND FINDINGS

SIMV + PS mode; rate set 17/minute; PS 10 cm H_2O; SIMV V_T set 0.75 liter; SIMV V_T exh 0.78 liter; PS V_T 0.435 liter; FIO_2 1.0; inspiratory flow 51 liters/minute; gas temperature 35°C; total rate 22/minute; $\dot{V}E$ 14.3 liters/minute; peak pressure 38 cm H_2O; plateau pressure 30 cm H_2O; set PEEP 10 cm H_2O; auto PEEP 11 cm H_2O; static compliance 41 mL/cm H_2O; effective airway resistance 9 cm H_2O per liter per second

LABORATORY FINDINGS

ABGs

pH 7.35, $Paco_2$ 44 mm Hg, Pao_2 350 mm Hg, HCO_3^- 23 mEq, $P(A-a)o_2$ 308 mm Hg; Pao_2/Fio_2 350; oxygen percent saturation (Sao_2) 100 percent (calculated); Spo_2 99 percent

Hematology

Hct 38 percent, Hb 12.7 g/dL, RBC 4.1 × 10⁶/mm³, WBC 10.4 × 10³, platelets 135 × 10³/mm³

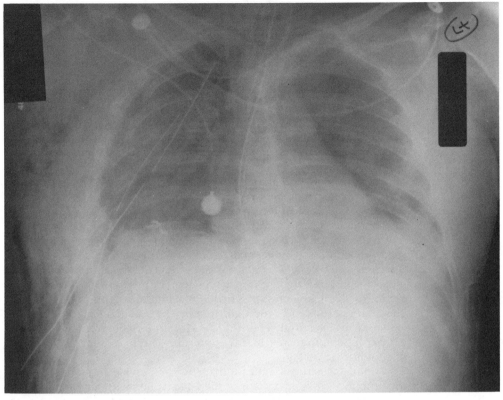

FIGURE 12–6 Portable chest radiograph of Ms. M shortly after admission to the trauma center.

Electrolytes and Chemistry
Na^+ 144 mEq/L, K^+ 4.1 mEq/L, Cl^- 100 mEq/L, glucose 116 mg/dL blood urea nitrogen (BUN) 18 mg/dL, creatinine 0.9 mg/dL
Toxicology
No ethyl alcohol or other drugs found
Microbiology
Blood, sputum, and wound smear and cultures pending

Questions

17. What do her airway care and breath sounds indicate? What would be recommended at this time?
18. How would you interpret her CVP?
19. How would you describe the radiographic findings?
20. How would you describe the ventilator settings, breathing patterns, pulmonary mechanics, and ABG findings? Are the ventilator settings appropriate for the patient's condition? What should be recommended at this time?
21. What do her other laboratory findings indicate?

Answers

17. Her airway is of an appropriate size and its position appears acceptable. Cuff pressure is effectively sealing the trachea at a safe pressure and high enough to help avoid silent aspiration of saliva around the cuff. Placement of a tracheostomy tube is not indicated at this time. Breath sounds indicate reduced ventilation of the right lung and retained secretions. The in-line aerosolization of albuterol is appropriate; however, its dosage may need to be increased or use of an in-line metered-dose inhaler (MDI) with a minimum of 4 to 10 "puffs" may be more efficacious. The sputum removed from the airway does not suggest pulmonary hemorrhage or infection at this time. Special attention to the airway, its maintenance, and sterile technique are necessary to help avoid complications.

18. The right heart filling pressure (CVP) indicates that she has an adequate blood volume at this time.

19. The portable AP chest radiograph taken shortly after admission to the trauma center (Fig. 12–6) shows subcutaneous emphysema in the lateral right hemothorax with generalized loss of lung volume. Ribs 3 through 8 are fractured along the right posterior and lateral margin with bilateral pleural effusions, right lung pulmonary contusion with air bronchograms, bilateral atelectasis, and abdominal compression of thorax. Two chest tubes are seen in the right thorax, the endotracheal tube is 3 cm above carina, a central venous line ends in the right atrium, and a nasogastric tube terminates in the stomach. There is no evidence of a pneumothorax.

20. The ventilator settings indicate that she is receiving substantial ventilatory support while in a state of mild tachypnea with an FIO_2 that may result in oxygen toxicity. The tidal volume setting of 0.75 liter (14 mL/kg) is appropriate for her frame size. She is triggering the ventilator at a rate beyond the set SIMV rate with 5 pressure-supported breaths. The pressure-supported tidal volumes should be increased (e.g., 0.6 liter) to improve their gas exchange effectiveness and reduce her rate. An alternative approach would be to return her to assist-control mode ventilation with sedation for better stabilization of her chest and reduction of her work of breathing. The peak and plateau pressures during volume-limited breaths are elevated as a result of the moderately reduced compliance and increased airway resistance. The PEEP is necessary to improve $\dot{V}/\dot{Q}$ matching, prevent further development of atelectasis, and allow FIO_2 reduction. Her respiratory pattern is not resulting in any additional auto PEEP, although she may start gas trapping if her rate increases. Her PaO_2 is excessive and requires a stepwise FIO_2 reduction with continuous pulse oximetry to maintain a targeted SpO_2 greater than 95 percent. The $P(A-a)O_2$ is significantly increased and indicates a diffusion defect, shunting, and/or $\dot{V}/\dot{Q}$ mismatching. Her arterial oxygen content is acceptable at 18 mL/dL. The $PaCO_2$ is normal but is requiring an elevated minute volume as a result of increased metabolic rate, dead space ventilation, or a combination of the two. The acid-base balance is acceptable.

21. The hematologic data indicate acceptable RBC count and hemoglobin concentration following massive transfusion. A mildly elevated WBC count is not uncommon after this degree of trauma and the stress response to it. The reduced platelet count is consistent with the DIC. The electrolytes and renal function are normal when considering the amount of blood and fluid that she has received. The slight hypergly-

cemia may be a result of glucocorticoid and catecholamine release secondary to the trauma and/or the IV fluids being given.

Following assessment of Ms. M's condition, her FIO$_2$ was gradually reduced to 0.50 over the next 2 hours and a third chest tube was placed in the left chest to drain the pleural effusion. Sputum cultures and sensitivity showed a heavy growth of Streptococcus pneumoniae *and she was started on appropriate antibiotics. Aerosolized bronchodilators were continued with a trial of modified Trendelenburg's position postural drainage. Postural drainage was discontinued after the first attempt when she became extremely short of breath and her pulse oximeter saturations dropped from 94 to 88 percent.*

For the next week her ventilatory requirements continued at the same level and she could not tolerate reduction of SIMV rate below 15/minute and pressure support below 10 cm H$_2$O without becoming excessively tachypneic, desaturated (pulse oximetry), tachycardiac, and hypertensive. Cyclic fever spikes and episodic atelectasis with infiltrates occurred during this period. These pulmonary changes required rigorous pulmonary hygiene and therapeutic bronchoscopy for removal of mucus plugs. One of the right chest tubes was eventually removed without recurrence of pneumothorax. Her abdominal wound required re-exploration and lavaging for a small abscess formation and the contents continued to be excessively swollen. Her nutritional status was maintained through regular central line alimentation and nasogastric tube feedings.

Eleven days after her accident her temperature rose to 39.3°C accompanied by tachycardia, tachypnea with obvious flail motion on the right side, and increasing FIO$_2$ requirements from 0.40 to 0.60 to maintain the oxyhemoglobin saturation greater than 92 percent. Breath sounds became progressively more coarse sounding with bilateral inspiratory and expiratory rhonchi and wheezes and diminished on the right. Sputum suctioned from her became purulent and somewhat foul smelling. A chest radiograph at this time shows increasing bilateral infiltrates with a loss of lung volume and no signs of pneumothorax (Fig. 12–7). The endotracheal tube, chest tube, central venous catheter, and nasogastric tube all appear in proper positions. Sputum smears showed 3+ gram-positive cocci and 1+ gram-positive bacilli. Her antibiotics were adjusted and airway care and aerosolized bronchodilators were intensified to help clear the retained secretions. She was still unable to tolerate chest physiotherapy. Over the next 48 hours her breath sounds, sputum production, and chest radiograph improved. Ventilatory support was gradually reduced to SIMV of 6/minute with PS of 12 cm H$_2$O and FIO$_2$ of 0.40. Over the next week this pattern of fever spike, breath sound changes, purulent sputum with heavy bacterial counts, and chest radiographic findings consistent with pneumonia was repeated two more times. In each case, her ventilatory support was increased and then reduced back to the same level. During this period her chest tubes were successfully removed. She was considered ready for removal from ventilatory support on the 11th day after admission to the trauma center and she was extubated. Shortly after extubation her respiratory rate climbed to 45 to 50/minute with obvious flail motion of the right hemithorax, heart rate increased to 140 to 150/minute, and oxyhemoglobin saturation declined to 88 percent despite use of 60 percent oxygen via high-flow oxygen therapy. She was reintubated and returned to SIMV of 12/minute and PS of 14 cm H$_2$O with an FIO$_2$ of 0.60. She stabilized rapidly and was able to tolerate reduction of her ventilatory support to PS ventilation alone with an FIO$_2$ of 0.30 over the next 2 days.

Twenty-three days after her initial injury she was again evaluated for extubation.

BEDSIDE FINDINGS

Ms. M is sitting up in bed, orally intubated, alert, and communicative through a writing tablet. She is spontaneously initiating every breath from the Siemens Servo 900C ventilator through a 7.5-mm internal diameter endotracheal tube. The airway

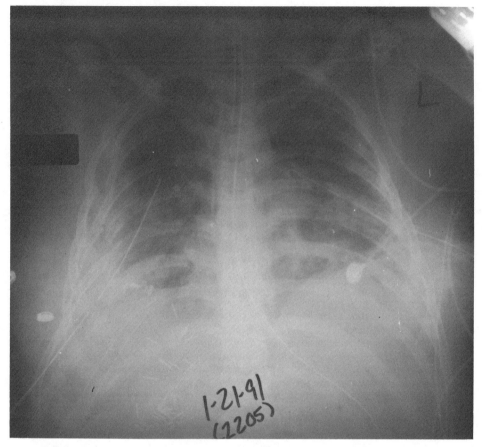

FIGURE 12–7 Portable chest radiograph 11 days after admission to the trauma center.

has 25 cm H₂O pressure in the cuff, no gas leakage is heard over the cuff site, and it is secured to the upper lip with waterproof tape and showing the 22-cm mark at the lip. The right hemithorax is still noted to have some flail motion when she makes vigorous efforts to breathe. Her breath sounds are generally diminished over the right lung with better aeration noted in the left lung with inspiratory and expiratory rhonchi heard bilaterally. Moderate amounts of mucoid sputum are periodically removed during airway care. In-line ventilator circuit delivery of 2.5 mg of albuterol diluted in 3 mL of saline continues every 4 hours and prn.

VITAL SIGNS, HEMODYNAMICS, AND URINE OUTPUT

Temperature 38.3°C; respiratory rate 23/minute (total rate observed while on ventilator); pulse 102/minute; systemic arterial blood pressure is 128/81 mm Hg; urine output continuing at about 70 mL/hour

CHEST RADIOGRAPH

Multiple rib fractures on the right, a few patchy infiltrates bilaterally in the process of clearing, and no signs of pneumothorax; endotracheal tube, central venous catheter, and nasogastric tube all appear properly positioned.

VENTILATOR SETTINGS AND FINDINGS

PS + PEEP mode; PS 10 cm H_2O; PS exhaled $\dot{V}T$ 0.425 to 0.635 liter; FIO_2 0.30; set PEEP 5 cm H_2O; gas temperature 34°C; total rate 23/minute; $\dot{V}E$ 12.7 liter/minute; peak pressure 15 cm H_2O

LABORATORY FINDINGS

ABGs

pH 7.42, $PaCO_2$ 38 mm Hg, PaO_2 96mm Hg, HCO_3^- 24 mEq, $PaO_2/F_{I}O_2$ 320, Hb 14 g/dL, SaO_2 98 percent (calculated), SpO_2 97 percent, CaO_2 18.6 mL/dL

Spontaneous Ventilation Study (following 5 minutes of breathing 40 percent oxygen via nonrebreathing valve)

Rate 36/minute; $\dot{V}E$ 11.2 L/minute; VT 0.31 liter, rate/VT 116; forced vital capacity (FVC) 0.68 liter; maximum inspiratory pressure (MIP) −20 cm H_2O; SpO_2 92 percent; pulse 129/minute; blood pressure 133/88 mm Hg
She became somewhat anxious toward the end of the trial and began to exhibit some flail motion of the right chest and increasing tachypnea (45/minute).

Questions

22. How would you interpret vital signs?
23. What do the current ventilator settings and breathing patterns indicate about her ventilator support?
24. What do the ABGs indicate?
25. How would you assess the spontaneous ventilation data?
26. What would you recommend at this time? Why?

Answers

22. Her vital signs indicate a mild stress response with the presence of mild tachypnea and tachycardia. Urine output and temperature are within normal limits.
23. She is currently in a spontaneous mode of pressure support ventilation with a low level of PEEP. Her respiratory pattern shows a mild tachypnea, acceptable tidal ventilation (7 to 11 mL/kg), and moderately elevated minute ventilation. Approximately 75 percent or more of her pressure support is overcoming the airway resistance imposed by the endotracheal tube. The FIO_2 is modestly elevated but well below a toxic level.
24. Her most recent ABG data indicate acceptable oxygenation with slight elevation of the $P(A\text{-}a)O_2$, consistent with persistent but improving $\dot{V}/\dot{Q}$ mismatching. The $PaCO_2$ indicates normal alveolar ventilation despite the elevated minute ventilation. The relatively high minute ventilation may be due to elevated metabolism or dead space or both. The acid-base indicate a normal balance.
25. The spontaneous ventilation data following a 5-minute trial with a nonrebreathing valve supplied with an FIO_2 of 0.40 show a marked tachypnea, elevated minute ventilation, and relatively shallow tidal ventilation. The ratio of rate to VT is markedly elevated and greater than 100, indicating a rapid and shallow respiratory pattern that is not predictive of successful spontaneous ventilation.[54] The best vital capacity was twice the tidal volume, indicating that she may not have an effective cough. The MIP is barely acceptable, consistent with a weakened ventilatory

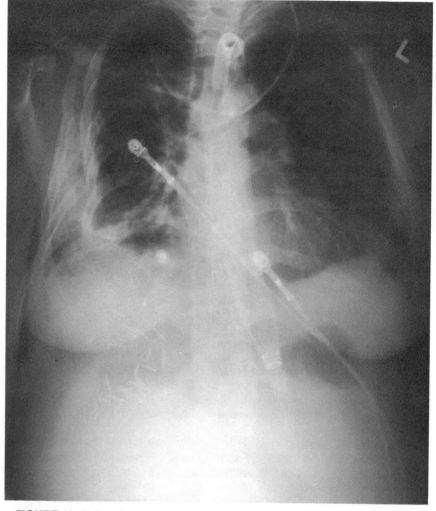

FIGURE 12–8 Portable chest radiograph 2 days after successful weaning from ventilatory support.

muscle capability. These measurements, when viewed together with her anxiety, desaturation of hemoglobin to 92 percent, increasing heart and respiratory rates, and the presence of a flail motion at the end of the trial, all indicate that she is not yet ready for spontaneous unsupported ventilation and extubation.

26. She should be returned to PS ventilation to stabilize her respiratory, cardiovascular, and psychologic status. It is clear that a more gradual approach to her weaning from ventilatory support will be necessary. The placement of a tracheostomy tube should facilitate her weaning and her secretion management and should prevent further laryngeal injury from the endotracheal tube.

A number of weaning strategies can be used. The patient may be given short trials (e.g., 10 to 30 minutes) of low-level PS (e.g., 5 cm H_2O) or CPAP three to four times/day with rest at night. The level of PS can be reduced as she develops more respiratory muscle endurance.

Her flail chest motion continues to retard her progress; however, this should gradually improve. Assessment of her abdominal wound; respiratory tract secretions; pain; and nutritional, psychologic, and fluid and electrolyte status should continue.

She was returned to PS ventilation and it was decided to attempt T-tube trials with adequate oxygen three times/day for 30 minutes, as tolerated. A 7.5-mm internal diameter cuffed tracheostomy tube was placed. T-tube trials continued over the next week until she was able to remain off the ventilator throughout the day and most of the night, without excessive dyspnea and flail motion. During this period she began first to stand at the bedside for a few minutes and then to take short walks in and outside her room while having ventilation assisted with manual bag ventilation. Thirty-two days after her accident she tolerated removal from the ventilator and her chest radiograph improved (Fig. 12–8). She did well on 30 percent oxygen via cool aerosol to a tracheostomy collar. Over the next 6 days she increased her ability to walk and her tracheostomy tube was intermittently plugged and the cuff deflated until she was decannulated. Forty days after the initial injury, Ms. M was discharged to her home.

REFERENCES

1. Statistical Abstracts of the United States: The National Data Book, ed 110. US Department of Commerce, 1990.

2. Trunkey, DD: Trauma care systems. Emerg Med Clin North Am 2:913, 1984.

3. Wilson, RF: Trauma. In Shoemaker, WC, et al (eds): Textbook of Critical Care, ed 2. WB Saunders, Philadelphia, 1989, pp 1230.

4. LoCicero, J and Mattox, KL: Epidemiology of chest trauma. Surg Clin North Am 69:15, 1989.

5. Kirsh, MM: Acute thoracic injuries. In Siegel, JH (ed): Truma—Emergency Surgery and Critical Care. Churchill Livingstone, New York, 1987, pp 863–882.

6. Gaillard, M, et al: Mortality prognostic factors in chest injury. J Trauma 30:93, 1990.

7. Wilson, RF, Gibson, DEB, and Antonenko, D: Shock and acute respiratory failure after chest trauma. J Trauma 17:697, 1977.

8. Marcus, NA, et al: Low-velocity gunshot wounds to extremities. J Trauma 20:1061, 1980.

9. Grimes, WR, Deitch, EA, and McDonald, JC: A clinical review of shotgun wounds to the chest and abdomen. Surg Gynecol Obstet 160:148, 1985.

10. Wilson, RF, Murray, C, and Antonenko, DR: Non-penetrating thoracic injuries. Surg Clin North Am 57:17, 1977.

11. Burke, JF: Early diagnosis of traumatic rupture of the bronchus. JAMA 181:682, 1962.

12. Wilson, JM, et al: Severe chest trauma: Morbidity implication of first and second rib fracture in 120 patients. Arch Surg 113:846, 1978.

13. Besson, A and Saegesser, F: Color Atlas of Chest Trauma and Associated Injuries. Vol 1. Oradell, NJ, Medical Economics, 1983.

14. Pate, JW: Chest wall injuries. Surg Clin North Am 69:59, 1989.

15. Sarkaran, S and Wilson, RF: Factors affecting prognosis in patients with flail chest. J Thorac Cardiovasc Surg 60:402, 1970.

16. Ashbaugh, DB, et al: Chest trauma: Analysis of 685 patients. Arch Surg 95:546, 1967.

17. Christensson, P, et al: Early and later results of controlled ventilation in flail chest. Chest 75:456–460, 1979.

18. Wilkins, EW: Non-cardiovascular thoracic injuries: Chest wall, bronchus, lung, esophagus, and diaphragm. In Burke, JF, Boyd, RJ, and McCabe, CJ (eds): Trauma Management. Year Book Medical, Chicago, 1988.

19. Van Way, CW: Advanced techniques in thoracic trauma. Surg Clin North Am 69:143, 1989.

20. Regel, G, et al: Occlusion of bronchopleural fistula after lung injury and treatment by bronchoscopy. J Trauma 29:223, 1989.

21. Pepe, PE, et al: Clinical predictors of the adult respiratory distress syndrome. Am J Surg 144:124, 1982.

22. Fuhrman, GM, Stieg, FH, and Buerk, CA: Blunt laryngeal trauma: Classification and management protocol. J Trauma 30:87, 1990.

23. Pate, JW: Tracheobronchial and esophageal injuries. Surg Clin North Am 69:111, 1989.

24. Ecker, RR, et al: Injuries of the trachea and bronchi. Ann Thorac Surg 11:289, 1971.

25. Ivantry, RR and Rohman, M: The injured heart. Surg Clin North Am 69:93, 1989.

26. Fulda, G, et al: Blunt traumatic rupture of the heart and pericardium: A ten-year experience (1979–1989). J Trauma 31:167, 1991.

27. Carasquilla, C, et al: Gunshot wounds of the heart. Ann Thorac Surg 13:208, 1972.

28. Doty, DB, et al: Cardiac trauma: Clinical and experimental correlations of myocardial contusion. Ann Surg 180:452, 1974.

29. Hilgenberg, AD: Trauma to the heart and great vessels. In Burke, JF, Boyd, RJ, and McCabe, CJ (eds): Trauma Management. Year Book Medical, Chicago, 1988.

30. Gewertz, B, O'Brien, C, and Kirsh, MM: Use of the intra-aortic balloon support for refractory low cardiac output in myocardial contusion. J Trauma 17:325, 1977.

31. Jones, JW, Hewitt, RL, and Drapanas, T: Cardiac contusion: A capricious syndrome. Ann Surg 181:567–574, 1975.

32. Parmley, LF, Manion, WC, and Mattingly, TW: Non-penetrating traumatic injury to the heart. Circulation 18:371, 1958.

33. Van Vugt, AB and Schoots, FJ: Acute diaphragmatic rupture due to blunt trauma: A retrospective analysis. J Trauma 29:683, 1989.

34. Symbas, PN and Gott, JP: Delayed sequela of thoracic trauma. Surg Clin North Am 69:135, 1989.

35. Hix, WR and Aaron, BL (eds): Residua of Thoracic Trauma. Mount Kisco, NY, Futura Publishing, 1987.

36. Champion, HR, et al: The trauma score. Crit Care Med 9:672, 1981.

37. Champion, HR, et al: A revision of the trauma score. J Trauma 29:623, 1989.

38. Trunkey, DD: Organization of trauma care. In Burke, JF, Boyd, RJ, and McCabe, CJ (eds): Trauma Management. Year Book Medical, Chicago, 1988.

39. Worthley, LIG: Thoracic epidural in the management of chest trauma: A study of 161 cases. Intensive Care Med 11:312, 1985.

40. Cicala, RS, et al: Epidural analgesia in thoracic trauma: Effects of lumbar morphine and thoracic bupivacaine on pulmonary function. Crit Care Med 18:229, 1990.

41. Dronen, S, Chadwick, O, and Novak, R: Endotracheal tip position in the arrested patient. Ann Emerg Med 11:116, 1982.

42. Jorden, RC, et al: A comparison of PTV and endotracheal intubation in an acute trauma model. J Trauma 25:978, 1985.

43. Gurevitch, MJ: Selection of the inspiratory:expiratory ratio. In Kacmarek, RM and Stoller, JK (eds): Current Respiratory Care. BC Decker, Philadelphia, 1988.

44. Tharatt, RS, Allen, RP, and Alberstson, TE: Pressure controlled inverse ratio ventilation in severe adult respiratory failure. Chest 94:755, 1988.

45.   Abraham, E and Yoshihara, G: Cardiorespiratory effects of pressure controlled inverse ratio ventilation in severe respiratory failure. Chest 96:1356, 1989.

46.   Enderson, BL, Farnham, JW, and Langdon, JR: Inverse ratio ventilation can improve oxygenation in respiratory distress syndrome (abstr). Crit Care Med 17:s152, 1989.

47.   Kanarek, DJ and Shannon, DC: Adverse effect of positive end expiratory pressure on pulmonary perfusion and arterial oxygenation. Am Rev Respir Dis 112:457, 1976.

48.   Glass, DD, et al: Therapy of unilateral pulmonary insufficiency with double lumen endotracheal tube. Crit Care Med 4:323, 1976.

49.   Branson, RD, Hurst, JM, and DeHaven, CB: Synchronous independent lung ventilation in the treatment of unilateral pulmonary contusion: A report of two cases. Respir Care 29:361, 1984.

50.   Ray, C: Independent lung ventilation. In Kacmarek, RM and Stoller, JK (eds): Current Respiratory Care. BC Decker, Philadelphia, 1988.

51.   Turnbull, AD, et al: High frequency jet ventilation in major airway or pulmonary disruption. Ann Thorac Surg 32:468, 1981.

52.   Kopec, IC, Van Dervort, AL, Carlon, GC: High frequency jet ventilation. In Kacmarek, RM and Stoller, JK (eds): Current Respiratory Care. BC Decker, Philadelphia, 1988.

53.   Zapol, WM, et al: Extracorporeal membrane oxygenation in severe acute respiratory failure: A randomized prospective study. JAMA 242:2193, 1979.

54.   Yang, LY and Tobin, MJ: A prospective study of the indexes predicting the outcome of trials of weaning from mechanical ventilation. N Engl J Med 324:1445, 1991.

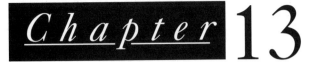

Chapter 13

Thomas P. Malinowski, BS, RRT

POSTOPERATIVE ATELECTASIS

INTRODUCTION

Atelectasis is a clinical condition characterized by regions of the lung that are collapsed or airless. Atelectasis is commonly seen after major surgery and can lead to severe respiratory dysfunction. In fact, postoperative atelectasis may lead to pneumonia and respiratory failure and is a common cause of an increased hospital stay.

Obesity, old age, smoking history, general anesthesia, and history of heart disease or lung disease increase the risk of developing postoperative atelectasis.[1] None of these risk factors is more significant than a past medical history that is positive for chronic lung disease (e.g., chronic bronchitis, emphysema).

ETIOLOGY

Three factors may combine or independently contribute to the development of atelectasis: inadequate lung distending force, obstruction of the airways, and insufficient surfactant.[2] All three of these factors may occur in the surgical patient, especially during the postoperative period.

Inadequate Lung Distention

Lung expansion depends on the ability of the respiratory muscles to generate negative intrapleural pressures and an intact chest cage. Factors that weaken the respiratory muscles or reduce the effect of normal negative inspiratory pressures will reduce lung inflation and encourage atelectasis.

For example, elderly patients and malnourished patients may be unable to generate the inspiratory force necessary for deep breathing and coughing. Patients with chest wall abnormalities (kyphosis and scoliosis) have limited lung expansion because of their thoracic cage malformation (Table 13–1). Diaphragmatic movement may be limited in obese patients or those with neuromuscular disease (see Chapter 15). Pulmonary fibrosis causes the lung to expand poorly in response to normal negative intrapleural pressures (see Table 13–2).

Numerous intraoperative factors may also affect lung distension. The diaphragm relaxes and displaces upward when patients are given anesthetics and paralytics.[3] Type, location, and duration of the surgical procedure also affect lung distension.[1,4,5] Upper abdominal procedures present the greatest risk for atelectasis, followed by thoracic, lower abdominal, and peripheral procedures. Postoperative pain is often associated with decreased respiratory effort and a reduction in pleural

217

Table 13–1 Factors that Decrease Ability to Generate Negative Pressures

Anesthesia
Pain
Reduction in lung volume
Diaphragmatic apraxia: phrenic neuropathy, myopathy
Chest wall disorders
Ascites
Malnutrition

and intra-abdominal pressures resulting in atelectasis after upper abdominal surgery.[1] Patients who have thoracic surgery are also at risk for postoperative atelectasis. Topical cooling of the left phrenic nerve, which commonly occurs during cardiac surgery, can cause inadequate diaphragmatic movement after heart surgery and contribute to left lower lobe atelectasis.[6] In the postoperative period the inadequate lung distension may persist for 7 to 14 days, especially when complications such as excessive pain or pleural effusion occur.[7]

Obstruction of the Airways

The development of postoperative atelectasis can also occur as a result of retained secretions in the bronchi.[2,8] Secretion retention occurs when mucociliary transport is diminished, cough is weak or absent, secretion volume is excessive, or hydration is inadequate. Anesthetic agents impair mucociliary activity and depress tidal volume and cough. Humidity is rarely added during anesthesia, and the anesthesiologist will frequently administer pharmacologic agents that, as a side effect, dry tracheobronchial secretions.[3] Pathologic conditions associated with excessive secretions and impaired mucus transport (i.e., smoking history, chronic bronchitis, asthma) will increase risk of secretion retention.[9] Mucus plugs lead to atelectasis with absorption of gases distal to the obstruction. This condition is enhanced during breathing of anesthetic gases or high inspired oxygen concentrations, as these gases are more readily absorbed into the pulmonary blood flow.[10,11]

Surfactant Depletion

An adequate quantity and quality of surfactant is necessary to maintain alveolar stability and prevent collapse. The quantity and quality of surfactant can be reduced with pulmonary edema, smoke inhalation, inhaled anesthetics, lung contusion, pulmonary embolus, adult respiratory distress syndrome (ARDS), high inspired oxygen concentrations, and prolonged breathing at low tidal volumes.[2] Cardiopulmonary bypass may cause an inadequate perfusion of the lung and alveolar epithelium, leading to insufficient release of surfactant.[12]

Table 13–2 Factors that Reduce the Effect of Normal Inspiratory Pressures

Reclining position
Pleural effusion
Pneumothorax
Pleural mass
Pulmonary fibrosis

PATHOPHYSIOLOGY

Atelectasis results in a decrease in functional residual capacity and lung compliance. This results in alterations in the distribution of the inhaled gas without corresponding changes in perfusion. As a result, ventilation-perfusion ratio ($\dot{V}/\dot{Q}$) mismatching occurs, which leads to hypoxemia. General anesthesia also inhibits hypoxic pulmonary vasoconstriction reflexes in the lung, which further contributes to $\dot{V}/\dot{Q}$ mismatching and hypoxemia.[12]

Surface tension forces hold collapsed alveoli shut so that higher distending pressures are needed to reinflate the affected regions of the lung. Unaffected lung regions are more compliant and easier to inflate. The more compliant regions receive more of the tidal volume than do the atelectatic areas and may be easily overinflated when large tidal volumes are used with mechanical ventilation.

CLINICAL FEATURES

Signs and symptoms of atelectasis vary with the amount of lung involved, the patient's previous health status, and duration of the problem. Dyspnea is the most common symptom associated with atelectasis, but this may not be present if the patient has minimal lung involvement and has been previously healthy. When the atelectasis involves larger portions of the lung or when the patient has a chronic lung disease, the dyspnea can become severe. A recent history of abdominal or thoracic surgery suggests that atelectasis is likely.

Tachypnea is commonly associated with atelectasis. Respiratory rates usually increase in proportion to the amount of lung involved with atelectasis. Decreased lung compliance results in the patient breathing smaller tidal volumes with minimal variations in the depth of the breath.[8,13] In order to maintain adequate gas exchange, the patient must breathe with a more rapid rate to compensate for the smaller tidal volume. Tachycardia and fever may indicate infection associated with retention of secretions.

Auscultation of breath sounds is often helpful in detecting the onset of atelectasis. Late-inspiratory crackles are heard on deep inspiratory efforts and represent the sudden opening of atelectatic regions. These inspiratory crackles are usually heard initially in the dependent regions of the lung and may clear after the patient takes several deep breaths. Bronchial breath sounds and bronchophony over the affected region indicate airway patency in the atelectatic area. Diminished or absent breath sounds indicate that the airways are plugged or collapsed in the affected region, which results in little or no ventilation into the affected area. Accessory muscle usage indicates a significant increase in the work of breathing, which is typically the result of a decreased lung compliance.

The chest radiograph is a helpful tool in the diagnosis of atelectasis.[2,8] Chest radiographs may reveal a reduction in lung volume and opacification that is not clinically apparent. Obliteration of typical radiographic shadows may indicate the location of involvement. For example, the right heart border is often obscured with right middle lobe atelectasis but is present with lower lobe atelectasis. Other signs of lung volume loss include elevation of the hemidiaphragm and mediastinal shifts toward the affected side.

Air bronchograms, frequently observed on the chest radiograph with atelectasis, are caused by collapse of the lung tissue around inflated airways. When present, air bronchograms indicate that the atelectasis is not due to mucus obstruction of the airways.

Arterial blood gases (ABGs) often reveal hypoxemia in the postoperative patient with atelectasis. The severity of hypoxemia does not necessarily correlate with the extent of atelectasis on chest radiograph. Profound hypoxemia may exist from microatelectasis that is not apparent radiographically. Hypoxemia frequently causes a mild respiratory alkalosis.

Because patients with pulmonary disease are at greater risk for postoperative complications, bedside spirometry is useful to identify high-risk patients before surgery. Spirometry is especially useful to assess patients with a significant smoking history or those scheduled for upper abdominal or thoracic surgery.[14] After surgery, bedside spirometry is also useful to detect the severity of the decrease in lung volumes (vital capacity and inspiratory capacity) associated with atelectasis. Severe decreases in vital capacity indicate that the simple techniques to correct atelectasis may not be sufficient (see farther on).

TREATMENT

The preoperative evaluation by the respiratory care practitioner (RCP) should identify factors that might contribute to the onset of postoperative complications. Patients with a long history of smoking or pulmonary symptoms should be evaluated with spirometry to identify whether obstructive or restrictive lung disease is present. Patients with moderate to severe chronic obstructive lung disease have a greater risk for postoperative respiratory failure. These patients will benefit from preoperative bronchial hygiene techniques and smoking cessation.

Once the diagnosis of postoperative atelectasis has been made, the severity of respiratory compromise will determine the therapy. If there is no significant respiratory distress and the patient is ambulating, treatment may not be needed. Patients with atelectasis who are distressed or not ambulatory should receive postoperative respiratory care.

Lung Inflation Techniques

Deep breathing and coughing are often as effective as any other of the more costly techniques for the treatment and prevention of atelectasis in the cooperative patient.[15] Incentive spirometry may benefit patients who require additional coaching, and it can serve as an indicator of improvement in pulmonary function.

Intermittent application of 10 to 15 cm H_2O continuous positive airway pressure (CPAP) or positive expiratory pressure (PEP) is often effective in the treatment of atelectasis.[16-18] Periodic application of CPAP (every 1 to 3 hours) is also frequently effective in clearing atelectasis and may be beneficial in those patients unresponsive to the simpler lung inflation therapies. It is also more effective for patients who are uncooperative or who have recurring or persistent forms of atelectasis. PEP therapy has been effective in improving postoperative pulmonary function when applied on an hourly basis.[17]

Intermittent positive-pressure breathing (IPPB) may be indicated in those patients unable to perform more simple maneuvers for lung inflation and whose vital capacity (VC) is less than 10 to 15 mL/kg. Volume-oriented IPPB can be instrumental in improving lung volumes and can help promote a more effective cough.[19]

Even though the complication rate is low, patients treated with positive-pressure therapy (CPAP, IPPB) should be closely monitored for the adverse affects of raised intrathoracic pressure (hyperinflation, reduced perfusion, barotrauma, and gastric inflation). The application of positive pressure must be used in conjunction with bronchial hygiene techniques when secretion retention is the cause of the atelectasis.

Secretion Removal

When the cause of the lobar atelectasis is retained mucus, treatment should be aimed at removal of airway secretions in addition to lung inflation. Encouraging the patient to generate an effective cough is often all that is necessary. If this therapy is not effective and radiographic evidence suggests the characteristic lobar atelectasis pattern (radiographic density, absence of air bronchograms, fissure displacement, mediastinal shift, diaphragmatic elevation, compensatory hyperinflation), then chest physiotherapy (CPT) may be indicated. Lobar atelectasis often responds to a vigorous, short course of CPT, often within 6 hours, and is often as effective as bronchoscopy at removing retained secretions.[20,21] If this program is inadequate, removal of central secretions by use of endotracheal suctioning or bronchoscopy is indicated.[22] Postoperative management of patients with chronic obstructive lung disease should also include bronchodilators to facilitate a better cough and secretion expectoration.

Mechanical Ventilation

Mechanical ventilation will be needed in some patients after major surgery especially if underlying chronic lung disease is present. In cardiac surgery patients mechanical ventilation is useful in the postoperative period until all hemodynamic parameters are stable.[12] In some cardiac surgery patients extubation can occur within a few hours after surgery but those with arrythmias, mediastinal bleeding, or decreased cardiac output will need mechanical ventilation for a longer period.[12]

Case Study

HISTORY

Mrs. M is a 67-year-old white woman who was admitted to the emergency room for complaints of dyspnea, chest pain, and diaphoresis. Further workup on this admission reveals a diagnosis of duodenal ulcer. On admission day she was taken to the operating room (OR), where a perforated prepyloric ulcer was repaired and purulent fluid removed from the peritoneal space. After surgery she returned to the surgical intensive care unit (ICU) and was maintained on continuous mechanical ventilation for 1 day. She was extubated on day 1 and placed on a 40 percent high-flow oxygen aerosol mask.

Two days after extubation and she began complaining of "not being able to catch her breath."

Her past medical history includes (1) systemic hypertension, which is adequately managed with a thiazide diuretic; and (2) a four-vessel coronary artery bypass graft procedure performed 2 years earlier. She denies any history of smoking, alcohol, or drug abuse.

Questions

1. What clinical conditions could cause the patient's acute dyspnea?
2. What is the significance of the anatomic location of the surgical procedure?
3. What physical examination procedures do you suggest should be done at this point?

Answers

1. Dyspnea may be due to an increased work of breathing associated with decreased lung compliance from pulmonary edema, atelectasis, or dia-

phragmatic compression from the abdomen. Other potential causes of dyspnea in this case would include pulmonary embolus and pneumonia.

2. There is a direct relationship between postoperative complications and the proximity of the surgical incision to the diaphragm. Upper abdominal surgery is much more likely to be associated with atelectasis than peripheral surgery.

3. Assessment of the respiratory rate, pulse rate, body temperature, breathing pattern, and breath sounds would help evaluate the patient's pulmonary status. Cardiac examination for S_3 or S_4 gallop, jugular venous distension, and hepatojugular reflex would help rule out pulmonary edema. Abdominal evaluation for excessive distension would help rule out diaphragm compression. Auscultation for a pleural friction rub and palpation of the calf muscles for tenderness would help rule out pulmonary embolism.

PHYSICAL EXAMINATION

General	*The patient is fatigued and in moderate respiratory distress. She is mildly diaphoretic, lying in a semi-Fowler's position in bed.*
Vital Signs	*Temperature 38.5°C; respiratory rate 38/minute; blood pressure 148/ 57 mm Hg; pulse 124/minute*
HEENT	*Pupils equal, round, and reactive to light and accommodation (PERRLA); tympanic membranes clear; no nasopharyngeal lesions, masses, or exudates present; alae nasi flaring with inspiration*
Neck	*Trachea midline and mobile to palpation; no stridor present; no carotid bruits, lymphadenopathy, thyromegaly, or jugular venous distension; sternomastoid muscles tense during inspiration*
Chest	*Symmetric chest expansion with rapid shallow breathing pattern; decrease resonance to percussion of lower lung fields*
Heart	*Regular rhythm with a rate of 124/minute; no murmurs, gallops, or rubs*
Lungs	*Late-inspiratory crackles heard in the bases, with diminished breath sounds in mid and upper lung fields*
Abdomen	*Distended, tender, with no bowel sounds heard*
Extremities	*No clubbing, cyanosis, or edema; capillary refill less than 3 seconds; pulses and reflexes +1 and symmetric.*

Questions

4. What pathophysiology is suggested by the rapid and shallow breathing pattern?
5. What is the cause of the late-inspiratory crackles in the bases? What characteristic of these crackles should the RCP identify?
6. What could be causing the patient's tachycardia?
7. Why is she using her accessory muscles to breathe?
8. What laboratory tests do you recommend at this point?

Answers

4. Rapid shallow breathing suggests that the patient is experiencing a significant drop in her lung compliance. This leads to breathing with smaller tidal volumes and a more rapid rate. Common causes of decreased lung compliance include pulmonary edema, atelectasis, and pneumonia.

5. Late-inspiratory crackles are caused by the sudden opening of many collapsed peripheral airways. This occurs when the patient with atelectasis inhales deeply enough to re-expand atelectatic regions. The RCP should determine whether the crackles diminish as the patient repeatedly inhales deeply. This would suggest that the crackles are due to atelectasis.

6. Tachycardia could be due to a number of causes: hypoxemia, inadequate pain management, fever, and anxiety. The patient has had cardiac disease in the past and may have an abnormal cardiac rhythm because of the heart disease.

7. The primary inspiratory muscle (the diaphragm) is much less effective for several weeks or months after abdominal surgery. Lungs are also less compliant and more difficult to expand after major surgery. Atelectasis may worsen the problem, and assistance may be needed from the accessory breathing muscles to maintain ventilation. This increases the total respiratory work exerted by the patient.

8. Laboratory tests that would be helpful are aimed at narrowing the list of problems that could cause the patient's current distress. Such tests include a chest radiograph, ABG analysis, complete blood count (CBC) and electrolyte evaluation, bedside spirometry, and an electrocardiogram (ECG).

LABORATORY EVALUATION

CHEST RADIOGRAPH

(Fig. 13–1).

ABGs

ph 7.46, $Paco_2$ 33 mm Hg, Pao_2 54 mm Hg on Fio_2 0.40, HCO_3^- 25 mEq

SPIROMETRY

Slow inspiratory capacity 1.0 liter; could not perform vital capacity maneuver

CBC

White blood cells 16,500/mm³ with 65 percent segs and 11 percent bands; red blood cells (RBC) 3.9 million/mm³; hemoglobin (Hb) 9.9 g/dL; hematocrit (Hct) 37%; platelets 155,000/mm³

CHEMISTRY

Na^+ 139 mEq/liter, K^+ 3.2 mEq/liter, Cl^- 102 mEq/liter, blood urea nitrogen (BUN) 17 mg/dL, total proteins 6.7 g/dL, albumin 3.2 g/dL, glucose 78 mg/dL

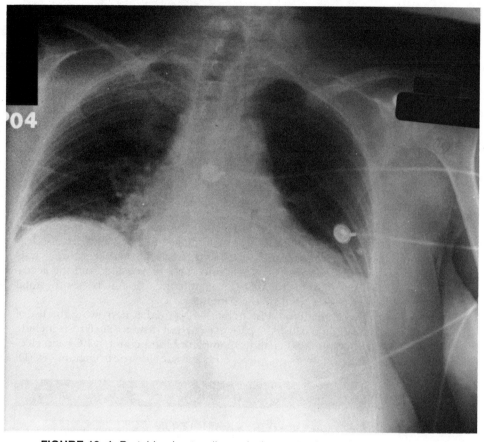

FIGURE 13–1 Portable chest radiograph demonstrating reduced lung volumes.

Questions

8. How would you interpret the ABG and spirometry results?
9. How do you interpret the chest radiograph and what is suggested by the findings on the chest radiograph?
10. How do you interpret the CBC and electrolyte values?
11. What are your therapeutic objectives for respiratory care?
12. What would be your treatment plan?
13. How would you evaluate the patient's response to therapy?

Answers

8. The ABGs reflect moderate hypoxemia with mild uncompensated respiratory alkalosis, suggesting that the patient is hyperventilating. The Pa_{O_2} of 54 mm Hg on 0.40 Fi_{O_2} suggests the hypoxemia is somewhat refractory to oxygen therapy. The spirometry results are consistent with a poor effort or a severely restrictive condition. The patient's inability to perform a vital capacity maneuver indicates significant fatigue.
9. The chest radiograph suggests poor inspiratory effort or reduced lung volumes. Obliteration of the right heart border is consistent with right middle lobe atelectasis. Presence of air bronchograms suggests a lack of mucus plugs in the affected regions.
10. The WBCs are elevated, consistent with infection. The increase in bands

indicates young WBCs have been recruited to fight an acute infection. Hb, Hct, and RBCs are reduced, indicating hemodilution or blood loss. This reduces oxygen-carrying capacity, requiring an increased cardiac output to maintain adequate oxygen delivery. The potassium is slightly reduced and should be replenished, especially if heart rhythm abnormalities develop. Circulating total proteins and albumin are reduced, which is a common finding after major surgery. This slightly reduces oncotic pressure, making the patient susceptible to fluid accumulation in the lungs.

11. The therapeutic goals are to re-expand collapsed areas of the lung via lung inflation techniques and to treat the hypoxemia.

12. Initial recommendations for treatment should focus on simple lung inflation techniques and correction of hypoxemia:

    (a) Incentive spirometry (IS) with multiple, maximal inspiratory capacity maneuvers should be performed hourly.

    (b) Lung volume improvement should be monitored.

    (c) Poor response to IS would warrant PEP mask therapy or intermittent CPAP, usually with initial pressures of 8 to 10 cm H_2O. Pressures may need to be increased if the initial settings do not prove effective.

    (d) Supplemental oxygen therapy should continue, with high-flow oxygen system at a specific FIO_2. A high-flow system will help ensure that inspired oxygen concentrations will not vary with changes in the tidal volume, pattern, or rate. Because the patient's ventilation ($PaCO_2$) is adequate, monitoring improvement in oxygenation can be done with intermittent pulse oximetry. A repeat ABG analysis is indicated if the clinical condition does not improve or deteriorates.

    (e) Hb and Hct should be monitored and transfusion should be suggested if values continue to drop.

    Patient compliance and proper coaching is extremely important to lung inflation therapy. Excessive secretions do not appear to be the cause of this patient's atelectasis, so CPT or bronchoscopy are not indicated.

13. The RCP should evaluate the patient's response to oxygen therapy by monitoring heart rate, respiratory rate, perceived dyspnea, pulse oximetry, and ABGs.

    The RCP can evaluate the response to lung inflation techniques by monitoring lung volumes (inspiratory capacity, tidal volume, slow vital capacity), chest radiograph, respiratory rate, breath sounds, and pulse oximetry or ABGs.

Initial treatment included incentive spirometry along with encouraging deep breathing and coughing. Six hours after initiating incentive spirometry, the patient remained alert and oriented but continued to complain of dyspnea. Her inspiratory capacity was 1.3 liters, respiratory rate 26/minute, and pulse 116/minute. She continued to be febrile, to use her accessory muscles of breathing, and to have diminished breath sounds in the bases with some inspiratory crackles. Pulse oximetry revealed a saturation of 92 percent on an FIO_2 of 0.45. A repeat of the chest radiograph is pending.

Questions

14. Are the therapeutic objectives being met?

15. What is your assessment of the patient's condition following incentive spirometry therapy for 6 hours?

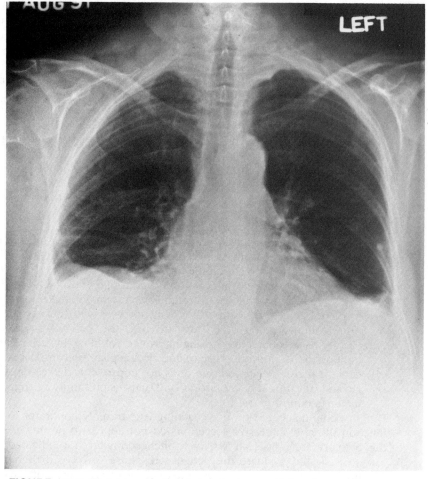

FIGURE 13–2 Portable chest radiograph demonstrating improvement with better lung expansion.

16. Do you suggest any changes in the treatment plan?
17. What is this patient at risk for, with regard to her pulmonary status?

Answers

14. The therapeutic objectives were to improve oxygenation and lung expansion. It appears that oxygenation has improved, although it remains less than optimal. Lung expansion has not improved significantly.

15. Assessment of the patient after 6 hours of incentive spirometry is persistent atelectasis. This assessment is based on the continued tachypnea, diminished breath sounds and crackles, and reduced inspiratory capacity.

16. Treatment at this point should include the application of intermittent CPAP or PEP therapy. This is needed because of the slow resolution of the atelectasis following incentive spirometry.

17. The patient is at high risk for respiratory failure. Respiratory failure could occur when the excessive work of breathing tires the respiratory muscles and results in fatigue. This would be recognized by deterioration of the ABGs, vital signs, and sensorium.

PEP mask therapy was started every hour for 15 breaths at 8 cm H_2O and increased to 12 cm H_2O. Four hours after initiating PEP, dyspnea improved, respiratory rate was 18/minute, and pulse oximetry was 97 percent on an F_{IO_2} of 0.40. A repeat of the chest radiograph demonstrated improvement (Fig. 13–2). PEP frequency was reduced to every 3 hours, and incentive spirometry maintained every hour while awake. The patient was switched to nasal cannula at 4 liters/minute, and 24 hours later transferred to a stepdown unit. Incentive spirometry and oxygen orders continued for 2 days after her transfer.

REFERENCES

1. Luce, JM: Clinical risk factors for postoperative pulmonary complications. Respir Care 29:484, 1984.

2. Johnson, NT and Pierson, DJ: The spectrum of pulmonary atelectasis: Pathophysiology, diagnosis, and therapy. Respir Care 31:1107, 1986.

3. Didier, EP: Some effects of anesthetics and the anesthetized state on the respiratory system. Respir Care 29:463, 1984.

4. Stein, M and Cassara, EL: Preoperative pulmonary evaluation and therapy for surgery patients. JAMA 211:787, 1970.

5. Wightman, JAK: A prospective survey of the incidence of postoperative pulmonary complications. Br J Surg 55:85, 1968.

6. Benjamin, JJ, et al: Left lower lobe atelectasis and consolidation following cardiac surgery: the effect of topical cooling on the phrenic nerve. Radiology 142:11, 1982.

7. Craig, DG: Postoperative recovery of pulmonary function, anaesthesia and analgesia. Anesth Analg 60:46, 1981.

8. Marini, JJ: Postoperative atelectasis: Pathophysiology, clinical importance, and principles of management. Respir Care 29:516, 1984.

9. Hodgkin, JE: Preoperative assessment of respiratory function. Respir Care 29:496, 1984.

10. Dale, WA and Rahn, H: Rate of gas absorption during atelectasis. Am J Physiol 170:606, 1952.

11. Webb, SJS and Nunn, JF: A comparison between the effect of nitrous oxide and nitrogen on arterial PO_2. Anaesthesia 22:69, 1967.

12. Matthay, MA and Wiener-Kronish, JP: Respiratory management after surgery. Chest 95:424, 1989.

13. Askanazi, J, et al: Patterns of ventilation in postoperative and acutely ill patients. Crit Care Med 7:41, 1979.

14. Stoller, JK: Pulmonary function testing as a screening technique. Respir Care 34:611, 1989.

15. Celli, BR, et al: A controlled trial of intermittent positive pressure breathing, incentive spirometry, and deep breathing exercises in preventing pulmonary complications after surgery. Am Rev Respir Dis 130:12, 1984.

16. Branson, RD: PEEP without endotracheal intubation. Respir Care 33:598, 1988.

17. Ricksten, SE, et al: Effects of periodic positive pressure breathing by mask on postoperative pulmonary function. Chest 89:774, 1986.

18. Ford, TG and Guenter, CA: Toward prevention of postoperative complications. Am Rev Respir Dis 130:4, 1984.

19. O'Donohue, WJ Jr: Maximum volume IPPB for the management of pulmonary atelectasis. Chest 76:683, 1979.

20. Marini, JJ, Pierson, DJ, and Hudson, LD: Acute lobar atelectasis: A prospective comparison of fiberoptic bronchoscopy and respiratory therapy. Am Rev Respir Dis 119:971, 1979.

   21.   Stiller, KB, et al: Acute lobar atelectasis: A comparison of two chest physiotherapy regimens. Chest 98:1336, 1990.

   22.   Mahajan, VK, Carton, PW, and Huber, GL: The value of fiberoptic bronchoscopy in the management of pulmonary collapse. Chest 73:817, 1978.

Chapter 14

N. Lennard Specht, MD

INTERSTITIAL LUNG DISEASE

INTRODUCTION

Interstitial lung disease refers to a group of diseases that cause inflammation and fibrosis of the lower respiratory tract. The term pulmonary fibrosis is also applied to these diseases because fibrosis of the lung is the ultimate result of interstitial lung disease. Many conditions lead to interstitial lung disease, including diseases that have no known etiology such as sarcoidosis, rheumatoid arthritis, and idiopathic pulmonary fibrosis. Causes of interstitial lung disease in which the etiology is known include diseases of inhalation such as asbestosis, silicosis, and hypersensitivity pneumonitis. Cancer chemotherapy, oxygen therapy, and radiation therapy may also cause pulmonary fibrosis.

The earliest descriptions of interstitial lung disease involved workers exposed to inorganic dusts. Hippocrates told stories of miners who had difficulty breathing. Dutch pathologists noted a sandy texture to the lungs in patients who had worked in mines. Nineteenth-century English medical literature contains many good descriptions of dust-related lung disease (pneumoconiosis).[1,2] Coal worker's pneumoconiosis generated a tremendous amount of publicity in the early 20th century. Worker safety concerns generated intense political debate and resulted in the "Black Lung Laws." These laws allow workers with coal worker's pneumoconiosis to be compensated financially for their lung disease.

Cutaneous sarcoidosis was first described in 1869 by two dermatologists. Sarcoid lung involvement was noted several decades later.[3] Idiopathic pulmonary fibrosis was first described in 1944—a recent discovery in comparison to those of other forms of interstitial lung disease.[4]

All forms of interstitial lung disease follow a common chain of events (Fig. 14-1). In this scheme the disease is initiated by an injury. The injury promotes a vigorous immune reaction and inflammation. Inflammation leads to destruction of lung tissue and is followed by a disorganized repair process. The disordered repair leads to pulmonary fibrosis and eventually to end-stage lung disease.

ETIOLOGY

An extremely large number of diseases may elicit interstitial lung disease. These diseases are usually classified according to the type of agent that causes the lung injury (Table 14-1). About one third of patients with interstitial lung disease have an identifiable agent responsible for inducing lung injury. Typical inorganic dusts that may induce interstitial lung disease include asbestos, silica (sand), coal, or talc. These agents injure the epithelium or endothelium of the lung by a direct

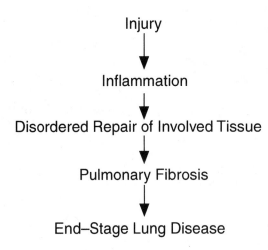

Injury

↓

Inflammation

↓

Disordered Repair of Involved Tissue

↓

Pulmonary Fibrosis

↓

End–Stage Lung Disease

FIGURE 14–1 Cascade of events thought to represent the steps leading from the initiation of interstitial lung disease and culminating with pulmonary fibrosis and end-stage lung disease. Each of these stages may be present simultaneously in a given patient.

toxic effect[5] or indirectly by leading to the production of toxic metabolites or by activating immune responses.[6] Perhaps the most infamous disease caused by the inhalation of inorganic dusts is coal worker's pneumoconiosis, which occurs in about 0.4 percent of people who regularly work with coal dust.[7]

Inhalation of organic dusts may create a form of interstitial lung disease known as hypersensitivity pneumonitis. Hypersensitivity pneumonitis is associated with repeated exposure to organic antigens. In susceptible patients, repeated exposure to the antigen leads to an abnormal allergic response that is destructive to the lung. Many organic antigens may cause hypersensitivity pneumonitis. One of the more notorious antigens is from a group of bacteria called *Thermophilic actinomycetes. T. actinomycetes* thrives at temperatures between 45°C and 60°C, temperatures that are present during vegetation decomposition. Repeated exposure to dusts from decomposing vegetation containing *T. actinomycetes* will precipitate the disease in susceptible individuals. A number of forms of hypersensitivity pneumonitis are named for organic materials that contain *T. actinomycetes* as they decompose. These forms include humidifier lung (air conditioning or humidifier ducts), bagassosis (sugar cane), mushroom worker's lung (mushroom compost), farmer's lung (hay), and grain handler's lung (grain). *T. actinomycetes* is only one group in a wide array of organisms that provide antigens that cause hypersensitivity pneumonitis. These organisms include various fungi, actinomycosis, bacteria, parasites, insects, and mammals.

Drug-induced interstitial lung disease is an important problem because the disease is frequently the result of therapy. Early recognition of drug-induced injury will allow discontinuation of the offending drug, will usually stop further injury,

Table 14–1 Classification of Interstitial Lung Disease

Known Etiology	Unknown Etiology
Inorganic dusts	Sarcoidosis
Hypersensitivity pneumonitis	Collagen vascular disease
	Idiopathic pulmonary fibrosis
Drugs	Other
Toxins	
Oxygen	
Radiation	
Infection	

and may reverse the disease process. A large array of drugs are known to induce lung injury (Table 14–2).

The majority of drugs that are well known for induction of interstitial lung disease are used in the treatment of cancer. Drug-induced lung disease is a major cause of morbidity and mortality in patients undergoing cancer chemotherapy.[8] Up to 20 percent of patients undergoing chemotherapy who develop diffuse infiltrative changes in their lungs have interstitial lung disease.[9] Many patients die as a result of chemotherapy-induced interstitial lung disease.[10] Most chemotherapy agents induce a pulmonary reaction within weeks of exposure, but some may result in lung disease many months after the last dose.

Amiodarone is a potent antiarrhythmic drug used for patients with serious cardiac arrhythmias that do not improve with other treatments. The development of amiodarone lung disease is related to the dose the patient receives.[11] Patients receiving high doses of amiodarone have a greater incidence of toxicity than those who receive a lower dose.[11] The incidence of pulmonary complications due to amiodarone is between 1 and 18 percent. Because of the risk for toxicity it is used only after most other antiarrhythmic agents have proven ineffective. If lung disease develops, it becomes a difficult decision whether to reduce or stop amiodarone and thereby risk sudden cardiac death or to continue the drug.

Nitrofurantoin is an antibiotic that is particularly effective for treating urinary tract infections. On rare occasions its use gives rise to interstitial lung disease. The pulmonary toxicity from nitrofurantoin is either an acute reaction that begins hours to a few days following the first dose or a chronic reaction that develops after months to years of drug use.

Illicit drugs, particularly narcotics such as heroin, produce an acute form of noncardiogenic pulmonary edema. Talc is occasionally mixed into illicit drugs either because it was used to dilute (cut) the drug or because the drug was prepared for injection from talc-containing tablets. The intravenous (IV) injection of talc creates a granulomatous reaction in small blood vessels and interstitium of the lung.

Oxygen at high concentrations over several hours or days may induce acute lung injury. Pathologic pulmonary changes develop in animals after 12 hours of exposure to 100 percent oxygen. Pulmonary edema develops after 48 hours of exposure to 100 percent oxygen. Adult respiratory distress syndrome (ARDS) follows the development of pulmonary edema.

The etiology of several forms of interstitial lung diseases is unknown. These

Table 14–2 Partial List of Drugs Associated with Development of Interstitial Lung Disease

Cancer chemotherapy
  Bleomycin
  Busulfan
  Cyclophosphamide
  Cytosine arabinoside
  Methotrexate
Antibiotics
  Nitrofurantoin
Anti-inflammatory agents
  Gold
  Aspirin
Cardiovascular drugs
  Amiodarone
Illicit drugs
  Heroin
  Propoxyphene

diseases include sarcoidosis, the collagen vascular diseases, and idiopathic pulmonary fibrosis. Although the initial injury that causes the process is unknown, all of these diseases are characterized by intense immune activity that results in destruction and fibrosis of the lung.

PATHOLOGY AND PATHOPHYSIOLOGY

The architecture of the lung can be viewed as a very delicate collection of small bubbles (alveoli). The bubbles connect to the trachea through a complex network of airways. The walls of the alveoli consist of an extremely thin layer of tissue and blood vessels. The walls of the alveolus are extraordinarily thin and provide little resistance to the diffusion of gas between the capillary and alveolar air. The epithelial cells responsible for most of the alveolar lining are the type I alveolar cells (pneumocytes). These cells are very flat with a large surface area that conforms to the shape of the underlying capillary bed. Scattered between the type I cells are a few type II cells that are much rounder and thicker; these are responsible for the secretion of surfactant. This fragile structure becomes the principal focus of the events that characterize interstitial lung disease (Fig. 14–1).

The pathologic appearance of the lungs in patients with early interstitial lung disease is characterized by inflammation. Some forms of interstitial lung disease develop characteristic patterns of inflammation on microscopic examination. The pattern of inflammation is used to assist in determining the underlying disease responsible for lung injury. However, most forms of pulmonary fibrosis are virtually indistinguishable by the time they reach end stage.

The initial event leading to interstitial lung disease is lung injury. In most cases of interstitial lung disease, no injuring agent is visible on microscopic evaluation. However, certain agents that create lung injury can be seen when the lung is examined microscopically. The inorganic dusts such as asbestos and talc are typically visible on microscopic section.

Following lung injury, patients with interstitial lung disease develop pulmonary inflammation. The alveolus is the most frequent site for inflammation but the vasculature and smaller airways may be involved as well. The inflammatory response is characterized by migration of neutrophils, eosinophils, lymphocytes, macrophages, and/or plasma cells into the alveolus and alveolar wall. The influx of immune cells is accompanied by fluid accumulation in the alveolar walls and alveolar air space. This immune reaction damages the alveoli. The flat type I pneumocytes are destroyed and replaced with the secretory type II cells. The alveolar walls become thickened and distorted by the inflammation. The alveoli are eventually destroyed as the disease progresses and are eventually replaced with fibrotic connective tissue and cystic air spaces. The cystic air spaces that result from this process are lined with cuboidal or columnar epithelium and do not participate in gas exchange.[12]

CLINICAL FEATURES

Medical History

The symptoms of lung involvement are similar regardless of the underlying cause. In addition, the symptoms of lung involvement are nonspecific and could suggest many other etiologies including obstructive lung disease, heart disease, or pulmonary vascular disease. The first symptoms of pulmonary fibrosis are usually progressive dyspnea on exertion or a nonproductive cough. Patients initially notice dyspnea only during heavy exertion. Lower levels of exertion induce breathlessness as the process advances. Dyspnea occurs at rest during very advanced stages of the disease.

Interstitial lung disease may lead to pulmonary hypertension and then right heart failure (cor pulmonale). Cor pulmonale causes edema fluid to accumulate primarily in the liver and lower extremities.

A careful history must include an employment record and a review of the patient's environment. A thorough review of the patient's past medical history with current and previous medications is also important. The goal of these questions is to determine whether the patient was exposed to agents known to cause interstitial lung disease. Evaluation and treatment may be greatly altered if the patient was exposed to such a substance.

Physical Examination

The physical examination in patients with interstitial lung disease is often very nonspecific. No abnormal findings are present early in the course of the disease. As the process progresses, tachypnea and inspiratory pulmonary crackles are present. A prominent pulmonic component of the second heart sound will occur if pulmonary hypertension is present. Distension of the jugular veins and edema of the lower extremities are signs of cor pulmonale. Clubbing of the digits is a frequent finding, particularly with asbestosis and idiopathic pulmonary fibrosis.

If the cause of pulmonary fibrosis is a systemic disease, then additional abnormalities specific to the disease can often be found on examination. For example, rheumatoid lung is almost always accompanied by arthritis. Patients with sarcoidosis may have a rash, swollen lymph nodes, or cardiac rhythm irregularities. A complete physical examination is vital because it may guide the clinician to the etiology of pulmonary fibrosis and it provides an indication of the severity of the disease.

Laboratory Data

Arterial blood gas (ABG) levels are normal early in the disease. As the process develops, the alveolar-arterial oxygen tension gradient [$P(A-a)O_2$] increases.[13,14] Hypoxemia during exercise is a frequent finding that may progress to hypoxemia at rest in advanced disease. Hypercapnia may occur during the terminal stages of pulmonary fibrosis.

Lung volumes and flow rates are initially normal, but both decrease throughout the course of the disease.[15] Pulmonary function testing usually shows a purely restrictive defect in most patients with interstitial lung disease. This is characterized by a decrease in forced vital capacity (FVC) and forced expiratory volume in 1 second (FEV$_1$). The loss of FEV$_1$ is proportional to FVC loss, so that the ratio of FEV$_1$ to FVC remains normal. Other measurements of lung volume such as total lung capacity (TLC) and residual volume (RV) are also usually reduced.

The compliance of the lungs decreases as lung involvement progresses. This is due in part to fibrosis of the pulmonary parenchyma and the formation of cystic air spaces.[16] Diffusion capacity of the lung (DLCO) is a good reflection of alveolar capillary surface area. Destruction of lung parenchyma results in a reduction in DLCO as interstitial lung disease progresses. An abnormal DLCO may be the earliest evidence of interstitial lung disease found on standard pulmonary function tests.[14,17]

Oxygen desaturation during exercise is a frequent finding in patients with interstitial lung disease and is usually the earliest detectable pulmonary abnormality.[13,14] Exercise desaturation is caused by worsening of ventilation-perfusion ratio ($\dot{V}/\dot{Q}$) matching and reduction in the red blood cell transit time through the alveolar capillaries.[16]

Interstitial lung disease diffusely effects both lungs; therefore, the typical chest radiograph shows diffuse involvement of both lungs. The chest radiograph is normal early in the course of interstitial lung disease. The initial chest roentgenograph abnormality is frequently a ground-glass appearance in the lungs.

Another radiographic presentation of this disease is diffuse pulmonary opacification (infiltrate). The pattern of opacities is characterized as small nodules (nodular), lines (reticular), or both (reticulonodular; see Fig. 14–2). Some chest radiographs contain specific findings that are suggestive of a particular disease process. For example, sarcoidosis is often associated with swelling of the lymph nodes in the hilum of the lung (hilar lymphadenopathy (Fig. 14–3)). Wegener's granulomatosis is associated with lower lobe cavities and nodules. Asbestosis is often associated with calcified pleural plaques (Fig. 14–4).

Most interstitial lung diseases cause a progressive increase in the opacities on the roentgenogram and culminate with the development of "honeycomb lung." The honeycomb appearance is created by the cysts that characterize the pathology of end-stage interstitial lung disease (Fig. 14–5).

Radioactive gallium-67 is absorbed in areas of inflammation. Gallium scans of the lungs frequently show uptake of the isotope in patients with interstitial lung

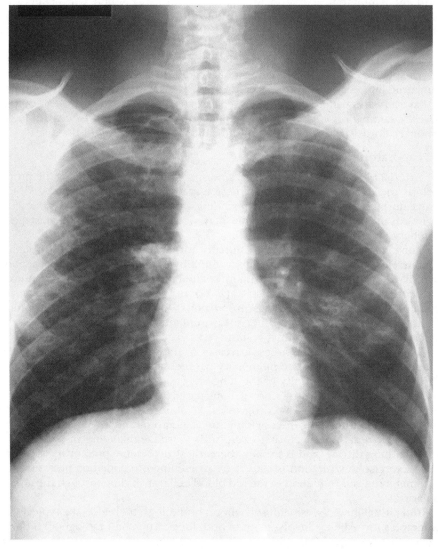

FIGURE 14–2 A diffuse reticular nodular pattern is visible diffusely throughout both lungs.

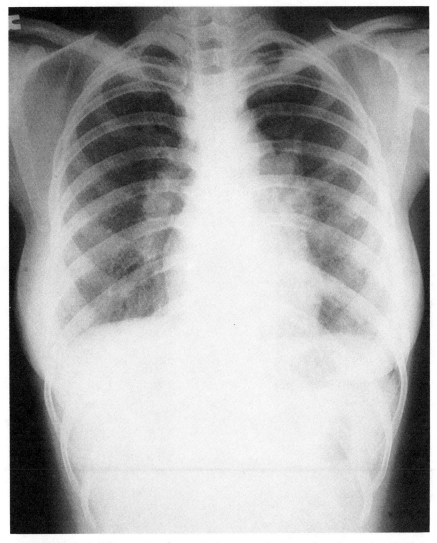

FIGURE 14–3 This chest radiograph shows a reticular pattern throughout both lungs. In addition, lymphadenopathy is visible in both hilar regions.

disease. The presence of inflammation may correlate with the presence of gallium-67 uptake in the lungs. Gallium scanning has been used to follow the effectiveness of therapy.[16,18]

Conformation of interstitial lung disease frequently requires a lung biopsy in addition to a meticulous history and physical examination, as well as laboratory and radiographic evaluations. Pulmonary fibrosis typically involves all lobes of both lungs. However, when the lung is examined microscopically, the stage of involvement is extremely variable from one area of the specimen to another. Portions of lung that reveal characteristic pathologic findings are often scattered among areas of normal lung and areas of end-stage fibrosis. In order to be certain that areas with characteristic changes are sampled, an open lung biopsy is usually required. Sarcoidosis is one disease that has such diffuse and characteristic pathologic changes that only very small pieces of lung are required to establish the diagnosis. These smaller specimens can be obtained with a bronchoscope using a technique called

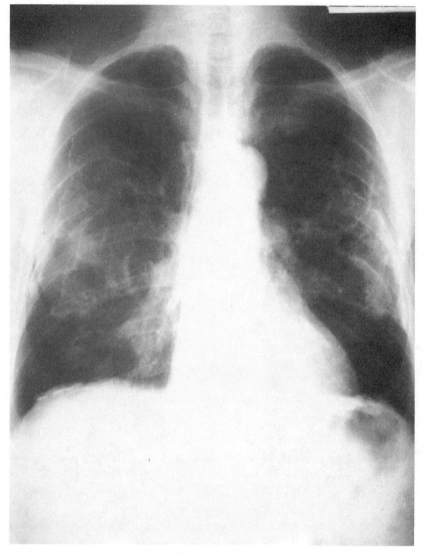

FIGURE 14–4 This chest radiograph discloses asbestos-related calcified pleural plaques. The plaques are easiest to see on the diaphragmatic surface as dense raised areas on both hemidiaphragms. Pleural plaques are also visible superimposed over the middle of both lungs. The plaques overlying the lung are more difficult to see than the diaphragmatic plaques because visualization is through the flat surface rather than the end of the plaque.

transbronchial biopsy. To perform transbronchial biopsy, the bronchoscope is positioned in a smaller airway and a forceps is passed beyond the view of the operator into the periphery of the lung. The forceps can then be used to take small biopsies of lung tissue.

Bronchoalveolar lavage is another diagnostic technique performed by passing a bronchoscope into a segmental or smaller bronchi. The area beyond the bronchoscope is washed with saline. The saline that is then aspirated back through the bronchoscope contains a small number of cells. The cells that are recovered include many from the alveoli and are representative of the cells associated with the inflam-

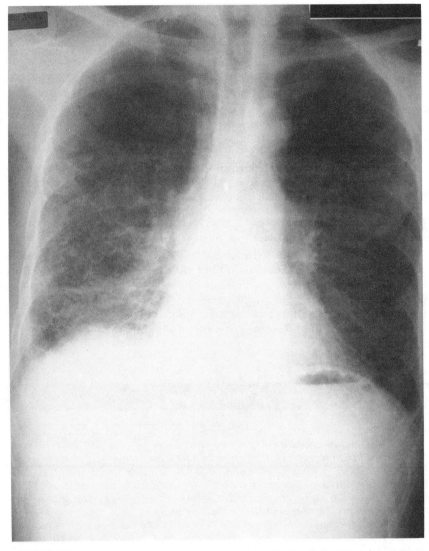

FIGURE 14–5 Dense reticular changes and cystic air spaces can be seen on this film—a pattern often called "honeycomb lung." This film is typical of end-stage pulmonary fibrosis.

matory process. The pathologic evaluation of these cells may provide data on the cause of the interstitial lung disease and may also be useful to follow the inflammatory activity of the lung during therapy.

TREATMENT

The events that cause interstitial lung disease begin with lung injury (Fig. 14–1), which leads to lung inflammation, which in turn results in irreversible pulmonary fibrosis and end-stage lung disease. The goal of therapy is to prevent further irreversible damage to the lung. This is achieved by prevention of further injury and suppression of the inflammatory response.

The most obvious treatment for lung injury induced by a known agent is preventing the patient from being further exposed to the injurious substance. For example, a person with busulfan-induced lung disease should take no more busulfan. A person with silicosis should no longer be exposed to further silica dust. Preventing further lung injury by avoiding any more exposure to the causative agent is often adequate treatment and arrests the disease.

Unfortunately, an injuring agent is identified in only about one third of patients with interstitial lung disease. If the source of injury cannot be removed, or if removal of the source of injury is insufficient to avoid disease progression, treatment is aimed at suppressing inflammation. The drug most commonly used to suppress inflammation initially is prednisone. In addition to prednisone, other immunosuppressive drugs such as cyclophosphamide[19] and azathioprine[20] are also used.

Exertional dyspnea associated with exercise hypoxemia is frequently improved by the addition of supplemental oxygen. Oxygen at rest is required in the latter stages of the disease when dyspnea at rest develops.

PROGNOSIS

The prognosis for patients with interstitial lung disease is extremely variable. A large number of diseases frequently do not alter life expectancy if treated early. These diseases include sarcoidosis, silicosis, hypersensitivity pneumonitis, and amiodarone toxicity. Other diseases are progressive and difficult to control even with aggressive therapy. These diseases include idiopathic pulmonary fibrosis, many forms of drug-induced lung disease, and some of the lung diseases associated with collagen vascular disease.

Case Study

HISTORY

RJ is a 28-year-old black man currently employed as a savings and loan computer analyst. He noticed increasing fatigue over the last several months, which progressed to the point that he stopped jogging and he felt listless and tired most of the time. This began as a flulike illness and left him with a nonproductive cough. He denied fever, chills, sore throat, coryza, headaches, or wheezing. He noted no sputum production, hemoptysis, or abnormalities in his feet or digits.

After further questioning he believed that the fatigue he experienced was probably dyspnea. He could walk indefinitely on level ground, but if he were to climb more than one flight of stairs he would have to stop to catch his breath. He did not awaken with breathlessness nor develop dyspnea at rest.

As a child he had had chickenpox but not measles or mumps. He has had no surgeries but had broken his leg in a skiing accident at age 22. RJ never smoked and used alcohol only socially. The only prescription medication he took was ampicillin once or twice for upper respiratory infections. He used aspirin for minor pain control, which was usually once a month.

His mother has hypertension and his father is healthy. His maternal grandfather has lung carcinoma and his maternal grandmother is well. Both of his paternal grandparents died in an automobile accident. He has two children; both are well. Two healthy birds are kept as pets in the house.

He works as a manager of a small group of computer technicians. He was not exposed to any dusts or fumes while he performed his duties. He had worked as a computer manager since graduating from college. While in college he had worked in a gas station pumping gas, and in high school at a local drive-through restaurant.

He is an avid sports fan and spends his leisure time watching professional sports. None of his hobbies place him at risk for the development of lung disease.

Questions

1. What is the principal problem RJ is complaining of? Is there anything in the history that helps us to characterize the problem?
2. What possible diagnosis could explain this man's dyspnea on exertion?
3. Do the jobs this man has performed place him at risk for lung disease? What jobs are typically related to exposure to inhaled inorganic dusts.
4. Though this patient denies the use of illicit drugs, what form of lung disease do these drugs cause?
5. What are your goals for the physical examination?

Answers

1. RJ's principal complaint is dyspnea. The dyspnea is present only on exertion and has been progressive.
2. The four major types of illness that can cause exertional dyspnea include (1) obstructive lung diseases such as asthma, emphysema, or chronic bronchitis; (2) interstitial lung disease; (3) pulmonary vascular disease such as primary pulmonary hypertension or chronic thrombotic obstruction of the pulmonary artery; (4) heart diseases such as ischemic or valvular heart disease.

    This patient lacks the typical symptoms of obstructive lung disease such as wheezing and experiencing episodic dyspnea at rest or that awakens him from sleep. He also lacks a history of previous cardiac problems that are typical of many patients with exertional dyspnea due to heart problems. There is no history of previous deep venous thrombosis to suggest chronic thrombotic obstruction of the pulmonary artery.

    Despite a careful history, none of these diagnoses can be excluded from consideration. The history does, however, clarify the problem we are dealing with and allows us to formulate a preliminary differential diagnosis.
3. RJ is young and has worked primarily as a manager. None of the jobs he describes are likely to have caused lung disease. A careful exposure history should also include a history of exposure to pets and hobbies. The birds that are kept in his home as pets are a possible source for hypersensitivity pneumonitis or infection.

    The most common forms of inorganic pneumoconiosis are coal worker's pneumoconiosis, asbestosis, and silicosis. Coal worker's pneumoconiosis is caused by repeated exposure to coal dust. This occurs in miners and people who load coal for shipment. Asbestosis occurs in workers who are exposed to dust from asbestos. These people have usually worked directly with asbestos as it is machined or installed. Asbestos is only hazardous when it is in the form of a dust that can be inhaled. Asbestos-containing products that do not shed dust are not dangerous. Silicosis occurs in miners, sand blasters, foundry workers, or anyone who deals with sand dust on a regular basis.
4. Illicit drugs may create lung disease in two ways: (1) by inducing noncardiogenic pulmonary edema or (2) by vasculitis induced by the IV injection of talc. Talc is sometimes used to dilute (cut) the active drug or may have contaminated the drug as it was extracted from talc-containing tablets.
5. The major goal of the physical examination is to help clarify the cause of RJ's dyspnea. Obstructive lung disease may be associated with increase in the anteroposterior (AP) diameter of the chest and wheezes over the lung. Interstitial lung disease is usually associated with pulmonary crack-

les. Pulmonary vascular disease is characterized by the signs of pulmonary hypertension. The physical examination findings in pulmonary hypertension are a loud pulmonic component to the second heart sound (P_2) and possibly right ventricular heave or lift. Patients with chronic heart disease may have an abnormal heart rhythm. Abnormal extra heart sounds such as a cardiac murmur and an S_3 or S_4 suggest valvular heart disease and heart failure, respectively.

PHYSICAL EXAMINATION ⎯⎯⎯⎯⎯⎯

Vital Signs   *Temperature 36.3°C; pulse 62/minute; respiratory rate is 14/minute; blood pressure 155/97 mm Hg*

General   *This is an athletic-appearing black man in no respiratory distress.*

HEENT   *Head normal; nose patent without discharge; pupils are equal, round, and reactive to light; mucous membranes moist without cyanosis*

Neck   *Carotid arteries have a normal contour and intensity; jugular neck veins not distended; trachea in midline of neck; swelling of submandibular salivary glands and several 1- to 2-cm lymph nodes in anterior cervical region*

Chest   *Configuration and expansion of the chest normal; diffuse fine inspiratory crackles throughout both lungs without wheezing found upon auscultation; normal resonance noted over all portions of the chest with percussion*

Heart   *Regular rate with no murmur or gallop; S_1 and S_2 have normal intensity and splitting; cardiac impulse is in the fourth interspace 1 cm medial to the midclavicular line*

Abdomen   *Soft, nontender; bowel sounds active; no masses or organ enlargement noted; abdominal wall rising with each inspiration*

Extremities   *No edema noted; no clubbing or cyanosis seen; extremities warm with good capillary refill*

Questions

6. What is your intepretation of the vital signs?
7. Interpret the pulmonary findings and state how they may affect your assessment of this patient.
8. Interpret the cardiac findings and state how they affect your assessment.
9. Does this patient have evidence of cor pulmonale?
10. What is the significance of the swelling of multiple structures in the neck?
11. Describe the normal relationship between the respiratory cycle and movement of the abdominal wall.
12. What pathology typically accounts for the fine inspiratory crackles heard in this patient? Are crackles commonly heard in patients with restrictive lung disease or obstructive lung disease?

13. Does the lack of cyanosis indicate that hypoxemia is not present?
14. What laboratory work would be most useful to determine the etiology of this person's dyspnea?

Answers

6. With the exception of the blood pressure, the vital signs are normal. The elevation of blood pressure may be due to hypertension or may be a response to stress in a healthy person. Treatment of hypertension of this magnitude is not necessary unless multiple measurements have shown chronic elevation of blood pressure.

7. It was noted that RJ had diffuse fine inspiratory crackles over both lungs, which is consistent with the diagnosis of interstitial lung disease or pulmonary edema from heart failure. Wheezing and increased AP diameter of the chest, signs of obstructive lung disease, are absent.

   The lung examination indicates that heart failure and interstitial lung disease are the most likely explanations for RJ's exertional breathlessness. It is still possible, though much less likely, that this represents an atypical presentation of obstructive lung disease or pulmonary vascular disease.

8. Results of the heart examination were normal. There were no extra heart sounds and no increase in P_2. The location of the cardiac impulse was normal.

   The lack of abnormal findings on cardiac examination decreases the likelihood but does not eliminate the possibility that RJ's dyspnea is related to pulmonary hypertension or heart failure.

9. Cor pulmonale is right heart failure that is the result of lung disease. Right heart failure causes systemic venous congestion characterized by distension of the jugular veins, pedal edema, and a hepatojugular reflux. In addition to systemic congestion, the heart examination is also abnormal when cor pulmonale is present. Right ventricular strain causes an abnormal pulsation (heave) over the lower left sternal border and an S_3 or S_4 that can be heard over this same area. RJ has none of these findings and therefore does not have cor pulmonale.

10. Swelling of lymph nodes (lymphadenopathy) may result from an infection or inflammatory process occurring either in the area drained by the lymph node or in the lymph node itself. Sarcoidosis is associated with cervical lymphadenopathy and enlargement of salivary glands.

11. The diaphragm is the major muscle of respiration. Contraction of the diaphragm causes it to descend, drawing air into the lungs. Diaphragmatic descent also causes the abdominal wall to rise during inspiration as seen in this patient. If a patient has a very high inspiratory muscle load or has diaphragmatic fatigue the diaphragm rises on inspiration. This paradoxic movement of the diaphragm causes the abdominal wall to fall on inspiration. This would be a sign of respiratory failure.

12. Inspiratory crackles are caused by sudden opening of peripheral lung units with inspiration. This finding is typical of patients with interstitial lung disease, atelectasis, or pulmonary edema.

13. A lack of cyanosis does not indicate that hypoxemia is not present.

14. The disease process that is causing RJ to experience dyspnea is probably an interstitial lung disease but this has not been proven. Pulmonary function testing including spirometry and DLco would help to determine if restrictive or obstructive lung disease is present and would also determine how severe the disease is.

A chest radiograph should be ordered to help classify the pulmonary disease. An ABG analysis should be ordered to determine RJ's ability to ventilate and oxygenate.

LABORATORY DATA

CHEST RADIOGRAPH

(Fig. 14–6)

ABG (ON ROOM AIR)

pH	7.45
Pao_2	65 mm Hg
$Paco_2$	32 mm Hg
bicarbonate	21 mEq/liter
$P(A-a)o_2$	44 mm Hg
O_2 content	17.5 mL/dL

COMPLETE BLOOD COUNT (CBC)

	Observed	Normal
White blood cells (WBCs)/mm³	9100	4,000–11,000
Red blood cells (RBCs) M/mm³	4.3	4.1–5.5

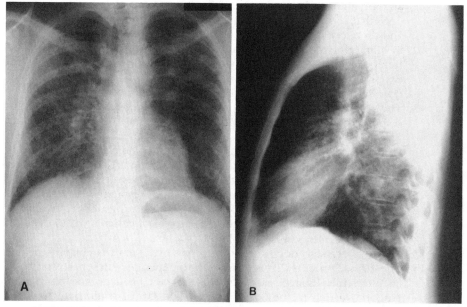

FIGURE 14–6 Chest radiograph of RJ at presentation. *A*, Posteroanterior (PA) view; *B*, lateral view.

	Observed	Normal
Hemoglobin (g/dL)	14.2	14–16.5
Hematocrit (%)	41	40–54
Differential		
Segmented neutrophils	69%	40–75%
Band neutrophils	9%	0–6%
Lymphocytes	17%	20–45%
Monocytes	3%	2–10%
Eosinophils	1%	0–6%
Basophils	1%	0–1%

CHEMISTRY

	Observed	Normal
Na^+ (mEq/liter)	142	137–147
K^+ (mEq/liter)	4.1	3.5–4.8
Cl^- (mmol/dL)	108	98–105
HCO_3^- (mEq/liter)	22	22–29
Blood urea nitrogen (BUN) (mg/dL)	19	7–20
Creatinine (mg/dL)	1.1	0.7–1.3
Calcium (mmol/liter)	2.5	2.1–2.55
Phosphate (mg/dL)	2.9	2.7–4.5
Uric acid (mg/dL)	6.9	4.5–8.2
Albumen (g/dL)	4.8	3.5–5.0
Protein (g/dL)	8.2	6.4–8.3

PULMONARY FUNCTION TESTING

	Value	Percent (%) of Predicted
Spirometry		
FVC (liters)	2.79	63
Slow vital capacity (SVC) (liters)	2.61	59
FEV_1 (liters)	2.12	67
FEV_1/FVC (%)	76	
FEF_{25-75} (liters/minute)	4.11	98
Body Plethysmography		
RV (liters)	1.20	118
TLC (liters)	3.99	74
Diffusion Capacity (DL_{CO})		
DL_{CO} (mL/min/mm Hg)	11.35	38

Questions

15. Please read the chest radiograph and correlate it with this patient's condition.
16. Evaluate and interpret this patient's ABG values.
17. Interpret the pulmonary function test. How do these tests affect possible diagnosis of interstitial lung disease or obstructive lung disease.
18. What testing may be helpful in determining whether this patient will be helped by supplemental oxygen?

19. What additional testing will be needed to determine the cause of this patient's disease?

Answers

15. The chest radiograph shows diffuse reticulonodular opacification of both lungs. There is bilateral hilar enlargement as well. The heart is of normal size and configuration. This chest radiograph is consistent with interstitial lung disease. The presence of hilar lymphadenopathy suggests the diagnosis of sarcoidosis.

16. Chronic respiratory alkalosis is demonstrated in these ABG values. The patient has mild hypoxemia with an increase in the $P(A\text{-}a)O_2$.

17. The reduction of lung volumes on spirometry suggests restrictive lung disease. The loss of FEV_1 is proportional to the loss of vital capacity (FEV_1/FVC is normal), suggesting restrictive lung disease. Measurements obtained from body plethysmography suggest restrictive lung disease. TLC is decreased. The normal RV indicates that some obstructive lung disease may also be present. The abnormal DL_{CO} indicates a loss of alveolar capillary surface area and strongly suggests that lung destruction is occurring.

    These findings are consistent with interstitial lung disease. The normal RV suggests that some obstructive lung disease is present. The obstructive lung disease is unlikely to be clinically relevant.

18. The initial ABG analysis does not indicate that supplemental oxygen is required. Patients with interstitial lung disease become desaturated upon exercise and may benefit from supplemental oxygen during exercise. Treadmill exercise testing with ABG samples and exhaled gas collection would determine whether RJ requires oxygen with exertion.

19. At this point there is strong evidence that RJ has a form of interstitial lung disease. It is important to determine the type of interstitial lung disease in order to devise an appropriate therapeutic plan. Lung biopsy is the most effective way to determine with accuracy what disease is responsible for RJ's symptoms.

    There are several reasons to suspect that RJ has sarcoidosis. Because sarcoidosis is the most likely diagnosis, transbronchial biopsy is the diagnostic test of choice.

ADDITIONAL DIAGNOSTIC DATA

The patient underwent pulmonary stress testing. He exercised for 8 minutes and 32 seconds using a modified Bruce protocol exercise test. He stopped because of extreme dyspnea. No cardiac abnormalities were noted on the electrocardiogram (ECG).

	Value	Percent (%) of Predicted
$\dot{V}O_2$max(mL/min)	1201	37
$\dot{V}CO_2$max (mL/min)	1528	
Respiratory quotient (RQ)	1.27	
Lowest O_2 saturation (percent)	81	

ABGs (ON ROOM AIR AT REST AND DURING PEAK EXERCISE)

Rest

pH	7.43
Pa_{O_2}	65 mm Hg
Pa_{CO_2}	33 mm Hg
HCO_3^-	22 mEq/liter
$P_{(A-a)O_2}$	44 mm Hg
O_2 content	17.5 mL/dL

Peak Exercise

pH	7.31
Pa_{O_2}	47 mm Hg
Pa_{CO_2}	28 mm Hg
HCO_3^-	14 mEq/liter
$P_{(A-a)O_2}$	67 mm Hg
O_2 content	15.6 mL/dL

A bronchoscopy with transbronchial biopsy and bronchoalveolar lavage were performed. The airways appeared normal on examination. A modest amount of bleeding was encountered following transbronchial biopsy. The transbronchial biopsy contained numerous noncaseating granulomas without infectious organisms. The pathologic diagnosis was sarcoidosis. The bronchoalveolar lavage showed numerous lymphocytes with alveolar macrophages and occasional neutrophils.

Questions

20. What is a plausible explanation for RJ's dyspnea on exertion?
21. Interpret the ABG analysis taken at peak exercise. What physiologic changes are responsible for each of the changes you see?
22. What is a respiratory quotient? What does RJ's respiratory quotient indicate?
23. How is a transbronchial biopsy obtained? What type of tissue will it provide for examination?
24. How is bronchoalveolar lavage obtained? What type of samples will it provide for examination?
25. Will oxygen therapy help relieve RJ's breathlessness? If oxygen is given to this patient, how should he use it?
26. What therapy should RJ receive for his sarcoidosis? What is the goal of that therapy?

Answers

20. There are many reasons for people with interstitial lung disease to experience dyspnea. RJ develops hypoxemia with exercise. This exertional desaturation may in part explain the breathlessness he develops when jogging.
21. There is profound hypoxemia. There is also a mixed acid-base disorder with a respiratory alkalosis and a metabolic acidosis. The hypoxemia in this case is caused by worsening of $\dot{V}/\dot{Q}$ matching and reduction in the RBC transit time through the alveolar capillaries.

    The drop in Pa_{CO_2} may be driven by hypoxia and acidosis. The fall in bicarbonate is due to the development of lactic acidosis from anaerobic metabolism of exercising muscle.

22. The RQ is the ratio of carbon dioxide produced to oxygen consumed. At rest, the respiratory quotient of a healthy person is about 0.8. With anaerobic metabolism, such as that during vigorous exercise, the amount of carbon dioxide produced exceeds the amount of oxygen consumed. When an individual makes a transition from aerobic to anaerobic metabolism, he or she is said to have crossed the "anaerobic threshold." RJ had an RQ of 1.27, which indicates that he crossed his anaerobic threshold.

23. Transbronchial biopsy is a technique for sampling alveoli and small airways without performing major surgery. A bronchoscope is used to locate the airway that leads to the portion of the lung that is to be sampled. Biopsy forceps are then passed several inches beyond the bronchoscope and the biopsy is taken from the small airways. The samples of tissue that are obtained are very small and are not adequate to diagnose many forms of interstitial lung disease. However, this technique is popular because it can easily diagnose sarcoidosis and does not require a general anesthetic or skin incision.

24. Like transbronchial biopsy, bronchoalveolar lavage is a bronchoscopic technique. The object of the lavage is to wash a small number of cells from the alveoli for pathologic examination. The bronchoscope is passed into the smallest airway it can enter. Several milliliters (50 to 200) of saline are injected into the bronchial lumen. The saline washes out to the small airways and is then aspirated back out through the bronchoscope. Unlike in biopsies, cells with no surrounding structure are obtained. This technique is useful to diagnose and stage interstitial lung disease, to diagnose certain lung infections (particularly *Pneumocystis carinii* pneumonia), and to diagnose some forms of lung cancer.

25. Yes, RJ has a marked tendency to develop desaturation with moderate exercise levels. The use of supplemental oxygen with exertion may help his exertional dyspnea. There is no need at this time to have him use oxygen 24 hours a day.

26. Sarcoidosis is one of the forms of interstitial lung disease that has no known cause. As a consequence, therapy cannot be directed at preventing further exposure to an injuring agent. Instead therapy is aimed at suppressing inflammation. Suppressing inflammation is usually done with corticosteroids, cyclophosphamide, or azathioprine, or a combination of these drugs. In sarcoidosis, therapy with corticosteroids such as prednisone is usually very effective at stopping progression of the disease.

FOLLOW-UP

One year after the initial diagnosis of sarcoidosis RJ felt much better. He took prednisone for 1 year, with improvement in his chest radiograph. He had less dyspnea on exertion and no longer required oxygen therapy. He continued to have a restrictive defect on spirometry and a reduction in his DLco, but these had improved.

Question

28. If the sarcoidosis had progressed to its end stage, what would RJ's lungs have been like radiographically and pathologically?

Answer

28. End-stage interstitial lung disease is characterized by replacement of normal lung tissue by cystic air spaces and fibrotic tissue. On radiograph, the cystic air spaces can be seen surrounded by fibrous connective tissue in a pattern called honeycomb lung (see Fig. 14–5).

REFERENCES

1. Morgan, WKC and Seaton, A: Occupational Lung Diseases, ed 2. WB Saunders, Philadelphia, 1984.

2. Becklake, MR: Pneumoconiosis. In Murray, JF and Nadel, JA: Textbook of Respiratory Medicine. WB Saunders, Philadelphia, 1988, pp 1556–1592.

3. Johns, CJ: Sarcoidosis. In Fishman, AP: Pulmonary Disease and Disorders. McGraw-Hill, New York, 1988, pp 619–641.

4. Hammon, L and Rich, AR: Acute interstitial fibrosis of the lung. Bull Johns Hopkins 74:177, 1944.

5. Stachura, I, Singh, C, and Whiteside, TL: Mechanisms of tissue injury in desquamative interstitial pneumonitis. Am J Med 68:733, 1980.

6. Fox, RB, et al: Pulmonary inflammation due to oxygen toxicity: Involvement of chemotactic factors and polymorphonuclear leukocytes. Am Rev Respir Dis 123:521, 1981.

7. Guidotti, TL: Coal workers' pneumoconiosis and medical aspects of coal mining. South Med J 72:456, 1979.

8. Batist, G and Andrews, JL: Pulmonary toxicity of antineoplastic drugs. JAMA 246:1449, 1981.

9. Cockerill, FJ, et al: Open lung biopsy in immunocompromised patients. Arch Intern Med 145:1398, 1985.

10. Rosenow, EC and Martin, WJ: Drug induced interstitial lung disease. In Schwarz, MI and King, TE (eds): Interstitial Lung Disease. BC Decker, Toronto, 1988, pp 123–137.

11. Kndenchyk, PJ, et al: Prospective evaluation of amiodarone pulmonary toxicity. Chest 86:541, 1984.

12. Flint, A: Pathologic features of interstitial lung disease. In Schwarz, MI and King, TE (eds): Interstitial Lung Disease. BC Decker, Toronto, 1988, pp 45–62.

13. Crystal, RG, et al: Idiopathic pulmonary fibrosis: Clinical, histologic, radiographic, physiologic, scintigraphic, cytologic and biochemical aspects. Ann Intern Med 85:769, 1976.

14. Fulmer, JD: The interstitial lung diseases. Chest 82:172, 1982.

15. Carrington, CB, et al: Natural history and treated course of usual and desquamative interstitial pneumonia. N Engl J Med 298:801, 1978.

16. Fulmer, JD: An introduction to the interstitial lung diseases. Clin Chest Med 3:457, 1982.

17. Crystal, RG, et al: Interstitial lung disease: Current concepts of pathogenesis staging and therapy. Am J Med 70:542, 1981.

18. Line, BR, et al: Gallium-67 scanning to stage the alveolitis of sarcoidosis: correlation with clinical studies, pulmonary function studies and bronchoalveolar lavage. Am Rev Respir Dis 123:440, 1981.

19. Johnson, MA, et al: Randomized controlled trial comparing prednisolone alone with cyclophosphamide and low dose prednisolone in combination in cryptogenic fibrosing alveolitis. Thorax 44:280, 1989.

20. Raghu, G, et al: Azathioprine combined with prednisone in the treatment of idiopathic pulmonary fibrosis: A prospective double-blind randomized placebo-controlled clinical trial. Am Rev Respir Dis 144:291, 1991.

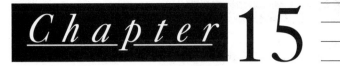

Chapter 15

N. Lennard Specht, MD
Robert L. Wilkins, MA, RRT

NEUROMUSCULAR DISORDERS

INTRODUCTION

The majority of our early experience with mechanical ventilation came from caring for patients with polio.[1,2] Neuromuscular disease remains a common problem confronting health care providers despite the advent of polio vaccination. Severe cases of neuromuscular disease frequently affect the respiratory pump and may lead to respiratory failure. For this reason respiratory care practitioners (RCPs) must be knowledgeable about and skilled at caring for patients with weakness of the respiratory pump.

The respiratory pump has four components:

1. Muscles of respiration
2. Respiratory center located in the central nervous system (CNS)
3. Nerves connecting the respiratory center to the respiratory muscles
4. Peripheral sensors that provide information such as oxygen and carbon dioxide concentrations to the respiratory center

A variety of neuromuscular diseases may affect one component of the respiratory pump and lead to respiratory failure. A review of the anatomy and physiology of the respiratory pump is helpful before discussing specific neuromuscular diseases.

RESPIRATORY CENTERS

The respiratory centers are located diffusely within the medulla and pons in the brainstem. Three major components form the respiratory centers. The medullary respiratory center is responsible for maintaining a regular rhythmic respiratory pattern. The apneustic center and the pneumotaxic center work together to regulate respiratory frequency and volume.[3]

The respiratory centers receive input from oxygen sensors in the carotid bodies, hydrogen ion sensors in the brainstem, mechanoreceptors in the lung, and the cerebral cortex. The respiratory centers interpret this information and produce a signal that is sent through peripheral nerves to the respiratory muscles. As the impulse leaves the brainstem it travels down the spinal cord and exits at numerous levels to travel through peripheral nerves to the neuromuscular junction and finally to the respiratory muscles.

CHEMORECEPTORS

There are two receptors (chemoreceptors) that sense the concentration of oxygen or carbon dioxide in the fluid around them. These receptors create neural impulses based on the concentration of oxygen or carbon dioxide. This impulse is then transmitted to the respiratory centers.

The oxygen chemoreceptors are located in the carotid bodies and the aortic bodies. The carotid bodies are located in the bifurcation of the common carotid arteries. The output of the carotid body increases as the Pao_2 drops.

The central chemoreceptors are located in the ventral surface of the medulla. These receptors are responsive to the concentration of hydrogen ions in the surrounding extracellular fluid. The extracellular fluid is largely controlled by the blood-brain barrier. This barrier strictly regulates the flow of ions and water into the brain. Three ions are the major determinants of cerebral spinal fluid (CSF) pH, bicarbonate, hydrogen, and carbon dioxide. Bicarbonate and hydrogen ion movement is carefully regulated by the blood-brain barrier. In contrast, CO_2 can freely cross the blood-brain barrier. The enhanced mobility of CO_2 makes the central chemoreceptors much more responsive to changes in blood CO_2 than to changes in blood pH.

NERVE TRANSMISSION

The three nerves that are most important to respiration are the phrenic, the intercostal, and the abdominal nerves (Fig. 15–1). The phrenic nerves arise from the cervical spinal cord at the C3 to C5 level. These nerves leave the spinal canal, travel through the neck and into the mediastinum and then over the pericardium, and insert into the diaphragm on either side of the heart.

The intercostal nerves arise from the thoracic spinal cord at levels T1 to T12. The intercostal nerves each course under a rib and supply innervation to the intercostal muscles. The abdominal nerves (muscular) arise from the thoracic and lumbar spine and innervate the abdominal wall muscles.

NEUROMUSCULAR JUNCTION

Each nerve contacts the muscle at a synapse called the neuromuscular junction. An impulse transmitted along a nerve reaches a nerve ending at the neuromuscular junction. The nerve ending releases acetylcholine when stimulated by a nerve impulse. The presence of acetylcholine is sensed by receptors on the muscle fiber. The muscle fiber contracts when these receptors are stimulated by acetylcholine. The acetylcholine is rapidly degraded by acetylcholinesterase to prevent excessive muscle stimulation.

RESPIRATORY MUSCLES

There are many muscles of respiration (Fig. 15–2). The diaphragm is the largest and most prominent inspiratory muscle. Other inspiratory muscles include the external intercostal, the scalene, and the sternocleidomastoid muscles. The expiratory muscles are the internal intercostal and abdominal wall muscles, including rectus abdominus, internal and external oblique, and transverse abdominus muscles.

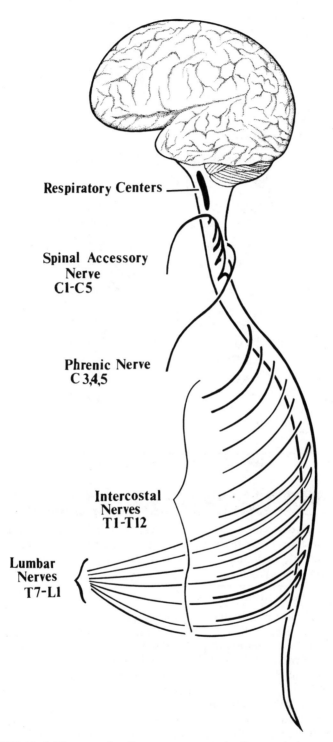

FIGURE 15–1 The neural pathways necessary for the respiratory pump.

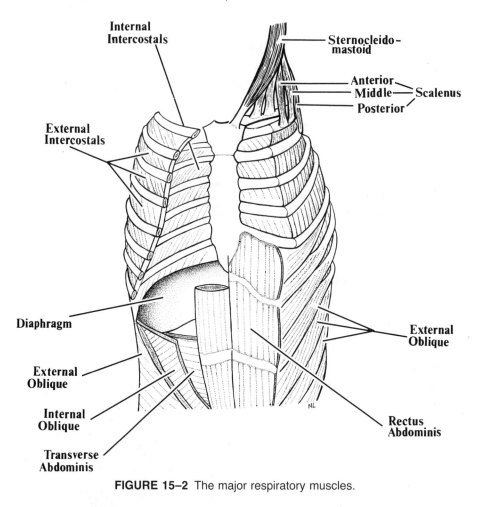

Internal
Intercostals

Sternocleido-
mastoid

Anterior
Middle — Scalenus
Posterior

External
Intercostals

External
Oblique

Diaphragm

External
Oblique

Internal
Oblique

Rectus
Abdominis

Transverse
Abdominis

FIGURE 15–2 The major respiratory muscles.

PATHOLOGY AND PATHOPHYSIOLOGY

The respiratory pump is an efficient system that evaluates respiratory requirements and translates these requirements into ventilation. However, the respiratory
pump is vulnerable to injury. Damage to even the smallest portion of the pump
may lead to respiratory failure.

Respiratory Centers

The diffuse location of the respiratory centers makes them relatively invul-
nerable to direct injury. In fact, the respiratory centers are frequently the only
neurologic function operating in patients with profound cerebral injury. However,
several disease processes appear to affect the respiratory centers. Several diseases
also are thought to result from abnormalities of the respiratory centers.

Central sleep apnea is characterized by lapses of breathing effort during sleep.
This disease primarily affects adults, particularly those with cerebral vascular disease. It is theorized that central sleep apnea is caused by inadequate respiratory
drive.[4] In many patients this inadequate respiratory drive is due to defects in the
central controller (Table 15–1).[5]

Primary alveolar hypoventilation is characterized by insufficient respiratory
drive in the absence of an obvious defect of the respiratory pump or lungs. These

Table 15–1 Neuromuscular Disorders

Location of Defect	Disorder
Central nervous system	Ondine's curse
	Central sleep apnea
	Primary alveolar hypoventilation
	Sedative hypnotic overdose
Neuronal pathway	Spinal cord injury
	Multiple sclerosis
	ALS
Neuromuscular junction	Myasthenia gravis
	Botulism poisoning
	Organophosphate poisoning
Muscular function	Muscular dystrophy
	Myotonic dystrophy

patients hypoventilate while awake and during sleep. They are able to lower their Paco$_2$ voluntarily to normal levels.

Sedative drugs, particularly narcotics, can suppress respiration by depressing the respiratory centers. Overdose of narcotics or barbiturates may lead to apnea.

Nerve Interruption

If signals from the respiratory centers to the respiratory muscles are interrupted, the respiratory pump will be affected. There are many common places where nerve damage can result in respiratory embarrassment.

Trauma is a frequent cause of nerve damage that affects the respiratory pump. Spinal cord transection commonly affects the respiratory pump. Nerves that arise from the spinal cord below the level of injury become nonfunctional. Therefore, muscles supplied by that nerve are also nonfunctional. Injuries to the cervical spinal cord create more difficulty than injuries to the thoracic and lumbar spine (Table 15–2). Damage to the midthoracic spine leads to loss of function of the abdominal and some of the intercostal muscles. Cervical spine injuries in the C6–C7 area lead to loss of function of all intercostal and abdominal muscles. A cervical spinal cord transection to C1–C3 will lead to apnea because all respiratory muscles are affected.

The phrenic nerve is the most important peripheral nerve that may be injured. Interruption of a phrenic nerve may occur during coronary artery bypass surgery. Cooling measures used to protect the heart from ischemia while the bypass grafts are being completed may cool the phrenic nerves excessively. Excessive cooling of the phrenic nerve causes interruption of the nerve and therefore, diaphragmatic paralysis. This paralysis is frequently temporary but may take months to resolve.

Nerves can also be interrupted by nontraumatic processes. Polio is a viral illness that destroys the motor neurons in the anterior horn of the spinal cord. The

Table 15–2 Respiratory Muscle Innervation

Spinal Cord Level	Peripheral Nerve(s)/Muscle(s)
C1–2	Spinal accessory/Sternocleidomastoid
C3–5	Phrenic/Diaphragm
C4–8	Cervical/Scalene
T1–12	Intercostal/Intercostal
T7–L1	Abdominal/Abdominal wall

destruction of motor neurons may involve nerves that innervate respiratory muscles. Paralysis of the respiratory muscles from polio may become so pronounced that respiratory failure and apnea develop. Respiratory failure from polio was a common occurrence in the 1930s.[1]

Amyotrophic lateral sclerosis (ALS) is a progressive fatal neurologic disease. Despite extensive research, no etiology for ALS has been discovered. As in polio, patients with ALS lose muscle function because of loss of motor neurons in the anterior horn of the spinal cord. Patients with this disease may also develop destruction of neurons in the cerebral cortex. Respiratory failure invariably develops in patients afflicted with ALS (Table 15–1).

Patients with Guillain-Barré syndrome (GBS) have a progressive ascending paralysis caused by an inflammatory destruction in the myelin sheath around peripheral nerves. Guillain-Barré is frequently preceded by a viral-type illness. The viral syndrome is followed by inflammation of spinal roots and peripheral nerves. The inflammation of the spinal roots causes destruction of the myelin sheaths. The loss of myelin sheaths causes the associated nerve to malfunction. Typically, after a few weeks the myelin sheath regenerates and the inflammation in the nerves resolves.

Neuromuscular Junction

The nervous impulse can be interrupted at the synapse of the neuromuscular junction. This interruption can be caused by failure of a nerve to release acetylcholine as in botulism poisoning. Destruction of acetylcholine receptors on the muscle as in myasthenia gravis will also lead to muscle weakness and potentially respiratory pump failure (Table 15–1). Certain toxins such as organophosphate insecticides and chemical warfare nerve gases block the breakdown of acetylcholine in the neuromuscular junction. Blocking the breakdown of acetylcholine causes muscle spasms, tetany, and respiratory failure.

Muscle Diseases

Several congenital abnormalities lead to progressive muscular weakness. Muscular dystrophies are examples of this type of disease. Muscular dystrophy leads to progressive muscle weakness and loss of function. Loss of muscle function eventually becomes so profound that respiratory failure develops. Patients with muscular dystrophy frequently die of respiratory failure or pneumonia unless chronic mechanical ventilation is instituted.

CLINICAL FEATURES

The patient with neuromuscular disease may not initially develop respiratory complications. Signs and symptoms of respiratory failure will occur, however, as the muscular weakness progresses to the point of involving the muscles of breathing. As the inspiratory muscles weaken, the patient's lung volumes decrease, and a rapid and shallow breathing pattern develops. The patient often complains of dyspnea, especially on exertion. Weakness of expiratory muscles leads to a poor cough and inability to clear excessive secretions from the airways. Retention of sputum in the lung may lead to mucus plugging, atelectasis, and pneumonia, which are common complications of neuromuscular disease.[6]

Initial arterial blood gas (ABG) findings may be normal in the patient with mild neuromuscular disease. With severe weakness of the respiratory muscles, the ABG values demonstrate hypoxemia, an increased $Paco_2$, and decreased pH. Hypoxemia is common because of ventilation-perfusion ratio ($\dot{V}/\dot{Q}$) mismatching and the increase in alveolar Pco_2 but typically responds to supplemental oxygen therapy. If the patient also has a complicating pneumonia, more severe hypoxemia may be present.

Bedside assessment of pulmonary function will reveal a reduced vital capacity

(VC). Severe disease is marked by a reduction in the VC below 1.0 to 1.5 liters in the adult. The maximum inspiratory pressure (MIP) decreases as the inspiratory muscles weaken. MIP is a useful tool for quantifying the degree of muscle weakness and for identifying trends in the course of the disease. A MIP measurement of less than -20 to -30 cm H_2O usually indicates severe weakness of the inspiratory muscles. Bedside clinicians should measure MIP against a closed mouthpiece after the patient has exhaled to residual volume. Exhaling to residual volume provides the inspiratory muscles with the best mechanical advantage for performing the MIP maneuver.[7]

GBS may occur at any age and has no discernible geographic or seasonal distribution. A preceding viral infection is commonly seen in patients diagnosed with GBS.[8] Initial symptoms often include weakness of the lower extremities and paresthesia (sensations of numbness or tingling) in the fingers and toes. The lower extremity weakness is usually symmetric and the weakness progresses to the muscles of the abdomen, diaphragm, arms, and face. The patient with GBS may experience difficulty swallowing and a poor gag reflex as the muscles of the throat become involved. This may lead to aspiration if the airway is not protected. Some patients with GBS develop hypertension or cardiac dysrythmias owing to involvement of the autonomic nervous system.[8] Cardiac dysrythmias may be serious enough to cause death if appropriate treatment is not implemented. Measurement of CSF protein level may be useful in making the diagnosis of GBS. CSF protein levels above 100 mg/100 mL are consistent with GBS.[9]

Myasthenia gravis may occur at any age but the incidence increases in early adulthood and in the elderly. In young adults, women outnumber men 2 to 1 in the incidence of the disease.[10] The patient with myasthenia gravis usually presents with weakness of certain muscles when used repeatedly. The extraocular muscles are often affected initially and cause the patient to experience blurred vision (**diplopia**) and droopy eyelids (**ptosis**). The symptoms may improve with rest and in fact may disappear following a good night of sleep. Some patients with myasthenia gravis experience gradual progression of the disease to other muscle groups including the pharyngeal, laryngeal, arm, trunk, and leg muscles. Respiratory symptoms usually do not develop in individuals with milder cases of myasthenia gravis; however, respiratory failure is likely when the diaphragm is affected by the disease. A number of factors (e.g., infection, surgery, menstruation, immunizations, certain drugs, and emotional distress) may precipitate a myasthenic crisis in a patient with a previously stable case.

The Tensilon test may prove useful when the diagnosis of myasthenia gravis is uncertain. This test requires intravenous (IV) injection of the patient with 10 mg of Tensilon (edrophonium). Muscle weakness will resolve temporarily within 20 to 30 seconds if myasthenia gravis is the cause.

The patient with ALS initially experiences progressive weakness of distal muscle groups such as the hands. The disease may cause asymmetric weakness, atrophy, and tremors. A characteristic feature of ALS is the development of muscle fiber twitching called fasciculations. ALS advances over a period of 2 to 7 years and eventually causes weakness of all four extremities as well as the breathing muscles. Dyspnea occurs at rest, and the patient begins having difficulty with coughing, swallowing, and talking as the disease progresses. Respiratory failure and death most often occur 3 to 4 years after the onset of symptoms.[11]

Respiratory symptoms of the patient with a spinal cord injury will vary with the location of the lesion. High cervical injuries above the level of C3 produce nearly complete respiratory muscle paralysis. In these cases the patient is unable to breathe effectively, talk, or cough. The lack of effective breathing causes the rapid onset of respiratory acidosis and hypoxemia. Breath sounds are very diminished or absent. The diaphragm is elevated and immobile. Bedside VC is at best 20 percent of predicted.[6] The patient with a spinal lesion at the level of C3 to C8 is quadriplegic but usually retains some use of the respiratory muscles. VC is markedly reduced immediately after the injury but improves somewhat over the initial 12 months. Dyspnea with exertion is common and may occur even at rest when a complicating pneumonia or atelectasis is present. ABG results usually demonstrate mild hypoxemia and normal $Paco_2$ during the daytime.[12] Disruption of the spinal cord below C8 does not usually cause significant reduction in lung volumes. A mid- to low-spinal-cord lesion often attenuates expiratory muscle function to the point that the patient's cough may be weak and ineffective. As a result, secretion retention and atelectasis is a potential complication.

TREATMENT

Neuromuscular disease may weaken the respiratory muscles and cause the patient to have difficulty clearing airway secretions. Bronchial hygiene techniques, including postural drainage, cough assistance, and aerosol therapy are often bene- ficial. Intermittent positive pressure breathing may be useful to prevent or treat atelectasis and dyspnea.

Careful monitoring of the vital signs, breathing pattern, ability to cough, VC, and MIP is essential to identify the need for ventilatory assistance. A decline in the ABG measurements is often a late clinical manifestation and should not be relied on to determine the need for mechanical ventilation. Intubation and mechanical ventilation is warranted if the patient demonstrates a respiratory rate greater than 30/minute, a VC less than 15 mL/kg, the inability to clear airway secretions, pro- gressive dyspnea, or an increasing $Paco_2$. Once the patient is intubated the RCP should keep the airway clear with postural drainage and suctioning. Tracheostomy is useful when long-term mechanical ventilation is needed, as in the case of a high cervical spine fracture. Tracheostomy is usually not used during the first 2 weeks of mechanical ventilation for reversible conditions such as GBS or myasthenia gravis. After 10 to 14 days of intubation, however, if the patient has not shown any signs of improvement, tracheostomy should be considered.

Clinicians caring for the patient with neuromuscular disease should anticipate complications such as pneumonia and pulmonary emboli. Antibiotics should be given if fever and pulmonary infiltrates develop. Prophylactic use of heparin is useful in reducing the incidence of deep venous thrombosis and pulmonary embolism.

Weaning from mechanical ventilation is reasonable when the patient is free of infection, is hemodynamically stable, and has significantly improved respiratory muscle function. Signs of improvement include a VC greater than 1.5 liter, an MIP greater than -30 cm H_2O, and a spontaneous tidal volume (VT) greater than 300 mL. Improvement in lung mechanics is not likely to occur in patients with high neck fractures or ALS.

Treatment of the patient with GBS is primarily supportive. Plasmapheresis has been used with some success and is reserved for the more severe cases. Plasma- pheresis requires removal of a portion of the circulating blood. The removed blood is centrifuged to separate the red blood cells (RBCs) from the plasma. The plasma is discarded and the RBCs are mixed with fresh plasma and reinfused into the patient. This process is continued until a major portion of the patient's plasma is replaced, causing dilution of the offending antibody. Corticosteroids are contro- versial and are not commonly used to treat the patient with GBS. Careful monitoring of the patient is crucial because respiratory failure represents the most immediate threat to life.[8,13] Mechanical ventilation is needed in about 25 percent of the cases.[14] After a period of stability the patient will typically begin to recover but several weeks or months are often needed for complete recovery. The prognosis is usually very good if serious complications do not occur.

Specific treatment of myasthenia gravis includes anticholinesterase medica- tions such as neostigmine. The patient with myasthenia gravis should be admitted to the hospital any time he or she experiences difficulty with breathing or swallowing. Careful monitoring of respiratory function is essential, as previously mentioned. Plasmapheresis and thymectomy (surgical removal of the thymus gland) have been used to treat more severe cases with some success.[15,16] Because patients with myasthenia gravis may have thymus gland enlargement, they may improve after thymectomy.

Treatment for the patient with ALS is nonspecific and supportive. Careful monitoring of respiratory function is important, as respiratory failure can occur with little warning. Intermittent mechanical ventilatory support using a negative-pressure body respirator may prove useful for the patient with more severe, chronic neuromuscular disease, as occurs with ALS. Nocturnal ventilation using a body respirator has the distinct advantage of not needing an artificial airway in place in order to achieve ventilation. This type of mechanical ventilation may allow the fatigued diaphragm to rest at night and subsequently results in better gas exchange and sleep during the night.[17,18] Nocturnal nasal-mask intermittent positive-pressure ventilation (NIPPV) represents an alternative to negative-pressure ventilation for patients with severe, chronic neuromuscular disease. NIPPV appears to be safe and effective and is less cumbersome to implement than is negative-pressure ventilation.[19]

Patients with spinal cord injury will need care according to the location of the lesion. Those who experience high neck fracture (above the level of C3) will need intubation and mechanical ventilation to survive. Once stabilized, tracheostomy is needed for long-term ventilatory assistance. Patients with fractures below C3 will need careful assessment to determine the extent of respiratory muscle paralysis. Most patients with neck fracture below the C3 level will not need continuous mechanical ventilation but may need nocturnal ventilatory support and assistance with secretion removal. In general, the lower the site of the neck fracture, the less respiratory care the patient will need.

Case Study No. 1

HISTORY

Ms. M is a 25-year-old white woman who came to the emergency room complaining of extremity weakness and difficulty with swallowing. The patient stated that 10 days earlier she had developed a fever, headache, and general malaise. At that time she visited her physician, who diagnosed her as having the flu. She was given acetaminophen for the headache and told to drink plenty of fluids and rest until the symptoms resolved. The next day she noticed dizziness, extremity weakness, and numbness. The extremity weakness had progressed to the point that she could not stand without assistance. She had noticed difficulty with swallowing over the past 24 hours and frequently choked. She stated that shortness of breath occurred with moderate exertion. She denied having dyspnea at rest, chest pain, cough, sputum, fever, or nausea.

Questions

1. What conditions are suggested by this medical history?
2. What is the significance of the patient having difficulty with swallowing?
3. What is the significance of the recent history of flu symptoms?
4. Should the patient be admitted? If so, why?

Answers

1. The symptoms suggest a neuromuscular disease such as myasthenia gravis, GBS, ALS, or flu with dehydration.
2. The difficulty with swallowing is significant because it suggests that neu-

romuscular control of the gag reflex may be in jeopardy, which could result in aspiration.

3. A recent history of flu symptoms is common in patients with GBS. Approximately 65 percent of patients with GBS have had a recent episode of respiratory or gastrointestinal flu within the past 8 weeks.

4. This patient should be admitted because of the difficulty with swallowing and because the respiratory muscles may weaken and result in a rapid onset of respiratory failure.

PHYSICAL EXAMINATION

General *The patient is alert, well oriented, and in no apparent distress. She is moderately obese and states that her height is 5 feet 4 inches and weight 155 lb.*

Vital Signs *Temperature 36.6℃, pulse 88/minute, respiratory rate 20/minute, blood pressure 150/110 mm Hg*

HEENT *Normocephalic with no signs of trauma; pupils equal, round, and reacting to light and accommodation (PERRLA); tympanic membranes intact; carotic pulses ++ bilaterally; trachea midline and without stridor; no ptosis noted, even upon repeated blinking*

Lungs *Clear breath sounds bilaterally; normal chest configuration; no evidence of trauma*

Heart *Irregular rate and rhythm without murmurs; normal S_1 and S_2 with no S_3 or S_4; point of maximal intensity (PMI) not palpable*

Abdomen *Obese, soft, nontender; positive bowel sounds; no hepatomegaly*

Extremities *Deep tendon reflexes of the extremities absent; noticeable weakness of legs and feet; grip weak in both hands; no evidence of cyanosis, edema, or clubbing; extremities warm to touch*

Questions

5. What are the key findings with the physical examination and what problems do they suggest?
6. What may explain the hypertension and irregular heartbeat?
7. Why did the examining physician ask the patient to blink her eyelids repeatedly?
8. What neuromuscular disease usually causes an ascending paralysis as seen in this case?
9. What laboratory and bedside test(s) would be useful in this case to identify the cause of the problem?
10. Should the attending physician administer the Tensilon test? What is the purpose of this test?

Answers

5. The key findings on the physical examination are the muscular weakness and loss of deep tendon reflexes of the extremities, and the irregular heartbeat and hypertension. The extremity weakness and loss of reflexes suggests that the neuromuscular system is not functioning properly.
6. The hypertension and irregular heartbeat may be the result of autonomic

nervous system involvement with the neuromuscular disease. It is also possible that the irregular heartbeat is the result of a heart condition not related to the neuromuscular disease.

7. Asking the patient to blink repeatedly is useful to check for myasthenia gravis. The eyelids will rapidly tire and begin to droop if myasthenia gravis is present. In this case myasthenia gravis is not the likely diagnosis, as the eyelids remained functional.

8. GBS typically causes an ascending paralysis as seen in this case.

9. Laboratory tests that would be useful include a CSF protein count, a bedside analysis of VC and MIP, complete blood count (CBC) and electrolyte measurement. A chest radiograph may be useful to assess the condition of the lungs. An ABG assessment is not needed at this point, as there is no evidence of respiratory complications.

10. The Tensilon test is useful to confirm the diagnosis of myasthenia gravis. In this case the evidence suggests that myasthenia gravis is not the cause of the patient's weakness and the Tensilon test would not be useful.

LABORATORY DATA

CBC

White blood cells (WBCs)	9.5
Segs	71%
Bands	6%
Lymphs	14%
Monos	8%
Basophils	1%
RBCs	4.2
Hemoglobin (Hb)	13 g/100 mL
Hematocrit (Hct)	38%

ELECTROLYTES

Normal, except for reduced CO_2 (21 mEq/liter)

MIP

−35 cm H_2O

BEDSIDE VC

2.4 liters (predicted normal = 3.6 liters)

CHEST RADIOGRAPH

Low lung volumes bilaterally with no evidence of infiltrates

Questions

11. How do you interpret the CBC results?
12. What could explain the reduced CO_2 on the electrolyte panel?

13. How do you interpret the bedside MIP and VC?
14. Is the chest radiograph consistent with the tentative diagnosis of neuromuscular disease? If so, why?

Answers

11. The CBC is normal.
12. The reduced CO_2 on the electrolyte panel represents reduced plasma bicarbonate. This is commonly seen in patients who have been hyperventilating long enough for the kidneys to compensate for a respiratory alkalosis by excreting plasma bicarbonate. A reduced plasma bicarbonate concentration is also seen when a metabolic acidosis is present.
13. The MIP and VC are reduced, which suggests that the respiratory muscles are probably affected by the disease and that careful monitoring of the patient is needed.
14. The chest radiograph finding of reduced lung volume is consistent with neuromuscular disease. As the inspiratory muscles weaken, the lung recoil is less opposed and the lung volumes tend to diminish.

The diagnosis at this point was neuromuscular disease, probably due to GBS. The patient was admitted to the intensive care unit (ICU) for careful monitoring. A spinal tap was done to measure the CSF protein level, which was found to be elevated. This provided more evidence to support the diagnosis of GBS. Plasmapheresis was started.

Four hours after admission the patient began complaining of shortness of breath after minimal exertion. Bedside assessment revealed a VC of 1.6 liters and a MIP of -20 cm H_2O. The patient's respiratory rate had increased to 36/minute and her pulse was 128/minute. Her blood pressure remained moderately elevated. ABGs at this point revealed pH 7.45, $Paco_2$ 30 mm Hg, Pao_2 89 mm Hg, Sao_2 95.9 percent; HCO_3^- 19 mEq/liter on room air

Questions

15. What is plasmapheresis and why is it used to treat GBS?
16. How do you interpret the changes in the VC and MIP measurements?
17. How do you interpret the ABGs?
18. What therapy is indicated at this point?

Answers

15. Plasmapheresis is the process of removing a portion of the patient's blood and centrifuging it to separate the blood cells from the plasma. The plasma is discarded and the remaining blood cells are mixed with fresh plasma and reinfused into the patient. The purpose of plasmapheresis is to dilute the offending antibody present in the plasma.
16. The VC and MIP are reduced significantly from the previous measurement. This suggests that the respiratory muscles are weaker and the patient is at high risk for respiratory failure.
17. The ABG demonstrates compensated respiratory alkalosis with adequate oxygenation on room air. The ABG results reflect adequate lung function. Respiratory failure, however, may occur in the very near future despite the relatively normal ABG results.
18. Based on the downward trend with regard to the respiratory muscle strength, increasing respiratory rate, and the increasing dyspnea, intubation and mechanical ventilation are indicated. It is usually better to

perform the intubation while the patient with neuromuscular disease remains somewhat stable. Once respiratory failure is present, attempts to intubate are often rushed and the patient is at greater risk for complications.

After explaining the procedure to the patient, she was intubated nasally and placed on mechanical ventilation. Initial settings were assist-control mode with a backup rate of 12/minute and a tidal volume of 800 mL, a fractional inspired oxygen (FIO_2) of 0.35, and no positive end-expiratory pressure (PEEP). A chest film confirmed appropriate placement of the endotracheal tube. ABGs 20 minutes after the initiation of mechanical ventilation with a mechanical rate of 16/min were pH 7.45, $Paco_2$ 32 mm Hg, Pao_2 105 mm Hg, HCO_3 20 mEq/liter, Sao_2 98 percent. The patient continued to complain of weakness and extremity numbness.

Questions

19. What changes in the ventilator settings do you suggest based on the ABG findings?
20. What complications should be anticipated in this case?
21. What should the patient be told about her prognosis?
22. Should a tracheostomy be performed to avoid permanent damage to the larynx by the endotracheal tube?

Answers

19. Because the oxygenation is more than adequate, a slight reduction in the FIO_2 from 0.35 to 0.30 is reasonable. A reduction in the mechanical minute volume would help increase the $Paco_2$ to normal range. This could be accomplished by reducing the tidal volume; however, a smaller tidal volume may promote atelectasis. Lowering the backup rate may decrease the minute volume, but only if the patient does not trigger the ventilator. Sedation may help reduce the patient's anxiety and reduce the hyperventilation. An alternative would be to switch the ventilator to the intermittent mandatory ventilation (IMW) mode (see Chapter 1). This would allow the patient to take spontaneous breaths between the mechanical breaths and should lower the overall minute volume. The IMV rate should be set high enough, however, to maintain adequate ventilation and allow the muscles to rest (e.g., 10 to 12 breaths/minute).
20. Complications in this case could include pulmonary embolus, atelectasis, pneumonia, cardiovascular compromise from the mechanical ventilation, and pneumothorax.
21. The patient should be told that a full recovery is expected. The larger majority of GBS patients recover fully within a few weeks or months.
22. At this point a tracheostomy is not needed. It is possible that the patient will recover enough to breathe on her own within a week or two. A tracheostomy should be considered if after 7 to 10 days the patient has not made any progress toward recovery.

Over the next week the patient was maintained on mechanical ventilation with an IMV rate of 10/minute and a mechanical tidal volume of 800 mL. Plasmapheresis was repeated daily. The patient's spontaneous tidal volume varied but usually was *in the range of 200 to 300 mL. On day 7 her MIP was −25 cm H_2O and she stated that she felt stronger. The bilateral extremity numbness was greatly reduced and her grip was noticeably stronger. Her vital signs remained stable except for an elevation in body temperature to 38.3 °C. Secretions suctioned from the endotracheal tube were white. The chest radiograph demonstrated bibasilar atelectasis. ABG findings on day 7 were pH 7.43, $Paco_2$ 36 mm Hg, Pao_2 84 mm Hg, Fio_2 0.30.*

Questions

23. What treatment should be given for the bibasilar atelectasis?
24. Should weaning from mechanical ventilation be started? Why or why not?

Answers

23. The bibasilar atelectasis should be treated with chest physical therapy and postural drainage. Frequent changes in position and occasional deep breaths with the volume ventilator may also be helpful. The sputum sample should be sent to the laboratory for Gram's stain and culture. If the sputum demonstrates numerous pus cells and bacterial growth, antibiotics should be started.
24. It appears that the patient is improving, but weaning from mechanical ventilation should not begin until the fever and atelectasis have cleared.

On day 14 the patient had a normal body temperature and the chest radiograph demonstrated significant clearing of the infiltrates. The weaning parameters at this point were VC 2.1 liters, MIP −35 cm H_2O, spontaneous VT 350 mL. The patient tolerated an IMV rate of 4/minute with normal ABGs. On the evening of day 14 the patient was extubated and she tolerated the procedure well. She stated that she still felt weak but much improved. Her cough was weak but improved daily. Her breath sounds remained clear and vital signs stable. Neurologic examination revealed improved deep tendon reflexes and nearly normal responses to stimuli. The patient was transferred from the ICU to the rehabilitation unit on day 18 and was sent home on day 21 without further complications.

Case Study No. 2

HISTORY

BR is a 62-year-old man with a 6-month history of ALS. Approximately 8 months earlier he had noticed weakness in his hands and legs. The initial problems he had recognized were in gripping objects like a cup or doorknob. He then had difficulty getting out of a chair. The disease had progressed rapidly over the last 6 months. He was now unable to walk, grip anything, or lift anything more 1 to 2 lb with his arms. Speaking had become more difficult but his mind was clear and he still communicated well with his family. His neurologist had referred him for an evaluation of his respiratory status.

BR was experiencing mild dyspnea, most notably when he talked or assisted in transferring himself to a wheelchair. His family had noted that he could not complete a sentence without stopping to catch his breath. When he was at rest and not talking he appeared in no distress. One month before this visit he had developed a right lower lobe pneumonia that was treated with amoxicillin and resolved.

There were no other significant problems identified in BR's past history. He was a dentist who had worked in practice until 8 months ago when the ALS was first discovered.

BR understood that his disease would lead to respiratory failure and was terminal. He felt that his quality of life was good enough at present that he would like to have ventilatory support if needed to prolong his life. In addition, if his ALS progressed to the point that BR felt that his quality of life did not warrant continued ventilatory support, he would like to discontinue mechanical ventilation at that time.

Questions

1. What part of the nervous system does amyotrophic lateral sclerosis affect and what is the etiology of the disease?
2. The initial sign of BR's muscle weakness was manifest by a weak grip. Is this pattern of weakness typical for proximal or distal muscle weakness?
3. Is it reasonable to provide mechanical ventilation for BR when his disease is progressive and terminal?
4. If you initiated mechanical ventilation for BR and he later decided he wanted to stop ventilatory support and die, should you assist him in discontinuing mechanical ventilation?
5. What characteristic muscle movements would you expect to see during your examination of the patient?

Answers

1. ALS is a degenerative disease of motor neurons that has no known cause. The disease specifically destroys the Betz neurons in the cerebral cortex and the motor neurons in the anterior horns of the spinal cord.
2. Weakness of the hands and feet are signs of distal muscle weakness. Distal muscle weakness at the onset of symptoms suggests that the disease is a neuromuscular disorder such as ALS or GBS. Proximal muscle weakness is characteristically seen in the arm and thigh. This weakness is most notable when a patient gets up from a chair. Proximal muscle weakness is characteristic of muscle diseases such as muscular dystrophy.
3. Yes, patients have the right to decide which therapies they are willing to undergo. Because BR is approaching respiratory failure, mechanical ventilation is a treatment option. Ideally, one of the roles of health care providers is to educate the patient regarding the benefits and costs of such therapy. It is important that discussion emphasize the discomfort associated with such therapy as well as the intrusion into his life. In addition, the patient needs to understand the nature and prognosis for the disease process that led to the requirement for this therapy. Only after patients have been fully educated in all aspects of their disease and the proposed therapy can they make an educated decision.
4. Yes, as in the discussion for question 27, the patient has the right to decide whether to initiate therapy and when to terminate therapy. It is probably wise to make certain that a decision of this importance has been thought through thoroughly by the patient and that the family understands and respects the decision before discontinuing mechanical support.
5. Patients with ALS develop muscle fasciculations, which are characterized by a visible twitching of muscle fibers from the affected muscles.

PHYSICAL EXAMINATION ————————————

General *The patient is sitting in a wheelchair and is in no respiratory distress. His vital signs are stable; his respiratory rate is 24/ minute.*

Head and Neck *No significant abnormalities*

Heart *Regular with a normal rate; both S₁ and S₂ normal; no murmur*

Lungs *A few fine inspiratory crackles heard over the bases of both lungs; weak cough.*

Abdomen *Soft, nontender; normal active bowel sounds; no masses palpated*

Extremities *Equal pulses in all extremities; no peripheral edema noted*

Neurologic *Alert, articulate; short sentences spoken, with pauses to take a breath every three to five words; cranial nerve function normal except weakness of sternocleidomastoid, trapezius, and facial muscles; sensory examination normal; extreme weakness of extremities revealed upon motor examination; legs move and gestures weak; fasciculations noted over forearm and thigh muscles*

Questions

6. In this setting, what is the most likely reason this patient has pulmonary crackles? Why do the crackles remain after coughing?
7. What tests are most important in determining when mechanical ventilation should be instituted?
8. Should the patient be admitted to the hospital at this time?

Answers

6. The principal pulmonary problem that patients with neuromuscular disease have is weakness of the respiratory pump. Weakness of respiratory muscles predisposes patients to develop difficulty in expanding lung units, so they develop atelectasis. In addition, these patients may have difficulty clearing secretions and develop atelectasis as a result of mucus plugging. In patients with neuromuscular disease the airway may not be protected; therefore, these individuals may aspirate and develop pneumonia.

   The profound respiratory muscle weakness that is common to patients with neuromuscular disease makes it difficult for the patient to breathe deeply and cough well enough to reverse atelectasis completely.
7. The test that is most commonly used to determine if patients with neuromuscular disease require mechanical ventilation is the measurement of VC. If the VC is less than 1 liter, then mechanical ventilation is usually indicated.
8. If mechanical ventilation becomes necessary the patient will then be admitted to train both the patient and family in the use of the ventilator and if necessary perform a tracheostomy.

LABORATORY DATA ══════════════

CHEST RADIOGRAPH

(Fig. 15–3)

ABGs (on room air)

pH	7.38
Pao_2	67 mm Hg
$Paco_2$	58 mm Hg
HCO_3^-	33 mEq/liter
$P(A\text{-}a)o_2$	10 mm Hg
O_2 content	16.8 mL/dL

CBC

	Observed	Normal
WBCs/mm³	5100	4,000–11,000
RBCs (M/mm³)	4.2	4.1–5.5
Hb (g/dL)	14	14–16.5
Hct (%)	41	37–50
Differential		
Segmented neutrophils	61%	38–79%
Band neutrophils	4%	0–7%
Lymphocytes	29%	12–51%
Monocytes	5%	0–10%
Eosinophils	1%	0–8%
Basophils	0%	0–2%

CHEMISTRY

	Observed	Normal
Sodium (mEq/liter)	141	136–146
Potassium (mEq/liter)	4.2	3.5–5.1
Chloride (mEq/dL)	93	98–106
Bicarbonate (mEq/liter)	37	22–29
Blood urea nitrogen (BUN) (mg/dL)	8	7–18
Creatinine (mg/dL)	0.5	0.5–1.1
Calcium (mmol/liter)	2.2	2.1–2.55
Phosphate (mg/dL)	2.9	2.7–4.5
Uric acid (mg/dL)	2.1	4.5–8.2
Albumin (g/dL)	3.9	3.5–5.0
Protein (g/dL)	7.2	6.4–8.3

SPIROMETRY

Forced vital capacity (FVC) 0.92 liters
Negative inspiratory pressure -12 cm H_2O

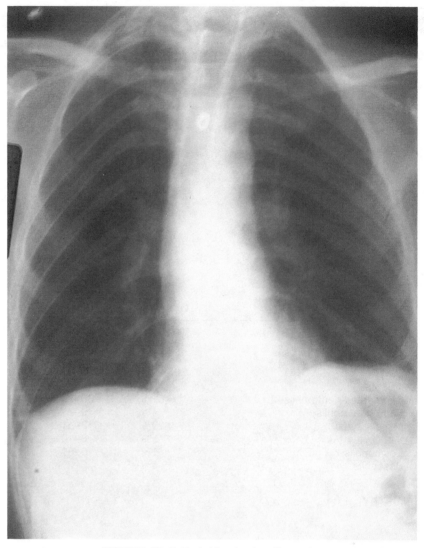

FIGURE 15–3 Portable chest radiograph.

Questions

9. Interpret the chest radiograph.
10. Interpret the results of the ABGs.
11. Interpret the spirometry results.
12. What treatment options would you recommend to the physician at this point?

Answers

9. The lungs are hyperinflated from previous COPD. A small amount of scoliosis is present in the spine.
10. The ABGs show a chronic respiratory acidosis. The alveolar-arterial oxygen gradient is normal.
11. The spirometry is consistent with severe profound respiratory muscle weakness.

12. With a chronic respiratory acidosis and profound respiratory muscle weakness this patient is in respiratory failure due to ALS. This patient wanted to begin mechanical ventilation when necessary. This is an appropriate time to admit the patient to begin mechanical ventilaton and to train the family members.

There are two different options in mechanical ventilation for patients with neuromuscular respiratory failure. One option is to perform a tracheostomy and initiate volume-cycled mechanical ventilation. A second option is to begin mechanical ventilation with nasal-mask intermittent positive-pressure ventilation (NIPPV). The second option has the advantage that no tracheostomy is required. At home, NIPPV or a negative-pressure body respirator may prove useful.

BR was admitted to the hospital. NIPPV was instituted for nocturnal use. The patient and family were instructed in the use of the ventilator and after a few days of stabilization on the new regimen the patient was discharged home.

For several weeks after the institution of NIPPV the patient felt more energetic and found breathing and talking easier. His ABGs improved with a normal Pa_{CO_2} using NIPPV and during the daytime.

Over the next several months he became progressively less functional as the ALS got worse. With the progression of ALS the ventilatory requirements increased and the symptoms of breathlessness worsened. He found that he required NIPPV 24 hours a day and could not easily talk or communicate with his family. The ALS had left him unable to perform even the simplest task in his own care. At this time BR decided that the cost of the NIPPV was greater than the benefits he was deriving. He did not want tracheostomy nor other, more invasive forms of mechanical ventilation. He decided he would stop using the NIPPV. He and his family fully understood the consequences of this step. After discussions with his family and care providers he stopped the ventilator on his own. He died a few minutes later.

REFERENCES

1. Petty, TL: The modern evolution of mechanical ventilation. Clin Chest Med 9:1, 1988.

2. Drinker, P and Shaw, LA: Apparatus for prolonged administration of mechanical ventilation. J Clin Invest 7:229, 1929.

3. West, JB: Control of ventilation. In West, JB (ed): Respiratory Physiology. Williams & Wilkins, Baltimore, 1985, p 113.

4. Phillipson, EA: Sleep disorders. In Murrary, JF and Nadel, JA (eds): Textbook of Respiratory Medicine. WB Saunders, Philadelphia, 1988.

5. Phillipson, EA: Control of breathing during sleep. Am Rev Respir Dis 118:909, 1978.

6. Rochester, DF and Findley, LJ: The lungs and neuromuscular and chest wall diseases. In Murray, JF and Nadel, JA (eds): Textbook of Respiratory Medicine. WB Saunders, Philadelphia, 1988.

7. Marini, JJ: Monitoring during mechanical ventilation. In Morganroth, ML (ed): Mechanical Ventilation. Clin Chest Med 9:73, 1988.

8. Derdak, S: Guillain-Barré. In Civetta, JM, Taylor, RW, and Kirby, RR (eds): Critical Care. JB Lippincott, Philadelphia, 1988, p 1251.

9. Andreoloi, TE (ed), et al: In Cecil's Essentials of Medicine. WB Saunders, Philadelphia, 1986, p 721.

10. Derdak, S: Myasthenia gravis. In Civetta, JM, Taylor, RW, and Kirby, RR (eds): Critical Care. JB Lippincott, Philadelphia, 1988, p 1257.

11. Fallat, RJ, et al: Spirometry in amyotrophic lateral sclerosis. Arch Neurol 36:74, 1979.

12. Ledsome, RJ and Sharp, JM: Pulmonary function in acute cervical cord injury. Am Rev Respir Dis 124:41, 1981.

13. O'Donohue, WJ, et al: Respiratory failure in neuromuscular disease: Management in a respiratory intensive care unit. JAMA 235:733, 1976.

14. Ropper, AH: Severe acute Guillain-Barre syndrome. Neurology 36:429, 1986.

15. Gracey, DR, Howard, FM, and Divertie, MB: Plasmapheresis in the treatment of ventilator-dependent myasthenia gravis patients. Chest 85:739, 1984.

16. Dau, PC: Respiratory failure in myasthenia gravis. Chest 85:721, 1985.

17. Holtackers, TR, Loosbrack, LM, and Gracey, DR: The use of the chest cuirass in respiratory failure of neurologic origin. Respir Care 27:271, 1982.

18. Curran, FJ: Night ventilation by body respirators for patients in chronic respiratory failure due to late stage Duchenne muscular dystrophy. Arch Phys Med Rehabil 62:270, 1981.

19. Leger, P, et al: Home positive pressure ventilation via nasal mask for patients with neuromuscular weakness or restrictive lung or chest-wall disease. Respir Care 34:73, 1989.

Chapter 16

Robert L. Wilkins, MA, RRT
James R. Dexter, MD, FCCP

BACTERIAL PNEUMONIA

INTRODUCTION

Pneumonia is an inflammation of the lung parenchyma; the term is used most often to describe inflammation from infection. Pneumonia can result from a large variety of infectious agents including bacteria, viruses, or fungi; however, this chapter will focus on bacterial pneumonia. This type of pneumonia continues to be a common medical problem despite the advent of antibiotics.

Each year approximately 1,200,000 people contract pneumonia in the United States and 50,000 die.[1] Pneumonia occasionally occurs in the hospitalized patient and in those cases is referred to as a **nosocomial** infection. Although other types of nosocomial infections (e.g., urinary tract) occur more often in hospitalized patients, pneumonia is the most common nosocomial infection causing death.[2] Pneumonia is more serious among hospitalized and elderly patients because their immune system is often functioning poorly.

ETIOLOGY

Normally the distal airways are sterile because of the wide variety of mechanical and chemical systems that protect the lungs from infectious agents (Table 16–1). These protective systems may become sabotaged when such factors as cigarette smoking, alcohol abuse, chronic lung disease, neuromuscular disease, or acute viral upper respiratory tract infection are present.[3] Neuromuscular disorders are partic-

Table 16–1 Summary of Protective Mechanisms of Respiratory System

Mechanical
   Filtration by nares
   Sneezing
   Gag reflex
   Cough
   Ciliary movement
Immunologic
   Phagocytosis by macrophages and leukocytes
   Immunoglobins such as IgA in secretions
   Cell-mediated immunity
   Opsonization by complement

Table 16–2 Factors That Predispose Patients to Pneumonia

Pulmonary factors	Systemic factors
Airway disease	Immunosuppression
Chronic bronchitis	Leukemia
Asthma	Chemotherapy
Bronchiectasis	AIDS
Obstructed bronchus due to tumor	Transplantation
Positive smoking history	Chronic systemic disease
Poor cough	Diabetes
Neuromuscular disease	Cirrhosis
Emphysema	Renal failure
Abdominal pain	Heart failure
Drug overdose	Iatrogenic procedures
Reduced gag reflex and aspiration	Intubation
Drug overdose	Mechanical ventilation
Alcohol abuse	Use of humidifiers and aerosol generators
Stroke	Lack of handwashing
Neuromuscular disease	Lack of sterile technique

ularly troublesome because they may reduce the effectiveness of the patient's cough and interfere with the protective reflexes of the upper airway that prevent aspiration.

The distal airways can become contaminated with potentially pathogenic organisms once the protective mechanisms are damaged. Infection is much more likely if the defense mechanisms of the lower airways are also compromised or if the organism is particularly virulent. Systemic disorders such as diabetes, cirrhosis, renal failure, malnutrition, acquired immune deficiency syndrome (AIDS), or cancer may compromise the patient's immune system and contribute to the onset of pneumonia (Table 16–2). Patients with AIDS frequently acquire *Pneumocystis carinii* pneumonia. The use of steroids also suppresses the patient's immune system and may contribute to the onset of pneumonia.

In addition to aspiration, potentially pathogenic organisms can enter the lung by inhalation and through the bloodstream. Inhalation of small droplet particles that carry organisms is not common when the upper airway is healthy and capable of filtering the inspired gas. If the upper airway is diseased or bypassed as with tracheostomy or intubation, organisms are more likely to be deposited in the lower airways. Systemic infections may result in the offending organism traveling to the lung via blood flow. Once the organism reaches the lung, pneumonia may result.

PATHOLOGY AND PATHOPHYSIOLOGY

Infections of the lung parenchyma incite an inflammatory reaction, which causes the outpouring of exudates and white blood cells to fight the infection. Interstitial and alveolar spaces are flooded with edema and exudative material. This inflammatory process causes the distal lung spaces to become dense and consolidated. Some cases of bacterial pneumonia are limited to small areas of lung parenchyma but others spread to surrounding tissue such as the pleura and pericardium.

Some bacterial organisms such as *Staphylococcus* and *Pseudomonas* are capable of permanently damaging lung tissue. The pneumonia is referred to as a **necrotizing** pneumonia in such cases.

Acute inflammation and consolidation of the lung leads to a reduction in ventilation and gas exchange in the affected region. Perfusion of the affected lung segments in areas that have poor ventilation results in severe ventilation-perfusion (V̇/Q̇) mismatching or shunt.

The lung consolidation associated with pneumonia reduces lung compliance in the affected region. This increases the patient's work of breathing and sensation of breathlessness. Lung volumes are typically reduced during the acute stages of pneumonia but usually return to normal once the infection resolves.

CLINICAL FEATURES

Medical History

The patient with bacterial pneumonia usually complains of fever, cough, and sputum production and may complain of shortness of breath and chest pain. Dyspnea is more common when the pneumonia involves multiple regions of the lung or when it is superimposed on a chronic pulmonary disease. Chest pain is usually pleuritic in nature. Systemic symptoms such as headache, skin rash, and diarrhea may be present with some types of pneumonia. The past medical history is often positive for a chronic systemic or pulmonary disorder in the patient with acute pneumonia.

Physical Examination

The patient often appears acutely ill at the onset of common bacterial pneumonia. Assessment of the vital signs often reveals a rapid pulse and breathing rate. Rapid breathing occurs with the drop in lung compliance and when fever or hypoxemia is present. Fever increases the metabolic rate of the patient, which increases demand on the heart and lungs to provide additional oxygen to the tissues.

Inspection may reveal cyanosis and use of the accessory muscles to breathe when the pneumonia is severe. A unilateral reduction in chest expansion may be seen with lobar pneumonia. This finding results from the poor expansion of the involved lobe associated with consolidation. Increased tactile fremitus and bronchial breath sounds are commonly found over the consolidated lung if the lobar bronchus associated with the affected region is patent.[4-6] Sound travels more readily through consolidated lung tissue, causing the turbulent flow sounds of the larger airways to be heard more easily over areas of consolidation. The breath sounds will be markedly diminished or absent if the bronchus is obstructed. Reduced resonance to percussion is present over areas of consolidated lung. Inspiratory crackles are often present. Coarse crackles imply excessive mucus, which is a common finding late in the course of bacterial pneumonia. A pleural friction rub may be present when pleural inflammation is complicating the pneumonia.

Laboratory Data

Examination of the peripheral blood sample will reveal leukocytosis in most cases of bacterial pneumonia. Acute bacterial infection stimulates the bone marrow to increase the neutrophils in the circulating blood. As the infection worsens, the number of immature white blood cells (bands) also increases. Leukopenia is seen in cases of severe bacterial pneumonia that overwhelm the immune system. A normal white blood cell (WBC) count is commonly encountered with *Mycoplasma* or nonbacterial pneumonias.

The chest radiograph is almost always abnormal when pneumonia is present. It provides information about the extent of lung involvement and the onset of complications such as pleural effusion. Radiographic changes associated with pneumonia include areas of increased density with air bronchograms. In some cases the pneumonia may involve the entire lobe (lobar pneumonia), whereas in others the infiltrates occur along the airways and have a patchy segmental distribution (bronchopneumonia) (Figs. 16–1 and 16–2). Necrotizing pneumonia produces areas of radiolucency seen in the areas of increased density. Viral pneumonia most often causes interstitial infiltrates throughout both lungs (Fig. 16–3). The chest radiograph may take as long as 3 months to clear completely in the patient with bacterial pneumonia.[2] Documentation of complete resolution of the infiltrate is not needed if the patient improves clinically unless he or she is at risk for bronchogenic carcinoma (e.g., cigarette smoker over the age of 40 years).

Arterial blood gases (ABGs) often reveal hypoxemia and respiratory alkalosis. Respiratory acidosis is uncommon unless the patient also has chronic obstructive pulmonary disease (COPD) or neuromuscular disease.

Microbiologic evaluation of sputum, which is done to identify the pathogen responsible for the respiratory infection, is best performed before initiating antibiotics. Unfortunately in many cases a legitimate sample from the lung is difficult to obtain or is contaminated with oral secretions as it passes through the mouth. Screening of the sputum sample is useful to identify significant contamination with oral secretions. Sputum samples should be discarded when 10 or more squamous

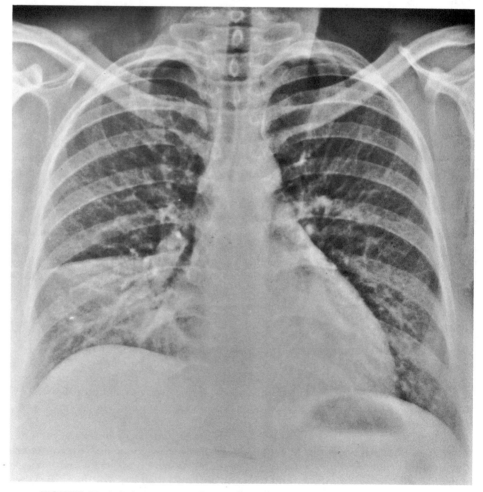

FIGURE 16–1 Lobar pneumonia as seen on posteroanterior (PA) chest radiograph. In this case the pneumonia is located in the right middle lobe.

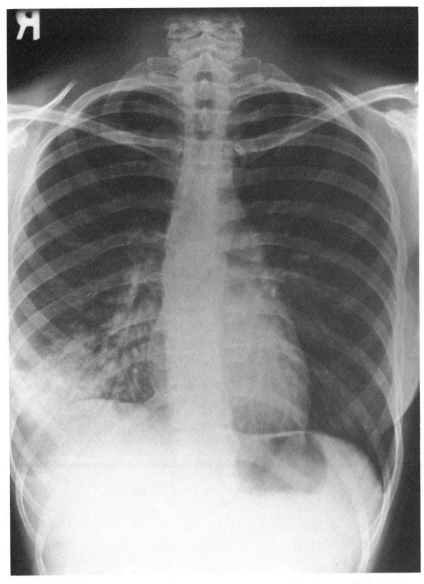

FIGURE 16–2 Bronchopneumonia as seen on a PA chest radiograph.

epithelial cells per low-powered field are present because this signifies that the sample is heavily contaminated by oral secretions. A good sample is recognized by identifying many (greater than 25 per low-powered field) polymorphonuclear WBCs in addition to few epithelial cells.[2] A Gram's stain and culture are more likely to be helpful when a good specimen has been obtained. The Gram's stain does not take long and often identifies the general category of bacteria present. It may allow the physician to start appropriate antibiotic therapy before the culture results are available. The culture may identify the specific pathogen responsible for the pneumonia, and the sensitivity identifies which antibiotics are most effective against the organism.

Because the sputum sample is difficult to expectorate for many patients, the attending physicians will occasionally employ invasive techniques. Although the

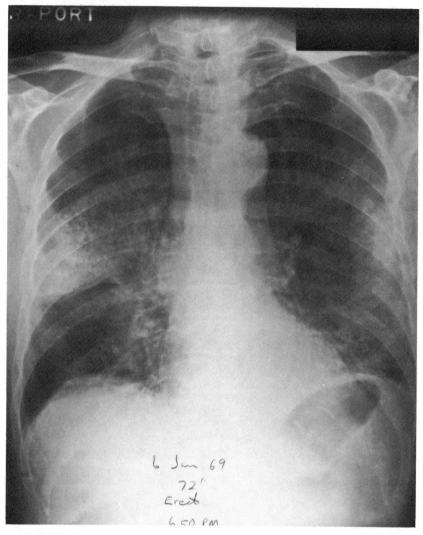

FIGURE 16–3 Viral pneumonia as seen on PA chest radiograph.

risk of these invasive procedures is greater than that of sputum expectoration, in some cases the potential benefit far outweighs the risk. Transtracheal and transthoracic aspiration, bronchoscopy, and open lung biopsy represent invasive techniques useful in obtaining a sputum specimen from the severely ill patient with pneumonia.

TREATMENT

Some patients may be treated for pneumonia as outpatients but those with severe cases should be attended to in the hospital. Severe cases generally require supportive care, which includes fluid and nutritional therapy. Oxygen is important when hypoxemia is present and 3 to 5 liters/minute by nasal cannula is adequate in most cases. Aerosol or humidity therapy can be useful when thick secretions are difficult to expectorate. Chest physical therapy is not useful in treating the typical case of bacterial pneumonia unless it is complicated by bronchiectasis.[7,8] Respiratory failure requiring mechanical ventilation is uncommon unless the pneumonia is superimposed on a chronic lung disease.

The attending physician should initiate the appropriate antibiotic as soon as possible, although several days of taking the drug are needed to reach its full effectiveness. In the patient who is not severely ill a short delay in the onset of the antibiotic therapy is reasonable while appropriate sputum and blood samples are obtained. Results of the preliminary diagnostic tests such as Gram's stain and chest radiograph may provide important clues as to the offending organism. If gram-positive elongated diplococci typical of pneumococci are seen, penicillin is the drug of choice. The presence of gram-negative coccobacilli on the sputum sample suggests that ampicillin or cephalosporin is the preferred agent. Once the culture results are available the most specific agent available to treat the offending organism should be given.

The patient admitted for pneumonia is at risk for developing a nosocomial infection, especially if the patient develops respiratory failure and needs ventilator therapy.[9-11] Careful handwashing between each patient and use of sterile technique during airway care are crucial to the prevention of the spread of organisms from one patient to another in the intensive care unit (ICU). This point is emphasized by the fact that many nosocomial pneumonias are caused by gram-negative organisms, which are spread most commonly in fluid and on people's hands. Gram-negative organisms are often relatively resistant to therapy, which makes treatment difficult and increases the risk of death.

Case Study

HISTORY

MC is a 60-year-old black woman who lives in a 1958 Nash Rambler. She earns money by collecting aluminum cans from along the road and trash dumpsters. She stated that she had been coughing up about one-quarter cup of white sputum each morning for the past 20 years. About 1 week earlier, she had noticed a sudden onset of shaking chills, fever, sweating, malaise, chest pain, and shortness of breath at rest. She also had begun coughing up rust-colored sputum that was thicker than her normal sputum production. MC admitted the current consumption of cigarettes and to a 45–pack-year smoking history. She admitted the occasional use of alcohol but denies orthopnea, ankle edema, nausea, vomiting, diarrhea, weight loss, dysuria, wheezing, or hemoptysis.

Questions

1. What are the key symptoms in this case and what disease do they suggest?
2. What is the significance of the place of residence and source of income?
3. What is the significance of the smoking history?
4. What is the significance of the patient's chronic sputum production?
5. What physical examination techniques are useful in this case and what purpose do they serve?

Answers

1. The key symptoms in this case are fever, sputum production, shortness of breath, and chest pain. These symptoms strongly suggest pneumonia.
2. The fact that MC lives in her car and earns money from collecting aluminum cans suggests that she may not have adequate nutritional intake. She is probably exposed to the elements and more prone than usual to develop pneumonia.
3. MC's smoking history is very significant and suggests that she is a candidate for lung cancer, COPD, and heart disease. Her current use of cigarettes adds to her susceptibility to pneumonia because smoking reduces the defense mechanisms of the lung.

4. The chronic sputum production is typical for patients with chronic bronchitis. Poor clearance of secretions in the lung makes infection, including pneumonia, more common.

5. The physical examination should begin with a general assessment and evaluation of the patient's vital signs. This will help assess the severity of MC's illness and provide a baseline for later comparison. The chest should be inspected for chest wall configuration and breathing pattern, percussed for resonance, palpated for tactile fremitus, and auscultated for the presence of bronchial breath sounds, adventitious lung sounds, and pleural friction rubs. This will help identify the presence of lung consolidation and determine any pleural involvement. The heart should be auscultated for evidence of failure (gallops) and murmurs. The extremities are examined for the presence of cyanosis, edema, or clubbing. The examiner should look for evidence of chronic obstructive lung disease.

PHYSICAL EXAMINATION

General
Chronically ill–appearing elderly patient in mild to moderate respiratory distress at rest. She is alert, oriented to person and place, and of nearly normal intellect with long-term memory better than short-term recall.

Vital Signs
Temperature 39°C; pulse 122/minute; respiratory rate 32/minute; blood pressure 110/60 mm Hg; height 150 cm; weight 65 kg

HEENT
Cyanosis of the lips and mouth

Neck
Supple with full active range of motion; trachea midline, mobile, and without stridor or wheezing; carotid pulsation are ++ and symmetric with no carotid bruits; mild supraclavicular and cervical lymphadenopathy present bilaterally; no jugular venous distension (JVD) noted.

Chest
Anteroposterior (AP) diameter slightly increased with diminished excursion noted on the right side with each inspiratory effort; diminished resonance to percussion and increased tactile fremitus noted over right middle lobe anteriorly

Heart
Regular rate and rhythm. No murmurs, gallops, or rubs are noted.

Lungs
Bronchial breath sounds noted over right middle lobe; clear breath sounds over entire left lung and right upper lobe; a pleural friction rub heard over right anterior chest wall

Abdomen
Normal appearance, without tenderness to palpation; bowel sounds present; no masses or organomegaly noted

Extremities
Cool, moist, and slightly dusky; cyanosis noted in the fingertips; no clubbing or edema present; pulses slightly diminished and symmetric.

Questions

5. What is the significance of the patient's poor short-term memory?
6. Interpret the vital signs.
7. What is the significance of an increase in AP diameter?

8. What explains the unilateral chest expansion?
9. What explains the decrease in resonance and increase in tactile fremitus?
10. What is the cause and significance of the bronchial breath sounds?
11. What is the significance of the pleural friction rub?
12. Why are the extremities cool, moist, and dusky?
13. What laboratory tests are useful in this case?

Answers

5. Poor memory is an indication of reduced mental acuity and may be related to a number of adverse events including hypoxia, alcohol abuse, sepsis, or chronic disease. Short-term recall is usually affected more severely than long-term recall.
6. The vital signs demonstrate fever, tachycardia, and tachypnea. The blood pressure is within normal limits, although on the low end of normal. These findings are consistent with a more severe case of acute pneumonia.
7. The increase in AP diameter is consistent with COPD. Because COPD is a common predisposing factor for pneumonia and because it may influence treatment, clinicians should be careful to note such findings.
8. A unilateral reduction in chest expansion is commonly seen in lobar pneumonia. The affected lobe does not expand with inspiration and lags behind the opposite side.
9. The decrease in resonance with percussion suggests that the tissue underlying the chest wall in the affected region is dense, which is common with pneumonia. Other conditions such as pleural effusion and lung tumors may cause the same finding. An increase in tactile fremitus is also consistent with lung consolidation. The vibrations generated at the larynx travel much better through dense lung tissue than through air-filled lung.
10. The bronchial breath sounds are consistent with lung consolidation. The turbulent flow sounds of the larger airways travel through consolidated lung more directly than through normal air-filled lung. The bronchus leading into the affected lung region must be patent to hear bronchial breath sounds over the affected region.
11. The pleural friction rub suggests that pleural inflammation is present. This finding indicates that the pneumonia is adjacent to the pleura.
12. The extremities are cool, moist, and cyanotic because of the release of catecholamines in response to stress. The catecholamines cause sweating and peripheral vasoconstriction, which reduces blood flow to the extremities. As a result, the hands and feet become sweaty, cool, and cyanotic.
13. Useful laboratory tests in this case would include a complete blood count (CBC), blood culture, chemistry profile, sputum Gram's stain with culture and sensitivity, an ABG analysis, and chest radiograph.

LABORATORY DATA

CBC (See Appendix for normal values.)

WBC 4000; segs 60 percent; bands 30 percent; lymphocytes 10 percent hemoglobin (Hb) 10.4 g/dL

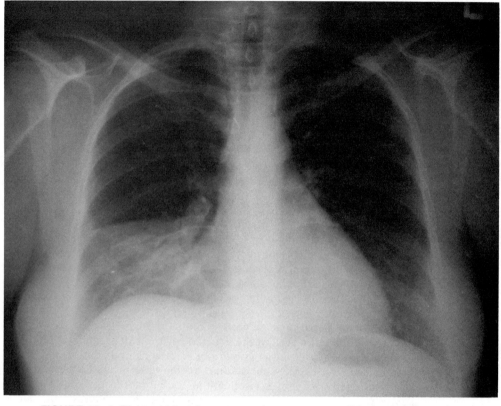

FIGURE 16–4 Right middle lobe pneumonia as seen on a PA chest radiograph.

ABGs

pH 7.47; P_{CO_2} 32 mm Hg; P_{O_2} 44 mm Hg; HCO_3^- 23 mEq

CHEST RADIOGRAPH

Right middle lobe consolidation; right heart border not visible (Fig. 16–4)

SPUTUM

Numerous gram-positive cocci with many WBCs and no epithelial cells

Questions

14. Interpret the CBC.
15. Interpret the ABG results. Explain why the P_{CO_2} and P_{O_2} are reduced.
16. What is the significance of the right heart border not being visible on the chest radiograph?
17. What is the significance of gram-positive cocci found on the sputum Gram's stain? What is the significance of the numerous WBCs and no epithelial cells?
18. Should this patient be treated as an outpatient, on the ward, or in the ICU?
19. What treatment should be provided?

Answers

14. The reduced WBC count in the presence of infection is consistent with an overwhelming infection. The WBC differential shows a large number of immature neutrophils called bands that are not usually called into action unless the infection is severe. The Hb is consistent with mild anemia.

15. The ABG measurements are consistent with acute respiratory alkalosis and moderate hypoxemia. The PO_2 would be lower if the patient were not hyperventilating. The patient may be hyperventilating in response to both hypoxemia and sepsis. The PO_2 is reduced due to $\dot{V}/\dot{Q}$ mismatching in the lung.

16. The inability to see the right heart border is evidence that the pneumonia is located in the right middle lobe. If the density was located in the right lower lobe the right heart border would probably be visible.

17. The gram-positive cocci found on the Gram's stain indicate that antibiotics such as penicillin derivatives and first-generation cephalosporins should be effective. The numerous leukocytes and lack of epithelial cells indicate a valid sputum sample representative of lower airway secretions with little oral contamination.

18. The patient should be admitted to the ICU, where she can be closely monitored. This is needed because she is at risk for respiratory failure and there is evidence (low WBC count) that the pneumonia is overwhelming the patient's immune system.

19. The patient should be given intravenous (IV) antibiotics, either a cephalosporin (Ancef) or a penicillinase-resistant penicillin (Nafcillin). Respiratory care should start the patient on oxygen with an FIO_2 of 0.40 to 0.50 and titrate her FIO_2 to an SaO_2 of approximately 90 percent. After her SaO_2 is stable, then a follow-up ABG analysis would confirm her ventilatory, acid-base, and oxygenation status. IV fluids are needed to maintain hydration as sepsis often decreases vascular tone and causes a relative hypovolemia. Sepsis-related decreases in vascular tone can result in profound hypotension and require large amounts of fluid. Central venous pressure monitoring would be important if hypotension develops.

MC was admitted to the ICU, where IV fluids and penicillin were administered. Oxygen was given by mask at an FIO_2 of 0.40 with a heated aerosol. A cardiac monitor was attached to her chest to allow continuous assessment of heart rate and rhythm. Repeat ABG 30 minutes after the start of oxygen therapy reveal pH 7.47; PCO_2 33 mm Hg; PO_2 53 mm Hg. Vital signs at this time were pulse 134/minute; respiratory rate 36/minute; temperature 38.2°C; and blood pressure 105/65 mm Hg. MC complained of increased dyspnea and cough. No change was noted in her right pleuritic chest pain. A blood sample was sent to the laboratory for culture.

Questions

20. Interpret the repeat ABG results.
21. What probably explains why the PaO_2 did not increase very much with the increase in FIO_2 to 0.40?
22. Why is the $PaCO_2$ not lower in response to the severity of the hypoxemia?
23. What is your assessment of the patient's condition in the ICU compared with his previous condition?

24. What treatment is indicated based on your updated assessment? Should the caregivers be concerned about oxygen-induced hypoventilation?

Answers

20. The acid-base status of the repeat ABG results has not changed significantly from that of the initial ABG results. Respiratory alkalosis with moderate hypoxemia continues.

21. Simple $\dot{V}/\dot{Q}$ mismatching causes hypoxemia that usually improves with supplemental oxygen therapy. Shunt is the likely explanation when the Pao_2 increases little or not at all in response to an increase in Fio_2. Pneumonia can lead to lung consolidation, which prevents air from entering the alveoli and coming in contact with blood in the pulmonary capillaries. An increase in Fio_2 will not increase the Pao_2 significantly unless the affected region is participating in gas exchange.

22. The $Paco_2$ is not lower in this case possibly because of the presence of COPD. A high work of breathing and a large physiologic dead space associated with COPD make it difficult for the patient to increase ventilation enough to reduce her $Paco_2$ more than the ABG now shows.

23. The patient's condition appears to be deteriorating. The fever increases her metabolic rate, which calls for increased ventilation and blood flow, thereby putting additional stress on the heart and lungs. Most patients do not tolerate respiratory rates greater than 30/minute for a prolonged time, and an increasing respiratory rate is evidence of respiratory distress. The patient is experiencing increased dyspnea, which also suggests that she may be tiring and on the brink of respiratory failure.

24. The Fio_2 should be increased in an effort to obtain a Pao_2 of 60 to 80 mm Hg. Given this patient's poor response to initial increases in the Fio_2 and the deteriorating vital signs, she will probably need intubation and mechanical ventilation to ensure adequate gas exchange. Oxygen-induced hypoventilation is not a concern in this case because the patient's previous ABG assessment reveals a reduced $Paco_2$. Adequate oxygenation should never be sacrificed to avoid an increase in the $Paco_2$ even if the $Paco_2$ were elevated.

MC's dyspnea and vital signs deteriorated further within the next hour. The cardiac monitor demonstrated frequent premature ventricular contractions and tachycardia with a rate of 144/minute. An endotracheal tube was placed and mechanical positive pressure ventilation was started when MC became confused and disoriented.

Questions

25. What is the significance of the patient's sudden confusion and frequent premature ventricular contractions seen on the electrocardiogram (ECG) monitor?
26. What mode of ventilation, tidal volume, rate, and Fio_2 would you recommend?
27. How should the intubation and mechanical ventilation be assessed?

Answers

25. The sudden confusion and premature ventricular contractions suggest that the patient has become more hypoxic or septic, or both, and that she has inadequate cerebral perfusion. This is a sign that the patient's cardiopulmonary system is failing.

26. The patient can be ventilated with assist-control or intermittent man-datory ventilation (IMV). A mechanical rate of 10 to 14 breaths/minute with a tidal volume of 650 to 900 cc (10 to 15 cc × 65 kg = 650 to 900 cc). An FIO_2 of 1.0 should be used initially because the patient is demonstrating signs of hypoxia.

27. The placement of the endotracheal tube can be assessed by listening for airflow at the tube orifice with the patient's respiratory efforts, auscul-tating for bilateral breath sounds on the lateral chest wall, listening for air entering the stomach with ventilator-driven breaths, and by a chest radiograph. The mechanical ventilation can be assessed by an ABG anal-ysis, by breathing pattern, and by vital signs.

MC was placed on a volume ventilator in the assist-control mode with a backup rate of 12/minute, a tidal volume of 800 cc, and an FIO_2 of 1.0. Initial auscultation revealed bilateral breath sounds with bronchial breath sounds over the right middle lobe. ABGs 20 minutes later revealed pH 7.46; PO_2 125 mm Hg; PCO_2 35 mm Hg; HCO_3^- 27 mEq. Initial vital signs on the ventilator were pulse 128/minute; respiratory rate 16/minute; blood pressure 100/68 mm Hg; and temperature 38.5°C. A repeat chest radiograph revealed appropriate placement of the endotracheal tube and no change in the right middle lobe infiltrate. A Foley catheter was placed and initial urine output was 25 mL for the first hour.

Questions

28. What changes in the ventilatory settings do you recommend based on the most recent assessment data?
29. What is the significance of the urine output of 25 mL for the first hour?
30. Is this patient at risk for nosocomial infection? If so, why? How can bedside clinicians reduce the risk?

Answers

28. The initial ABG analysis shows a relatively high PaO_2 on an FIO_2 of 1.0. The oxyhemoglobin dissociation curve demonstrates that nearly as much oxygen is carried by blood with a PaO_2 of 60 mm Hg as by blood with a PaO_2 greater than 100 mm Hg. An FIO_2 of 1.0 puts the patient at risk for oxygen toxicity and it should be titrated down to achieve a saturation of approximately 90 percent (PaO_2 of about 60 to 65 mm Hg). Because the PCO_2 is within the normal range, no change in the tidal volume or rate is needed.

29. The initial urine output of 25 mL/hour suggests that the patient has poor renal perfusion or is low on blood volume. A normal urine output is approximately 60 mL/hour. IV fluid therapy is usually provided as initial therapy for patients with low urine output or low blood pressure asso-ciated with sepsis. Evidence that fluids might not be appropriate would include elevated jugular venous pressure, a gallop heart rhythm (S_3 or S_4), hepatojugular reflex, and peripheral edema.

30. The patient is at high risk for nosocomial infection because of the com-promised immune system, intubation, and mechanical ventilation. Care-ful handwashing by all bedside clinicians before caring for each ICU patient is very important to prevent spread of bacteria from one patient to the next. The use of sterile technique for suctioning the airway is also important.

Over the next 24 hours MC improved steadily. Her body temperature dropped to 37.5°C and her pulse rate reduced to 95/minute. A repeat CBC revealed a WBC of 6000 with 65 percent segs and 20 percent bands. IV penicillin and fluids were continued. ABGs at this time were pH 7.44; P_{CO_2} 39 mm Hg; P_{O_2} 72 mm Hg; F_{IO_2} 0.50.

On day 3 the patient's weaning parameters were good, and she was weaned from mechanical ventilation without difficulty. Her vital signs were normal except for a respiratory rate of 28/minute. The endotracheal tube was removed, and she tolerated spontaneous breathing well. She was placed on a heated aerosol by mask with an F_{IO_2} of 0.50 after extubation. A repeat chest radiograph on day 3 demonstrated that the right middle lobe infiltrate was less dense. The patient was switched to a nasal cannula at 3 liters/minute, which she tolerated well. After the patient's temperature was normal for 24 hours the IV antibiotics were discontinued and oral antibiotics started. The patient was discharged on day 5 on oral penicillin. A follow-up visit with her physician was scheduled for 1 week later.

Questions

31. What risk factors for pneumonia existed in this patient?
32. How long might it take for the infiltrate to completely clear on the chest radiograph? Should this patient have follow-up chest radiographs to document complete resolution of the pneumonia? If so, why?

Answers

31. The risk factors for pneumonia in this patient include positive smoking history, COPD, possible alcohol abuse, and malnutrition.
32. The infiltrate seen on the chest radiograph with bacterial pneumonia generally clears in 2 weeks in young healthy patients but may take as long as 3 months to clear in older patients with lung disease. Yes, this patient should have follow-up chest radiographs to document complete resolution of the pneumonia. She is also at high risk for bronchogenic carcinoma (see Chapter 17). This is needed because the infiltrate may be caused by airway obstruction from bronchogenic carcinoma and in such cases the infiltrate will not clear completely with antibiotics. A nonresolving pneumonia requires further evaluation, most likely with bronchoscopy.

REFERENCES

1. Spence, TH: Pneumonia in the adult. In Kirby, RR and Taylor, RW (eds): Respiratory Failure. Year Book Medical, Chicago, 1986, pp 349–364.
2. Johnson, CC and Finegold, SM: Pyogenic bacterial pneumonia, lung abscess, and empyema. In Murray, JF and Nadel, JA (eds): Textbook of Respiratory Medicine. WB Saunders, Philadelphia, 1988.
3. Weinberger, SE: Principles of Pulmonary Medicine. WB Saunders, Philadelphia, 1992, p. 264.
4. Loudon, RG: The lung exam. In Braman, SS (ed): Clinics in Chest Medicine, Pulmonary Signs and Symptoms. WB Saunders, Philadelphia, Vol 8, No 2, June 1987, p 268.
5. Wilkins, RL and Hodgkin, JE: The history and physical exam. In Burton, GG, Hodgkin, JE, and Ward, JJ (eds): Respiratory Care, ed 3. JB Lippincott, Philadelphia, 1991, pp 211–232.
6. Seidel, HM: Mosby's Guide to Physical Exam. CV Mosby, St Louis, 1987.
7. Britton, S, Bejstedt, M, and Vedin, L: Chest physiotherapy in primary pneumonia. Br Med J 290:1703, 1985, p 264.

8.   Eid, N, et al: Chest physiotherapy in review. Respir Care 36:270, 1991.

9.   Crawford, GE: Infectious disease problems in respiratory failure. In Kirby, RR and Taylor, RW (eds): Respiratory Failure. Year Book Medical, Chicago, 1986, pp 365–386.

10.   Craven, DE and Steger, KA: Pathogenesis and prevention of nosocomial pneumonia in the mechanically ventilated patient. Respir Care 34:85, 1989.

11.   Celis, R, et al: Nosocomial pneumonia: A multivariate analysis of risk and prognosis. Chest 93:318, 1988.

Chapter 17

Gregory A.B. Cheek, MD

LUNG CANCER

INTRODUCTION

Lung cancer, also called bronchogenic carcinoma, is now the most common fatal malignant lesion in both men and women in the United States. In 1989 there were an estimated 155,000 new cases and 142,000 deaths (or 6 percent of all United States deaths) due to lung cancer.[1] Despite advances in methods of diagnosis and therapy, overall survival for lung cancer has changed little over the past 30 years. About 1 in 10 patients lives beyond 5 years from the time of diagnosis.[2] Earlier diagnosis and more effective therapy become ever more important as the worldwide incidence of lung cancer rises.

The term "malignant" denotes the lethal behavior of abnormal tissue that serves no useful purpose and spreads unchecked at the expense of healthy tissue. This chapter discusses those malignancies that arise within the lung itself (called **primary malignancies**), but not those that arrive in the lung from other tissues (called **metastatic malignancies**).

ETIOLOGY

Most scientists, except perhaps those employed by the tobacco industry, agree that cigarette smoking causes lung cancer. There is a strong association between smoking exposure and the incidence of bronchogenic carcinoma. Ten percent of all smokers get lung cancer and about 83 percent of all lung cancer patients smoke or have smoked.[1] The risk of lung cancer is related to the number of cigarettes smoked, the duration (in years) of smoking, the age at initiation of smoking, the depth of inhalation, and the tar and nicotine content in cigarettes smoked. There is a 10- to 25-fold greater risk of lung cancer among smokers than among non-smokers.[3] The risk of developing lung cancer gradually declines for about 13 years after one quits smoking but never quite reaches nonsmoker risk level.[4]

A nonsmoker in the vicinity of a smoker inhales "sidestream" smoke that contains higher concentrations of carcinogens than smoke inhaled by the smoker. There is about a twofold increased risk of lung cancer in individuals exposed to passive smoke.[5,6] Exposure to certain irritant fibers, ionizing radiation, and fumes from various chemicals has also been linked to an increased incidence of lung cancer. These agents include asbestos, chromium, nickel, uranium, vinyl chloride, bischloromethyl ether, and decay products of radon gas.[7] Many of these materials potentiate the effect of cigarette smoke in the induction of bronchogenic carcinoma. Asbestos exposure in nonsmokers has been associated with a fivefold increase in

Table 17–1 Relative Risk of Lung Cancer

Patient History	Risk Ratio*
Never smoked; no significant industrial contact	1
Cigarette smoker	
<½ pack/day	15
½–1 pack/day	17
1–2 packs/day	42
>2 packs/day	64
Cigar smoker	3
Pipe smoker	8
Ex-smoker	2–10
Nonsmoking female exposed to husband's smoke	1.4–1.9
Asbestos worker	
Nonsmoker	5
Cigarette smoker	92
Uranium miner	
Nonsmoker	7
Cigarette smoker	38
Relatives of lung cancer patients	
Nonsmokers	4
Smokers	14

*The risk ratio is the relative risk of developing lung cancer compared to the risk of comparable individuals without the listed exposure.

Source: Adapted from Murray, JF and Nadel, JA: Textbook of Respiratory Medicine. WB Saunders, Philadelphia, 1988, p 1177, with permission.

the incidence of lung cancer. Asbestos exposure in cigarette smokers is associated with a 92-fold increase in the incidence of lung cancer (Table 17–1).[8,9]

Other risk factors may include air pollution, cigar or pipe use, and lung scars. The reducing type of pollutants (e.g., sulfur dioxide, carbonaceous particulate matter) are thought to be carcinogens, whereas oxidants (e.g., hydrocarbons, nitrous oxides) are not. A familial predisposition to lung cancer increases individual susceptibility to lung cancer. Those who have close relatives with lung cancer are up to three times more likely to develop lung cancer than the general population.[10] Sarcoidosis is associated with a threefold increase in incidence of lung cancer.[11]

PATHOLOGY

The four major histologic types of lung cancer are epidermoid or squamous cell carcinoma (25 percent), adenocarcinoma (30 percent), large-cell carcinoma (15 percent), and small-cell carcinoma (25 percent).[12] The clinical effect of small-cell cancer is much different from that of the other three forms of lung cancer, so that lung cancers are usually classified in terms of small-cell and non–small-cell cancers.

Squamous cell carcinoma is named for the appearance of the cells that resemble cells of the skin (epidermis). These cells usually contain the skin protein called keratin. Squamous cell carcinomas arise most often from the bronchial lining and may grow to obstruct air passages.

Adenocarcinoma resembles poorly formed glandular tissue. It may be difficult to determine whether an adenocarcinoma is a primary lung cancer or a metastatic malignancy from elsewhere in the body. Many organs in the body develop adeno-carcinoma that may metastasize to the lungs.

Large-cell carcinomas are characterized by a collection of poorly formed large cells that have abundant cytoplasm. These tumors may exhibit glandlike structure and produce some mucin.

Small-cell carcinomas are characterized by very small cells with scant cyto-plasm. Small-cell carcinoma is a very rapidly growing tumor that usually metastasizes to distant tissue (e.g., brain, liver, bone) while the tumor is quite small.

Lung cancer may affect lung function in a variety of ways, depending on the size and location of the tumor. Small peripheral lung tumors may not impair lung function in a noticeable way. Larger tumors may invade the lung parenchyma and reduce lung volume in an amount proportional to the size of the growth. Cancerous growths may obstruct a major airway and result in pooling of secretions and little or no gas exchange distal to the obstruction. The affected lung region will typically become atelectatic and susceptible to pneumonia.

CLINICAL FEATURES

A complete medical history and physical examination is essential when evaluating a patient for lung cancer. Emphasis is placed on identifying symptoms commonly associated with cancer (Table 17–2) and staging the extent of the disease.

The clinical presentation of lung cancer depends on several variables, including the cell type, growth rate, where in the lung it originates, and the integrity of the host immune system. Approximately 15 percent of patients are asymptomatic at the time of diagnosis (i.e., incidental nodule seen on chest radiographs).[3] Symptoms due either to local intrathoracic or to distant metastatic effects of tumor are present in about 70 percent of all lung cancer patients on presentation.[13]

Table 17–2 Clinical Manifestations of Bronchogenic Carcinoma[13]

Cough	74%
Weight loss	68%
Dyspnea	58%
Chest pain	49%
Sputum production	45%
Hemoptysis	29%
Malaise	26%
Bone pain	25%
Lymphadenopathy	23%
Hepatomegaly	21%
Fever	21%
Clubbing	20%
Neuromyopathy	10%
Superior vena cava syndrome	4%
Dizziness	4%
Hoarseness	3%
Asymptomatic	12%

Source: Adapted from Doyle, LA and Aisner, J: Clinical presentation of lung cancer. In Roth, JA, Ruckdeschel, JC, and Weisenburger, TH (eds): Thoracic Oncology. WB Saunders, Philadelphia, 1989, p 53.

Pulmonary symptoms associated with lung cancer may include a change in cough or sputum production, hemoptysis, wheezing, dyspnea, stridor, chest pain, or fever. These findings may provide the first clue that lung cancer is present and often are the result of the cancer obstructing airways and lymphatics.

Cough and sputum production are not specific symptoms, as the majority of lung cancer patients suffer from chronic bronchitis and emphysema due to cigarette smoking. However, a change in the character of the cough, a change in the quality and quantity of sputum, or unresponsiveness to previously effective therapy (i.e., bronchodilators, antibiotics, and steroids) should raise suspicion of a tumor.

Shortness of breath may be associated with lung cancer when the tumor obstructs a large airway. Large pleural effusions or paralysis of a hemidiaphragm resulting from phrenic nerve involvement may contribute to the patient's complaint of dyspnea.

Hemoptysis associated with lung cancer is caused by ulceration of the bronchial mucosa. The quantity of blood is usually small but sometimes may be massive and life threatening. Hemoptysis usually prompts the patient to seek immediate medical attention and should raise suspicion for endobronchial tumor.

Chest pain in lung cancer may indicate local invasion of the pleura, ribs, and nerves. It may be dull, constant, and debilitating or intermittent and sharp, varying with the respiratory cycle. It may localize to the chest wall or radiate to the midback or scapula, shoulder, or arm on the side of the tumor. Chest pain may decrease as pleural effusion develops.

Physical examination of the patient with lung cancer may be relatively normal when the tumor is small and located peripherally. Auscultation may reveal wheezing if an airway is partially obstructed. The wheezing is usually monophonic, is localized, and does not disappear after a cough. Wheezing may be heard on inhalation and exhalation. Percussion will reveal diminished resonance over lung tissue affected by a large tumor, pleural effusion, or pneumonia (consolidation). Careful examination may reveal distant metastasis to skin or regional lymph nodes. Clubbing of the fingers or toes or both may indicate hypertrophic pulmonary osteoarthropathy (paraneoplastic syndrome) caused by subperiosteal new bone formation of the extremities associated with lung cancer.

Physical examination may also reveal evidence of tumor spread, which precludes surgical resection. Hoarseness suggests left vocal cord paralysis caused by recurrent laryngeal nerve compression by tumor. Facial edema suggests compression of the superior vena cava by tumor. Tumor compression of the cervical sympathetic nerve plexus causes Horner's syndrome. Horner's syndrome is ptosis (drooping eyelid), myosis (pinpoint pupil), and anhydrosis (lack of sweating of the cheek). Arm and shoulder pain suggests superior sulcus tumor invading the brachial nerve plexus (Pancoast's syndrome combined with Horner's syndrome).[14] Bone pain suggests metastasis to the bone. Change in mental status, emotional status, or coordination suggests brain metastasis.

METASTATIC DISEASE

Clues to metastatic disease may include chest wall or distant bone pain, seizures from brain metastasis, stroke from tumor emboli, paraplegia from spread to spinal cord, or weight loss associated with liver metastasis.

Patients with advanced lung cancer may present with the following:

1. Nonspecific systemic symptoms
2. Signs and symptoms of intrathoracic spread
3. Signs and symptoms of extrathoracic extension
4. Classic systemic paraneoplastic syndromes

Nonspecific Systemic Symptoms

Nonspecific systemic symptoms include weight loss, anorexia, nausea, vomiting, and weakness. Systemic symptoms do not necessarily mean that the tumor is nonresectable but they are generally a poor prognostic sign.

Intrathoracic Spread

Signs of tumor spread or metastasis within the chest include (1) pleural effusion, (2) superior vena cava syndrome, (3) brachial neuritis, (4) hoarseness, (5) pericardial effusion, and (6) diaphragm elevation.

1. Pleural effusion is a collection of fluid in the pleural space around the lung. It may be caused by direct extension of the lung tumor to the pleural surface, by blockage of lymphatic ducts, or by pneumonia associated with malignancy. Tumor cells invading lymphatics obstruct normal lymph flow in the lung and result in the accumulation of fluid in the pleural space.

2. Superior vena cava syndrome is caused by tumor compression or direct invasion of the great veins in the thoracic outlet. It is associated with dyspnea, headache, and periorbital, facial, neck, and upper trunk edema. Collateral circulation across the upper thorax and neck is usually prominent and very distended.

3. Brachial neuritis is typically caused by a superior sulcus tumor (most often squamous cell carcinoma located in the lung apex; may be pleural based) called Pancoast's tumor that grows through the parietal pleura and invades the brachial plexus. Involvement of the last cervical and first thoracic (C7 to T2) segment of the sympathetic nerve trunk results in a triad of clinical findings called Horner's syndrome (see physical examination for definition).

4. Pressure on the recurrent laryngeal nerve where it encircles the aortic arch from tumor or enlarged lymph nodes causes nerve disruption resulting in hoarseness.

5. Pericardial effusion (fluid in the sac around the heart) is a serious complication of thoracic cancer caused by metastasis or direct tumor extension into the pericardium and epicardium. It causes neck vein distension, cardiac arrhythmias, and cardiac tamponade (fluid compressing on the heart muscle preventing it from pumping blood, which may be fatal).

6. Unilateral hemidiaphragmatic paralysis with paradoxic motion (upward motion on rapid inspiration) on fluoroscopy may occur as a result of phrenic nerve involvement.

Extrathoracic Spread

Symptoms of extrathoracic spread or distant metastases depend on the sites involved. Common sites of spread include lymph nodes, brain and spinal cord, liver, adrenal glands, bone, bone marrow, and skin. Bone and central nervous system (CNS) spread usually results in symptomatic disease, whereas liver and adrenal gland metastases may be asymptomatic.

DIAGNOSIS

The 5-year survival rate for all patients with carcinoma of the lung is only about 10 percent.[2] This dismal statistic reflects the fact that disease is advanced in most patients when first detected. Unfortunately, routine frequent screening with sputum cytology and chest radiographs has not proved to alter the mortality rate from lung cancer and is not cost effective.[15] There are no official recommendations for screening patients for lung cancer, except for a high clinical suspicion, based on risk factors previously discussed.[16]

The aim of diagnostic procedures is twofold: (1) to confirm the clinical diagnosis by cytology or histology, and (2) to establish the extent of dissemination (stage) of the disease in order to determine the most suitable treatment (i.e., surgical, or irradiation or chemotherapy or both).

Radiographic Data

The chest radiograph may demonstrate asymptomatic lung cancer but is almost always abnormal when the patient is symptomatic. A tumor nodule must be about 2 to 3 mm before it is visible on chest radiograph and greater than 1 to 2 cm before fluoroscopic guided transthoracic needle aspiration biopsy has a reasonable chance of making the diagnosis.[17]

A common dilemma associated with small pulmonary nodules is whether the nodule is a small bronchogenic cancer or a benign granuloma. Clues to the probability of malignancy include growth rate, margin configuration, and presence of calcification. Malignant tumors grow at a rate that doubles the number of cells in the tumor at least every 400 days and no more often than every 30 days.[18] Careful measurement is important because a tumor or granuloma is a three-dimensional sphere, and doubling its volume only changes its diameter by a factor of 1.27. Tumor margins are most often irregular and indistinct because tumors invade neighboring tissue. Granulomas will often develop around a central area of inflammation and develop very smooth, distinct borders. Tumors may rarely develop significant calcification but granulomas develop central, well-defined calcification. A rare benign tumor called hamartoma is noted for developing a pattern of calcification in a "popcorn ball" configuration.

The heart and other thoracic structures obscure large portions of the lung tissue and it is important to evaluate both a frontal and side view before calling a chest radiograph "normal." The four most common types of bronchogenic carcinoma (squamous, adenocarcinoma, small-cell, and large-cell) usually present with slightly different chest radiographic patterns, but there is so much overlap that only biopsy and histologic examination provide reliable evidence about the cell type.

Obstruction of a main or segmental bronchus may be associated with atelectasis. Atelectasis is collapse of lung alveoli distal to an obstructing lesion causing volume loss in a segment of lung and a shift of the mediastinum toward the lesion best seen on maximal inspiratory chest radiograph (Fig. 17–1). Obstruction may also cause a refractory pneumonia (Fig. 17–2).

Laboratory Studies

Other diagnostic tests that may reflect local, metastatic, or paraneoplastic effects of lung cancer include serum chemistry, complete blood count (CBC), liver function, arterial blood gas (ABG), and the 12-lead electrocardiogram (ECG). Hyponatremia occurs in the presence of ectopic (hormone produced by tumor cells) antidiuretic hormone (ADH), most often from small-cell carcinoma. Hypercalcemia in lung cancer occurs either from metastatic tumor spread to bone or from a parathyroid hormonelike substance most often from squamous cell carcinoma. Alkaline phosphatase may be elevated in the presence of bone or liver metastases. Liver dysfunction may occur because of intrahepatic spread and/or extrahepatic obstruction from metastatic disease. Anemia (low hemoglobin), thrombocytopenia (low platelet count), or leukoerythroblastic (immature blood cell forms resembling leukemia) peripheral blood pattern and even pancytopenia (low count of all blood cell types) may occur from metastatic spread of tumor to bone marrow. The ECG may show low voltage or pulsus alternans (amplitude of QRS waveform varies with

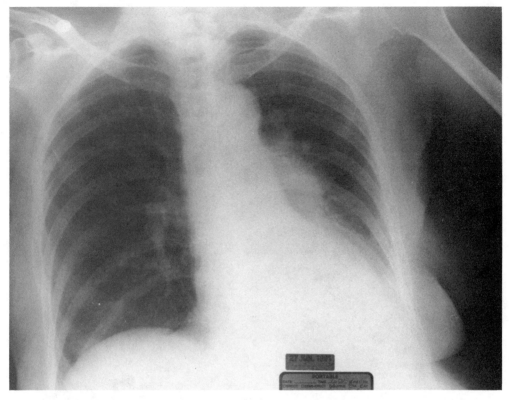

FIGURE 17–1 Chest radiograph demonstrating tumor obstruction of left lower lobe bronchus ("cutoff sign") leading to atelectasis distal to obstruction and mediastinal shift toward the lung volume loss.

respiration) from pericardial effusion or a conduction block from metastatic disease. A murmur may indicate marantic endocarditis (noninfectious vegetations on heart valves) or spread of tumor via pulmonary vein to form an intracardiac mass. Pulmonary function tests may indicate restrictive disease owing to lymphatic spread. ABGs may show hypoxemia resulting from ventilation-perfusion abnormalities or shunting.

Diagnostic Procedures

Methods available for diagnosing bronchogenic carcinoma include sputum cytology, fiberoptic bronchoscopy, transbronchial needle or forceps biopsy, percutaneous transthoracic needle aspiration biopsy (also termed fine-needle aspiration), thoracentesis, pleural biopsy, thoracoscopy, mediastinoscopy, and thoracotomy (wedge resection/lobectomy/pneumonectomy). Each method has its inherent benefits, risks, and limitations.

Sputum cytology is most useful in diagnosing central squamous cell carcinomas. Potential problems in accurately interpreting sputum cytology specimens include

1. Inadequate specimen without alveolar macrophages (less than 3 to 4/high-power field [hpf]) or greater than 5 to 10 epithelial cells/hpf
2. Degeneration of malignant cells before examination
3. Purulent samples

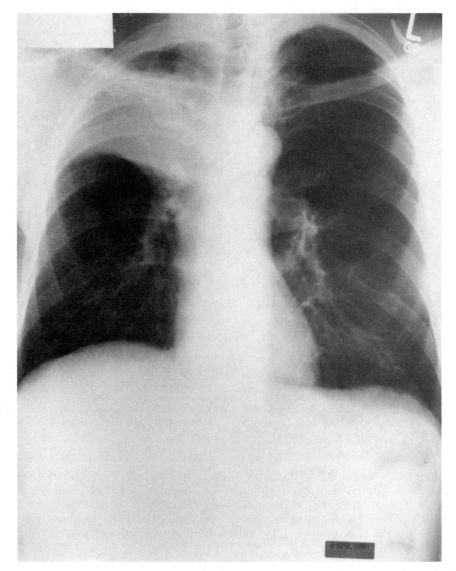

FIGURE 17–2 Chest radiograph demonstrating right upper lobe pneumonia and atelectasis from tumor obstruction of a major airway.

4. Inexperience of cytologist-technician (bronchial squamous cell metaplasia frequent in chronic bronchitis makes distinction of malignancy difficult)
5. Asthma patients may produce cell clumps that resemble adenocarcinoma[19]
6. Lipoid pneumonia and pulmonary infarction, which may produce cellular changes easily confused with malignancy[19]

Cytologic evaluation of sputum offers little help to patients with peripheral lesions or solitary nodules.

Flexible fiberoptic bronchoscopy used under local anesthesia with or without intravenous (IV) sedation is an invaluable tool for diagnosing bronchogenic carcinoma. The extent and operability of the tumor are assessed by observing the site of the tumor, extent of tumor infiltration, narrowing of the airway, and widening of the carina. When lesions are visible endobronchially, bronchial washings have a diagnostic yield of approximately 80 percent; bronchial brushings and bronchial mucosal forceps biopsy samples provide diagnosis of tissue in nearly 98 percent of visualized tumors.[15] False-negative results may occur in deeper submucosal lesions owing to the inability to grasp and sample these tissues. Under fluoroscopic control, transbronchial forceps biopsies, brushings, and washings can diagnose more peripheral, parenchymal lesions up to 60 percent of the time. Blind transbronchial fine-needle aspiration biopsies are commonly directed toward submucosal lesions or known areas of adenopathy evident on computerized tomography (CT) of the chest.[17]

The use of percutaneous transthoracic needle aspiration biopsy (TNAB) is most suitable for peripheral pulmonary nodules. Tumors located away from mediastinal vascular structures and emphysematous bullae are most suitable for this technique. Fluoroscopic guidance is adequate for those nodules 2 cm or greater in diameter and visible on both frontal and lateral chest radiographs. For lesions as small as 2 cm the diagnostic accuracy is about 95 percent for malignant lesions.[3] Nodules smaller than 2 cm in diameter are usually aspirated under CT guidance. The needle is of fine bore (often 25 gauge). Tumors up to 12 cm deep can be reached by this method. The incidence of pneumothorax is from 15 to 35 percent and is more common in emphysematous patients. Only 5 to 10 percent of patients with TNAB require any kind of thoracostomy tube placement for lung re-expansion following biopsy.[20] Bronchoscopy carries less risk of pneumothorax (less than 5 percent with transbronchial biopsy[21]) and is often performed before TNAB. A TNAB may be indicated before thoracotomy to confirm that a lesion is not small-cell carcinoma. Also, in a patient who is a poor surgical candidate it may provide a cytologic diagnosis and obviate the need for exploratory thoracotomy.

A positive pleural fluid cytology proves the spread of malignancy to the pleural space. Definitive diagnosis may be obtained from a cell block of centrifuged pleural fluid or positive histology from pleural biopsy. Thoracentesis and pleural biopsy combined provide up to a 90 percent yield in patients with malignancy.[3] Most malignant pleural effusions are exudative.

Thoracoscopy improves the diagnostic yield of exudative pleural effusions. Biopsy specimens are taken under direct vision with much lower risk than thoracotomy and a diagnostic yield of 93 to 96 percent for malignant pleural effusions.[22]

Mediastinal lymph nodes are involved at initial presentation in about half of lung cancer patients.[23] Patients with evidence of mediastinal lymphadenopathy (lymph nodes 1 cm and greater) and central or large (greater than 6 cm) peripheral lesions should have a diagnostic mediastinoscopy before having a thoracotomy. Anterior cervical mediastinoscopy allows direct visualization and biopsy of mediastinal nodes with less risk than an exploratory thoracotomy. Its use has decreased the percentage of unnecessary exploratory thoracotomies.[24]

STAGING

Staging the extent of lung cancer is essential in selecting appropriate therapy and avoiding unnecessary surgery. The modified staging classification system developed by the American Joint Committee and the Union Contre le Cancer in 1986 provides a nomenclature that is accepted by specialists around the world. This system is based on the TNM (T = primary *t*umor; N = regional lymph *n*odes; M = distant *m*etastasis [spread of cancer to distant site identified on biopsy]) system. T describes the size of the tumor (Table 17–3). N describes the lymph node buds involved (Table 17–4). M is either present (M1) or absent (M0) (Table 17–5).

TNM classification is then used as a basis from which to formulate five stages of severity of lung cancer (Table 17–6). This system is primarily used in the management of non–small-cell lung cancer. In stages I and II the cancer is considered

Table 17–3 Definition of Primary Tumor (T) Characteristics in Lung Cancer According to TNM System

Descriptor	Definition
TX	Tumor proved by the presence of malignant cells in bronchopulmonary secretions but not visualized on chest radiograph or by bronchoscope, or any tumor that cannot be assessed as in a retreatment staging
T0	No evidence of primary tumor
TIS	Carcinoma in situ
T1	A tumor that is 3.0 cm or less in greatest dimension, surrounded by lung or visceral pleura, and without evidence of invasion proximal to a lobar bronchus at bronchoscopy
T2	A tumor >3.0 cm in greatest dimension, or a tumor of any size that either invades the visceral pleural or has associated atelectasis or obstructive pneumonitis extending to the hilar region; at bronchoscopy, the proximal extent of demonstrable tumor must be within a lobar bronchus or at least 2 cm distal to carina
T3	A tumor of any size with direct extension into the chest wall, diaphragm, or mediastinal pleura or pericardium without involving the heart, great vessels, trachea, esophagus or vertebral body, or a tumor in the main bronchus within 2 cm of the carina without involving the carina
T4	A tumor of any size with invasion of mediastinum or involving heart, great vessels, trachea, esophagus, vertebral body or carina or presence of malignant pleural effusion

Table 17–4 Definition of Nodal Involvement (N) in Lung Cancer by TNM Classification

Descriptor	Definition
N0	No demonstrable metastasis to regional lymph nodes
N1	Metastasis to lymph nodes in the peribronchial or ipsilateral hilar region, or both, including direct extension
N2	Metastasis to ipsilateral mediastinal lymph nodes and subcarinal lymph nodes
N3	Metastasis to contralateral mediastinal lymph nodes, contralateral hilar lymph nodes, ipsilateral or contralateral scalene or supraclavicular lymph nodes

Table 17–5 Definition of Distant Metastasis (M) in Lung Cancer by TNM Classification

Descriptor	Definition
M0	No (known) distant metastasis
M1	Distant metastasis present; specify sites

Table 17–6 TNM Stage Grouping for Lung Cancer

Stage	TNM Subsets		
	T	N	M
Occult cancer	TX	N0	M0
0	TIS	Carcinoma in situ	
I	T1	N0	M0
	T2	N0	M0
II	T1	N1	M0
	T2	N1	M0
IIIA	T3	N0	M0
	T3	N1	M0
	T1–3	N2	M0
IIIB	Any T	N3	M0
	T4	Any N	M0
IV	Any T	Any N	M1

surgically resectable. Stage IIIA cancer may be surgically curable but the perioperative risk is higher and the survival benefit marginal. Cancers in stages IIIB and IV are not surgically resectable and often receive radiation therapy with or without chemotherapy.

TREATMENT AND PROGNOSIS

The majority of lung cancer patients present with metastatic disease and have a poor prognosis. The choice of therapy and survival rate are related to the histologic cell type of the tumor and the stage of the disease at the time the physician makes the diagnosis.

One of the most important indices of long-term survival is the patient's performance status at the time lung cancer is diagnosed. The performance status is an objective assessment of the effect that the cancer has on the patient's ability to carry on with daily activities and work. Two scales are widely used in the United States: the Karnofsky Performance Scale and the Eastern Cooperative Oncology Group (ECOG) or Zubrod Performance Scale.[24] A poor performance status with a low-stage lung cancer indicates the cancer may actually be more widespread than believed or the patient's physiologic status is such that he or she will not tolerate therapy well. There is a very strong relationship between performance index and survival.

Surgery

Surgical resection provides a cure in 60 to 80 percent of patients with stage I non–small-cell lung cancer (NSCLC).[12] A segmented wedge resection may be adequate in those with small tumors (stage I) and poor pulmonary reserve. Patients with stage I NSCLC and inadequate pulmonary reserve or severe concurrent medical problems are candidates for radiation therapy and have an anticipated cure rate of about 20 to 30 percent.[12] Radiotherapy does not improve cure rate after surgical resection of stage I NSCLC.[12]

Surgery is the only curative modality for stage II and IIIA NSCLC. The treatment of choice is lobectomy or pneumonectomy with resection of regional and mediastinal lymph nodes, depending on the tumor size and location. Although 15 to 25 percent of patients who undergo surgical resection for stage II or IIIA NSCLC have local tumor recurrence, radiotherapy is not used because of its cost, toxicity, and lack of proven benefit on survival.

Stage IIIB (locally advanced unresectable disease) is treated with radiation therapy especially when symptoms of pain, hemoptysis, or airway obstruction are present. Chemotherapy combined with radiotherapy has not substantially improved survival rates. Chemotherapy alone has generally provided relatively brief partial remissions.

Radiation Therapy

Radiation therapy can be an effective form of primary treatment in NSCLC or can be beneficial in the palliation of hemoptysis, bronchial obstruction, and bone pain from metastatic disease. However, it is not a comparable alternative to surgical therapy for cure. Candidates include those patients who have inoperable NSCLC due to advanced stage or medical reasons. They should have a good performance scale status and be able to tolerate pulmonary fibrosis. Complications include radiation pneumonitis and fibrosis, esophagitis, pericarditis, and damage to the spinal cord. Preoperative radiation is recommended only for superior sulcus (Pancoast's) tumor.

Chemotherapy

Chemotherapy is not used as a primary form of treatment for NSCLC but is recommended for small-cell lung cancer (SCLC) and in clinical trials of adjuvant therapy (additional chemotherapy after surgery) for NSCLC. Chemotherapy can be given before surgery (neoadjuvant therapy) or after surgery when resected hilar or mediastinal lymph nodes contain metastatic cancer. Despite the administration of newer drugs in higher concentrations, a long-term response can only be achieved in 5 to 10 percent of patients with NSCLC.[25]

Adverse side effects of chemotherapy depend on the drug regimen chosen. The most common side effects include bone marrow suppression, nausea, vomiting, renal and liver toxicity, and neuropathy. Some agents will cause severe tissue necrosis if leaked into the skin around the IV catheter site. Bone marrow suppression will cause the patient to be neutropenic (low white blood cells) and susceptible to numerous bacterial, viral, and opportunistic infections. Nausea and emesis will lead to weight loss and a miserable quality of life unless treated. Arrhythmias, red urine, and permanent cardiac dysfunction may result from the use of some agents.

SMALL-CELL DISEASE

Limited Disease   Chemotherapy is much more effective for small-cell cancer than for non–small-cell cancer. The overall response rate (remission of tumor growth or shrinkage of primary tumor mass or both) with limited small-cell disease ranges from 70 to 90 percent, with a long-term remission rate of 40 to 50 percent.[12] Concurrent radiotherapy of the thorax may decrease incidence of local recurrence. Prophylactic cranial radiation is used because metastasis to the brain occurs frequently and chemotherapy does not cross the blood-brain barrier.

Extensive Disease   Systemic chemotherapy results in an overall response rate of 60 to 80 percent.[12] Unfortunately, response rates are temporary and chemotherapy is palliative. The median survival rate ranges from 9 to 12 months.[12] Prophylactic cranial irradiation and early chest irradiation have no value in patients with extensive disease. Radiotherapy is important for palliation of brain and bone metastases.

Preoperative Evaluation

Among patients undergoing thoracotomy for diagnosis or cure, several parameters must be measured to estimate the patient's risk of perioperative pulmonary complications. One of the most important is pulmonary function. Postoperative survival depends on adequate preoperative pulmonary reserve. The desired postoperative forced expiratory volume in 1 second (FEV_1) is greater than 0.8 liter. In patients with borderline or poor lung function, a differential lung perfusion study helps to predict postoperative effective FEV_1. The percent of flow to the "good" lung that is to remain is multiplied by the preoperative FEV_1 to estimate postoperative FEV_1. This estimate is most helpful when large portions of lung are to be removed. Exercise testing is performed in some patients considered high risk for surgery (i.e., preoperative FEV_1 less than 40 percent predicted and arterial P_{CO_2} greater than 45 mm Hg) to measure oxygen consumption at peak exercise. In several studies a peak oxygen consumption value of greater than 15 mL/kg per minute carries a significantly lower risk for perioperative cardiopulmonary complications and death than does a lower value.[26,27]

Case Study

HISTORY

A 65-year-old man presents with fever, chills, progressive dyspnea, and cough. The cough had produced one-quarter cup of yellow-green sputum each day for 2 weeks and had been blood-tinged for 2 days. He has had decreasing exercise tolerance for the past 6 months but never sought medical attention. He had noticed a 30-lb weight loss over 6 months. He had smoked two packs of cigarettes per day for 40 years but quit 4 months ago because "they didn't taste good anymore." He stated that he has had difficulty swallowing solids for 4 months and hoarseness for 3 months. He had been seen in the emergency room 2 days earlier for a diagnosis of "pneumonia" and given a course of oral antibiotics.

Surgical *Transurethral resection of the prostate (TURP) 2 years earlier; basal cell carcinoma of the lip removed 1 year earlier*

Medications *Amoxicillin 500 mg three times/day, metaproterenol inhaler two puffs every 4 hours as needed*

Exposure *Worked in the boiler room on a ship in the Navy for 3 years during the Korean War, then as a sandblaster in a shipyard for 2 years; denies tuberculosis (TB), fungal disease, or exposure*

Occupation *Car mechanic and garage manager*

Questions

1. What risk factors for bronchogenic carcinoma in this man's history can you identify? How many pack-years has he smoked?
2. What symptoms in the history suggest lung cancer?
3. Would old granulomatous disease increase the risk of lung cancer?
4. What could the following symptoms indicate in a patient suspected of having cancer?
   (a) Chest pain
   (b) Bone pain
   (c) Hoarseness
   (d) Dysphagia (difficulty swallowing)
   (e) Weakness of extremities or change in mental status

Answers

1. Age is a significant risk for lung cancer.[28]

    Tobacco smoking is the most significant risk factor for bronchogenic carcinoma. Pack-years is calculated by multiplying the packs smoked per day times the number of years smoked. Ten percent of smokers get lung cancer and about 80 percent of all lung cancer patients smoke or have smoked.[1] This patient has a 80–pack-year smoking history.

Asbestos exposure (working in boiler room without protective respiratory apparatus) is a risk factor. Concurrent smoking and asbestos exposure vastly increase the risk for developing lung cancer, up to 90-fold.[8,9] Exposure to silicates (sandblasting) also increases the risk of lung cancer in smokers.

2. Change in cough and sputum production may be a sign of lung cancer.

    Hemoptysis has many causes, including acute bronchitis, tuberculosis, pulmonary embolus, trauma, or tumor, but tumor is a likely cause of the bleeding in this case.

    Progressive dyspnea may be due to large airway obstruction from a tumor or worsening of underlying emphysema. Other possible causes for the dyspnea include pleural effusion, diaphragmatic paralysis, pulmonary embolus, or pericardial effusion.

    Unexplained weight loss should prompt a search for hidden malignancy.

3. Old granulomatous disease is associated with a slightly higher risk of lung cancer, especially if extensive scarring is present.

4. (a) Lung tissue does not have pain receptors; therefore, chest pain usually indicates spread of the lung cancer to parietal pleura, ribs, or other chest wall structures.

    (b) Bone pain may indicate bone metastasis or osteoarthropathy.

    (c) The recurrent laryngeal nerve travels from the neck around the aorta and back to the vocal cord. Compression of the recurrent laryngeal nerve by tumor or enlarged para-aortic lymph nodes may cause hoarseness. It is evidence that the tumor has involved vital structures and is not resectable.

    (d) Dysphagia (difficulty swallowing) may indicate esophageal compression from mediastinal adenopathy or invasion by lung tumor.

    (e) Arm or leg weakness or change in mental status suggest metastasis to the brain. Tumor in the brain may be manifest initially by relatively subtle signs, gradually progressing to clear evidence of mental, emotional, or physical dysfunction.

PHYSICAL EXAMINATION

General Lethargic, thin, chronically ill–appearing white man who appears older than stated age, with mild respiratory distress; patient alert but mildly confused (disoriented to place and time) and unable to provide coherent history

Vital Signs Temperature 37.6°C, pulse 102/minute, respirations 22/minute, blood pressure 110/50 mm Hg; height 5 feet 8 inches, weight 120 lb

HEENT Pupils equally round and responsive to light and accommodation, no ptosis, fundoscopically normal; tympanic membranes clear bilaterally, edentulous; no jugular venous distension, facial edema, or adenopathy

Chest Chest wall: nontender
Heart: Regular rhythm, no murmur, gallop, or rub; point of maximum impulse (PMI) below xiphoid process

Lungs: Markedly decreased breath sounds over lower right lung with inspiratory coarse crackles; localized monophonic expiratory wheeze in the right midlung; no pleural rub; right lower lobe dull to percussion

Abdomen   *Soft, nondistended, with bowel sounds active; slightly enlarged liver at 4 cm below the right costal margin*

Extremities   *Abnormally small muscle mass, no edema or cyanosis; mild enlargement of distal fingertips*

Questions

5. What do the vital signs and general appearance indicate?
6. What does the decreased resonance to percussion over the right lower lobe indicate?
7. What does the monophonic wheeze indicate?
8. What would be the significance of facial edema?
9. What would be the significance of ptosis (drooping of the eyelid)?

Answers

5. Low-grade fever is consistent with pneumonia. Respiratory rate is elevated, indicating compromised respiratory mechanics, compromised gas exchange, psychogenic stress (anxiety), or a combination of these. There is no evidence of accessory respiratory muscle use or paradoxic breathing to indicate diaphragmatic fatigue (pending respiratory failure). Weight loss in conjunction with tumor is a poor prognostic sign. Confusion and lethargy suggest cerebral metastasis or hypoxia.
6. Dullness to percussion indicates lung consolidation.
7. The localized right monophonic wheeze indicates partial airway obstruction of a single, large conducting airway in the right lung.
8. Tumor-related facial edema is most often caused by compression of the superior vena cava by enlarging tumor.
9. Eye ptosis is a sign of Horner's syndrome, which is caused by tumor compression of the sympathetic nerves (from lower cervical and upper thoracic spinal nerves).

DIAGNOSTIC DATA

CHEST RADIOGRAPHS

(Figs. 17–3 and 17–4)

ESOPHAGOGRAMS

(Figs. 17–5 and 17–6)

CHEST CT

(Fig. 17–7)

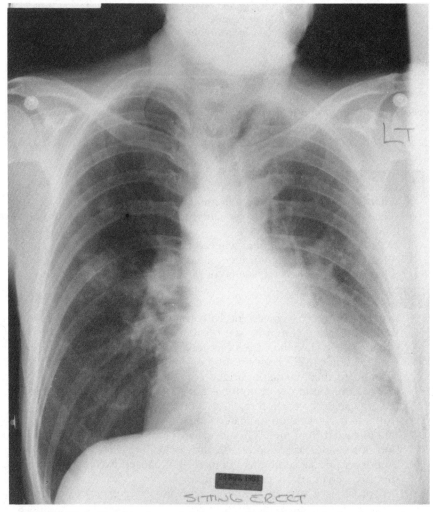

FIGURE 17–3 Chest radiograph taken the day before admission (emergency room visit) shows right lower lobe pneumonia with patchy infiltrate in the left lower lobe.

LABORATORY DATA

ABGs ON ROOM AIR

pH 7.38, Pa_{CO_2} 48 mm Hg, Pa_{O_2} 60 mm Hg, HCO_3^- 28 mEq/liter, Sa_{O_2} 94 percent.

ELECTROLYTES (See Appendix for normal values.)

Na^+ 144, K^+ 3.7, Cl^- 108, total CO_2^- 29, blood urea nitrogen (BUN) 20, creatinine 0.9

CBC (See Appendix for normal values.)

White blood cells 16,500/mm³, granulocytes 64 percent, bands 14 percent, lymphocytes 12 percent, monocytes 4 percent, eosinophils 2 percent, basophils 1 percent;

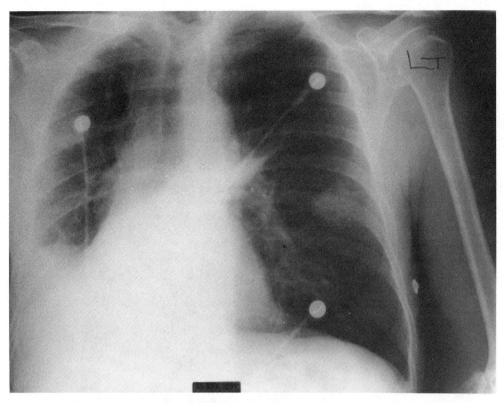

FIGURE 17–4 Chest radiograph (frontal view) demonstrates considerable atelectasis of the right middle and lower lobes with right pleural effusion due to obstruction of right bronchus intermedius. Evidence of bilateral metastatic disease most likely represents bronchogenic carcinoma. (Radiograph on day of admission.)

hemoglobin (Hb) 12.1 g/dL, platelets 415,000/mm^3; Ca^{++} 12.5 (8.5 to 10.5 mg/dL); liver function tests normal; lactate dehydrogenase 240 (100 to 190 IU/liter), total protein 5.2 (6 to 8 g/dL), albumin 3.0 (3.5 to 5.5 g/dL)

SPUTUM GRAM'S STAIN FOR CULTURE AND SENSITIVITIES

4+ polymorphonuclear neutrophils (pus), 3+ gram-negative rods, 1+ budding yeast with hyphae; epithelial cells less than 3 to 5/hpf

SPIROMETRIC STUDIES (2 MONTHS BEFORE THIS VISIT)

Prebronchodilator forced vital capacity (FVC) 3.4 (68 percent predicted), FEV$_1$ 1.7 liters (55 percent predicted) and FEV$_1$/FVC 50 percent; Postbronchodilator FVC 3.6 liters (72 percent); FEV$_1$ 1.9 liters (60 percent); FEV$_1$/FVC 53 percent.

Questions

10. Interpret the ABG values.
11. What do the chest radiographs tell you about this individual's pulmonary condition?

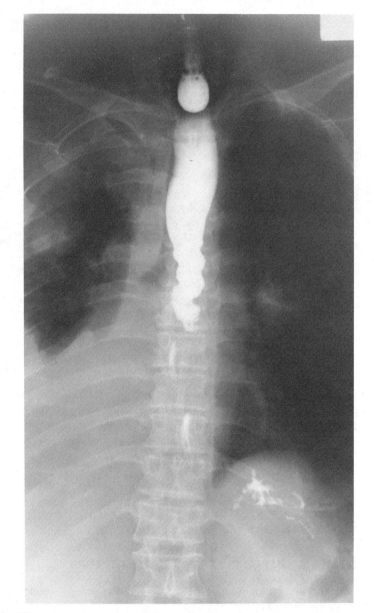

FIGURE 17–5 Frontal view of an esophagogram reveals high-grade obstruction of midesophagus, likely due to extensive mediastinal adenopathy or tumor invasion.

12. What did the CT scan and esophagogram add to the information provided by the chest radiograph?
13. What pulmonary abnormality do the pulmonary function data suggest in this patient?
14. What is the significance of the elevated serum calcium?
15. What evidence indicates pneumonia in this case?
16. What diagnostic procedure would be most appropriate at this time?
17. Should the patient be hospitalized?

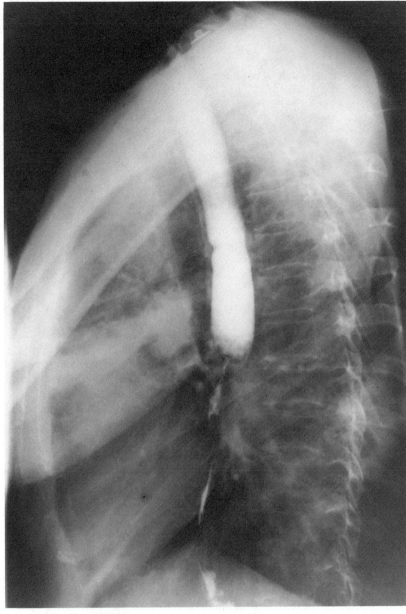

FIGURE 17–6 Lateral view of Figure 17–5.

10. The ABG is consistent with mild hypoxemia on room air. The acid-base status indicates compensated respiratory acidosis.
11. Comparison of the admission chest radiograph to that of the day before reveals a right bronchus intermedius obstruction, likely from tumor. There is also evidence of a cavitating metastasis to the left lung.
12. The CT scan of the chest demonstrates a mass in the right middle lobe and probable mediastinal and left lung metastases. Tumor appears to

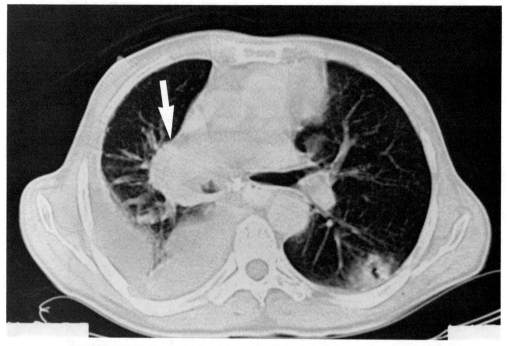

FIGURE 17–7 Computerized tomography of the chest shows a right hilar mass greater than 5 cm *(arrow)*. A cavitary metastatic lesion is seen in the posterior left lung. There is evidence of pretracheal lymphadenopathy with 2.5- to 3-cm lymph nodes. A moderate right pleural effusion is also visualized.

have involved the esophagus by esophagogram (Figs. 17–5 and 17–6), causing high-grade obstruction to food passage. Overall stage of cancer appears to be more advanced.

13. The pulmonary function data indicate moderate obstructive pulmonary disease. The mild decrease in lung volumes may be due to air trapping or tumor. The patient demonstrates minimal improvement with bronchodilator therapy.

14. The elevated serum calcium may be responsible for the patient's confusion and lethargy. Squamous cell carcinomas are the tumors most commonly associated with hypercalcemia.

15. Indicators of pneumonia in this patient are the elevated white blood cell count with increased band cells (left shift to earlier white cell forms produced in response to significant infection), fever, pulmonary opacification on chest radiograph, and sputum Gram's stain positive for pus cells with predominance of gram-negative rod organisms.

16. Bronchoscopy would quickly distinguish between a common pneumonia and a cancer partially obstructing a bronchus causing a postobstructive pneumonia. Not every patient with pneumonia needs bronchoscopy. In this patient with evidence of an obstructing lesion, weight loss, and a monophonic right lower lobe wheeze, bronchoscopy should have a high diagnostic yield for malignancy.

Sputum cytology is much less sensitive than bronchoscopy but may provide a specific tumor diagnosis with central airway lesions in up to 40 to 50 percent of the time.[14] It provides little information about the extent of tumor.

17. The patient should be hospitalized because of the presence of pneumonia, hypercalcemia, and symptoms suggesting lung cancer. The lung cancer alone would not require hospital admission but the combination of pneumonia and hypercalcemia requires IV drug therapy and close observation: antibiotics for the pneumonia and IV saline and furosemide (a diuretic to assist in urinary dumping of calcium) for the treatment of severe hypercalcemia. Staging of the cancer is necessary, as well as assessing the patency of the right bronchial airways. If an airway is found to be partially obstructed by a tumor, laser therapy may be useful to open the airway (laser fulguration).

The patient was given IV antibiotics for the pneumonia and IV saline plus furosemide (Lasix) for the hypercalcemia. Flexible fiberoptic bronchoscopy was performed after 2 days of therapy. Bronchoscopy showed tumor totally obstructing the right bronchus intermedius with mucosal spread to within 2 cm of the carina. The scope could not be passed beyond the lesion and the patient was deemed not to be a laser fulguration candidate. Specimens of the tumor demonstrated squamous cell carcinoma.

Questions

17. What is the TNM classification of this lung cancer, and what stage is this tumor? (See Tables 17–3, 17–4, 17–5, and 17–6 for the classification systems.)
18. Is this patient a surgical candidate?

Answers

17. The TNM classification is T4 (greater than 3 cm in diameter by chest CT, within 2 cm of carina, and involvement of esophagus); N2 (2 cm mediastinal lymphadenopathy); M1 (evidence of metastasis to contralateral lung). T4N2M1 = stage IIIB.
18. Surgical resection is not an option for stage IIIB lung cancer. Palliative therapy with radiation to shrink the tumor and reduce the symptoms of local and distant spread can be offered.

FOLLOW-UP

Two months after starting external-beam irradiation therapy to thorax and mediastinum, the patient returned to the emergency room for a sudden onset of massive hemoptysis. The patient coughed up about 800 mL of bright red blood over 30 minutes. He was taken to the operating room for emergency rigid bronchoscopy. The airway was cleared of blood, a large clot was removed from the right mainstem bronchus, and tamponade with packing was successful. The packing was removed after about 15 minutes, and there was no further bleeding. After recovery from bronchoscopy, he was sedated with morphine to prevent cough and transferred to the intensive care unit for observation. The patient enrolled in an outpatient hospice program. Six weeks later the patient developed postobstructive pneumonia (Fig. 17–8), was treated with oral antibiotics, and kept comfortable with supplemental oxygen and narcotics, but later expired at home from respiratory failure due to pneumonia and sepsis.

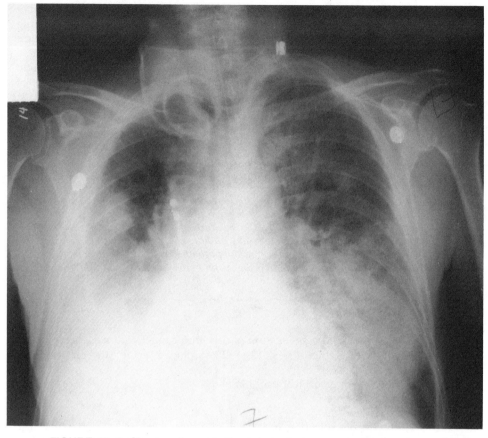

FIGURE 17–8 Chest radiograph (frontal view) shows pneumonia advanced to the left lower lobe with progressive postobstructive pneumonitis in the right lower and middle lobes.

REFERENCES

1. Silverberg, E and Lubera, JA: Cancer statistics. Cancer 39:3, 1989.

2. Khouri, NF, et al: The solitary pulmonary nodule: Assessment, diagnosis and management. Chest 91:128, 1987.

3. Filderman, AE, Shaw, C, and Matthay, RA: Bronchogenic carcinoma. In Brandstetter, RD (ed). Pulmonary Medicine. Medical Economics, Oradell, NJ, p 525, 1989.

4. Wynder, EL: The etiology, epidemiology and prevention of lung cancer. Semin Respir Med 3:135, 1982.

5. Hirayama, T: Passive smoking and lung cancer: Consistency of association. Lancet 2:1425, 1983.

6. Weiss, ST: Passive smoking and lung cancer. What is the risk? (editorial) Am Rev Respir Dis 133:1, 1986.

7. Cothern, CR: Indoor air radon. Rev Environ Contam Toxicol 111:1, 1990.

8. Warnock, M and Churg, A: Association of asbestos and bronchogenic carcinoma in a population with low asbestos exposure. Cancer 35:1236, 1975.

9. Hammond, EC, Selikoff, IJ, and Seidman, H: Asbestos exposure, cigarette smoking, and death rates. Ann NY Acad Sci 330:473, 1979.

10. Samet, JM, Humble, CG, and Pathak, DR: Personal and family history of respiratory disease and lung cancer risk. Am Rev Respir Dis 134:466, 1986.

11. Brincker, H and Wilbek, E: The incidence of malignant tumors in patients with sarcoidosis. Br J Cancer 29:247, 1974.

12. Buzaid, AC and Murren, JR: A progress report: Treating lung cancer. Contemp Int Med Sept. 1990, pp 78–90.

13. Doyle, LA and Aisner, J: Clinical presentation of lung cancer. In Roth, JA, Ruckdeschel, JC and Weisenburger, TH (eds): Thoracic Oncology. WB Saunders, Philadelphia, 1989, p 53.

14. Pancoast, HK: Superior pulmonary sulcus tumor; tumor characterized by pain, Horner's syndrome, destruction of bone, and atrophy of hand muscles. JAMA 99:1391, 1931.

15. Frost, JK, et al: Early lung cancer detection: Results of the initial (prevalence) radiologic and cytologic screening in the Johns Hopkins study. Am Rev Respir Dis 130:549, 1984.

16. Martini, N, Zaman, MB, and Melamed, M: Early diagnosis of carcinoma of the lung. In Roth, JA, Ruckdeschel, JC, and Weisenburger, TH (eds). Thoracic Oncology. WB Saunders, Philadelphia, 1989, pp 133–141.

17. Wang, KP and Terry, PB: Transbronchial needle aspiration in the diagnosis and staging of bronchogenic carcinoma. Am Rev Respir Dis 127:344, 1983.

18. Lillington, GA: Management of solitary pulmonary nodules. Dis Mon, May, 1991, Mosby Year Book, St Louis, pp 271–318.

19. Koss, LG: Diagnostic Cytology, ed 3. JB Lippincott, Philadelphia, 1979, pp 534–606.

20. Chaffey, MH: The role of percutaneous lung biopsy in the work up of a solitary pulmonary nodule. West J Med 148:176, 1988.

21. Fletcher, EC and Levin, DC: Flexible fiberoptic bronchoscopy and fluoroscopically guided transbronchial biopsy in the management of solitary pulmonary nodules. West J Med 136:477, 1982.

22. Menzies, R, and Charbonneau, M: Thoracoscopy for the diagnosis of pleural disease. Ann Int Med 114:271, 1991.

23. Bruderman, I: Bronchogenic carcinoma. In Baum, GL and Wolinsky, E (eds): Textbook of Pulmonary Diseases, ed 4. Little, Brown, Boston, 1989, pp 1197–1237.

24. Carr, DT and Holoye, PY: Bronchogenic carcinoma. In Murray, JF and Nadel, JA (eds). Textbook of Respiratory Medicine. WB Saunders, Philadelphia, 1988, pp 1174–1250.

25. Faber, LP: Lung cancer. In Holleb, AI, Fink, DJ, and Murphy, GP (eds). American Cancer Society Textbook of Clinical Oncology. American Cancer Society, Atlanta, 1991, p 194.

26. Morice, RC, et al: Exercise testing in the evaluation of patients at high risk for complications from lung resection. Chest 101:356, 1992.

27. Olsen, GN: Preoperative physiology and lung resection: Scan? Exercise? Both? (editorial) Chest 101:300, 1992.

28. Cummings, SR, Lillington, GA, and Richard, RJ: Estimating the probability of malignancy in solitary pulmonary nodules. Am Rev Respir Dis 134:449, 1986.

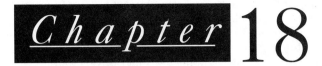

Chapter 18

Robert L. Wilkins, MA, RRT

James R. Dexter, MD, FCCP

SLEEP APNEA

INTRODUCTION

Sleep apnea is repeated pauses in breathing, or apneas, during sleep. Because short pauses in breathing are normal during sleep, true clinical sleep apnea is defined as a lack of breathing for at least 10 seconds that occurs more than 30 times in 7 hours of sleep.[1] Some experts use the apnea index to determine if sleep apnea is present. The apnea index is a measurement of the number of apnea episodes per hour of sleep. An apnea index of 5 or more is a diagnostic criterion for the presence of sleep apnea. The apnea index also provides an indication for the degree of sleep apnea; 5 to 20 apneas per hour of sleep indicates mild sleep apnea; 21 to 40 per hour indicates moderate sleep apnea; and more than 40 per hour indicates severe sleep apnea. Other indications for the severity of sleep apnea include the degree of clinical symptoms such as excessive daytime sleepiness.

There are three different types of sleep apnea. **Obstructive sleep apnea (OSA)** is present when the drive to breathe is intact but the upper airway intermittently becomes obstructed during sleep. Once the upper airway is obstructed, the respiratory muscles try harder and harder to move air. Eventually the patient partially awakens and clears his or her airway, and ventilation resumes. **Central sleep apnea** indicates that the drive to breathe is absent intermittently during sleep. As the patient's effort to breathe stops, the muscles of breathing fail to contract and airflow into the lungs ceases. **Mixed apnea** is present when the patient has both obstructive and central sleep apnea episodes during sleep. This chapter emphasizes OSA, as it dominates the clinical picture.

In addition to apneas, individuals with abnormal respiratory activity during sleep can have **hypopneas**. Hypopneas are similar to apneas; however, they represent a discrete episode of hypoventilation during sleep in which the arterial oxygen saturation (Sao_2) drops significantly. With hypopneas, ventilation continues but the quantity is not enough to meet the metabolic needs of the body. The respiratory disturbance index is the number of apneas plus the number of hypopneas per hour of sleep. A respiratory disturbance index greater than 10 is abnormal.[1]

To measure objectively the problems occuring during sleep, the patient is typically monitored in a sleep center. At the sleep center the patient sleeps in a laboratory where breathing, pulse oximetry, eye movements, electroencephalogram (EEG), electrocardiogram (ECG), and leg movements are monitored. Throughout the night of sleep a recording of all parameters is made and the patient is observed by a sleep technician. The recording is made by a polygraph machine (multichannel recorder) and the resulting printout is called a **polysomnogram**.

The multiple sleep latency test (MSLT) identifies the degree of daytime sleepiness (hypersomnolence). This test is performed during the day by asking the rested patient to nap in a quiet darkened room every 2 hours five times throughout normal waking hours. The patient is allowed to sleep only about 10 to 20 minutes if he or she should fall asleep. During the brief period of sleep or rest the patient is monitored by similar parameters used to record night-time sleep. The amount of time from when the patient reclines in bed to when sleep occurs is a measurement of **sleep latency**. A daytime sleep latency of less than 5 minutes is abnormal and indicates that excessive daytime somnolence is present. Two common causes of excessive daytime sleepiness are sleep apnea and narcolepsy.[1]

SLEEP AND BREATHING

To understand sleep-related breathing disorders, it is helpful to appreciate normal sleep physiology. Normal sleep comes in two types: nonrapid eye movement (NREM) and rapid eye movement (REM). NREM sleep consists of four stages that represent progressively deeper sleep. A combination of EEG tracings and sleep behavior distinguishes the two types of sleep and the different stages of NREM sleep.

The normal sleeper enters stage 1 NREM sleep upon becoming drowsy (Fig. 18–1). This represents the lightest level of sleep. During stage 1 sleep the individual is easily arousable and, in fact, often alternates between being awake and being in stage 1 sleep. After a short time (normally 5 to 7 minutes) of stage 1 sleep, the normal sleeper slips into stage 2 sleep, which is characterized by EEG evidence of sleep spindles and K complexes (Fig. 18–2). The deepest stages of sleep that follow are known as **delta** or **slow-wave** sleep (stages 3 and 4). The EEG high-amplitude delta waves characteristic of slow-wave sleep signify the deepest level of sleep, from which the patient is difficult to arouse.

After approximately 90 minutes of NREM sleep, the normal sleeper enters REM sleep.[2] REM sleep, also called active sleep, is the sleep stage in which the sleeper probably experiences dreaming. REM sleep is characterized by increased cerebral activity as noted on the EEG recording and by a general increase in autonomic activity (Fig. 18–3). Heart rate, blood pressure, and respiratory rate may vary significantly during REM sleep because of the physiologic changes in the body associated with the onset of this stage of sleep. REM sleep typically continues for

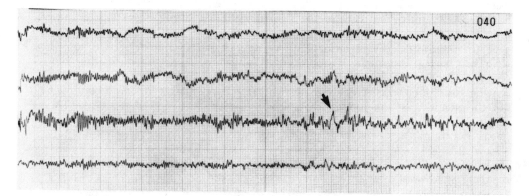

FIGURE 18–1 Electroencephalogram (EEG) tracing (lines 3 and 4) of a patient during sleep, demonstrating the onset of stage I sleep (*arrow*).

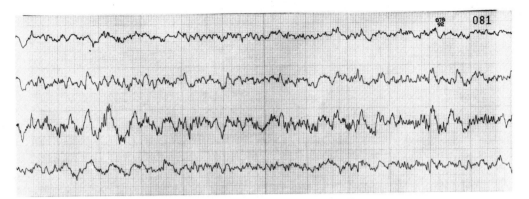

FIGURE 18–2 EEG tracing (lines 3 and 4) demonstrating stage II sleep.

10 to 20 minutes, after which NREM sleep returns. The normal adult sleeper alternates between NREM and REM sleep about every 90 minutes throughout the night, experiencing four to five REM episodes each night.

REM and NREM sleep both cause significant changes in breathing, even in individuals without disease.[3,4] Typically the individual in NREM sleep develops irregular breathing during the lighter stages of sleep (stages 1 and 2) similar to Cheyne-Stokes respiration. This is due to the decrease in respiratory drive associated with the loss of the stimulatory effect of wakefulness and decreased metabolic rate associated with sleep.[3-5] As the deeper stages of NREM sleep occur, the metabolic respiratory control system regulates breathing, and overall respiratory drive is more stable. As a result, breathing is typically very regular during delta sleep; however, overall ventilation is reduced compared with that during wakefulness. Specifically, minute ventilation is 1 to 2 liters/minute lower, Pao_2 5 to 10 mm Hg lower, and $Paco_2$ 2 to 8 mm Hg higher during NREM deep sleep.[5]

During REM sleep the respiratory drive is irregular owing to the transient decrease in ventilatory response to chemical and mechanical stimuli. As a result, short apneas of 15 seconds or less are common in normal sleepers during REM sleep.[5]

REM and NREM sleep cause a general decrease in the tone of the skeletal muscles throughout the body. This decrease in muscle tone is believed to affect

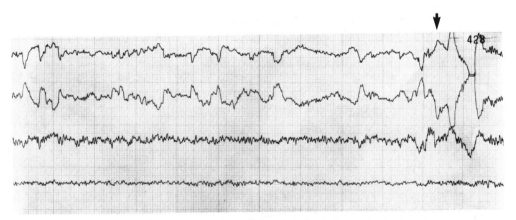

FIGURE 18–3 Electrooculogram (EOG) tracing of the left and right eyes (lines 1 and 2), demonstrating the onset of rapid eye movement (REM) sleep (*arrow*).

A

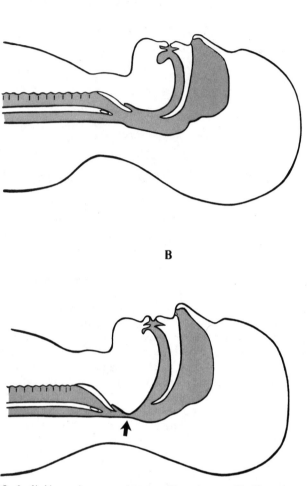

B

FIGURE 18–4 *A)* Normal upper airway with patency. *B)* Obstructed upper airway typical for the patient with obstructive sleep apnea (OSA) (*arrow*).

the accessory muscles of breathing and may contribute to the decreases in ventilation seen during certain stages of sleep.[5] In addition, the influence of sleep on the upper airway is similar and typically results in a general loss of muscle tone and an increase in airway resistance with onset of deep NREM or REM sleep (Fig. 18–4). In most sleepers these physiologic changes are not significant and go unnoticed. In others, however, the onset of sleep marks the beginning of sleep-related breathing problems.

ETIOLOGY

Precipitating factors associated with OSA include obesity, macroglossia (enlarged tongue), micrognathia (a small lower jaw), or enlarged tonsils. Those with anatomic defects of the upper airway represent a minority of the patients with OSA. Most experts consider obesity to be a major contributing factor of OSA.

Ironically deep sleep plays a key role in the onset of OSA. As the patient enters deeper stages of NREM sleep or REM sleep, the muscles of the upper airway tend to relax and allow the surrounding tissues to block the airway (Fig. 18–4). As the patient with OSA generates an inspiratory effort during sleep, the subatmospheric pharyngeal pressure creates enough vacuum to overcome the forces maintaining airway stability. This causes the upper airway to occlude and the onset of apnea despite continued efforts to breathe.

PATHOPHYSIOLOGY

The effects of sleep apnea on gas exchange follow a predictable pattern. With the onset of apnea, the Pao_2 begins to fall while the $Paco_2$ rises. The degree of hypoxemia and hypercapnia is primarily a result of the length of the apneic episode although the baseline blood gas values before the onset of apnea are also important.

The hypoxemia and hypercapnia eventually arouse the patient from a deeper stage of sleep to a lighter stage. This arousal causes the muscle tone of the upper airway to return and allows airflow to resume. Once ventilation resumes, the arousal response diminishes and the patient returns to a deeper stage of sleep. This allows the entire cycle to begin again and it may literally repeat itself hundreds of times each night. As a result, sleep is very fragmented and the deeper periods of sleep are minimal or absent.[2] The patient awakes the next morning feeling unrefreshed and exhausted despite not being able to recall any arousals during the night.

The repeated episodes of significant hypoxemia during sleep typically result in dramatic changes in the patient's hemodynamic system.[2] With the onset of hypoxemia, bradycardia typically occurs. The bradycardia is vagally mediated and proportional to the degree of hypoxemia. Bradycardia is somewhat beneficial because it reduces myocardial oxygen consumption during a period of significant hypoxemia.[2] Once breathing resumes, the patient will experience tachycardia as the vagal parasympathetic tone is diminished and sympathetic neural activity increases in response to the hypoxia.

Systemic and pulmonary artery blood pressure tends to rise during apneic episodes. The magnitude of hypertension appears to be related to the degree of oxyhemoglobin desaturation seen during apnea. Systemic and pulmonary blood pressure typically decreases back to baseline values soon after ventilation resumes. Only a minority (10 to 15 percent) of patients with OSA go on to develop sustained pulmonary hypertension and right heart failure. Although the cause-and-effect relationship between OSA and sustained systemic hypertension is not clear, 60 percent of OSA patients have hypertension.[5]

In addition to fluctuations in heart rate, other dysrythmias have been documented in patients with OSA. Sinus pauses, premature ventricular contractions, heart block, and ventricular tachycardia have been seen in OSA patients during sleep. These dysrythmias are believed to be primarily related to the onset of significant hypoxemia. Dysrythmias may be responsible for sudden death in patients with OSA.[2]

CLINICAL FEATURES

Medical History

Patients with OSA commonly complain of excessive daytime fatigue and sleepiness.[1,2,6] Initially the patient with hypersomnolence may fall asleep only during any quiet functions such as reading or watching television. As the condition worsens, the excessive sleepiness may encroach upon the majority of daytime activities (e.g., conversation, driving, eating) and can be a serious problem. The daytime hypersomnolence is probably the result of sleep fragmentation associated with numerous arousals from apneic episodes during sleep. When the sleep apena is severe, the excessive daytime sleepiness is a constant problem; however, in milder cases patients often report fluctuations in the degree of daytime fatigue.[2]

The fluctuation in symptoms seen in milder cases of OSA sometimes relates to the amount of time the patient spends sleeping in the supine versus the lateral position. For most patients the upper airway obstruction is more significant in the supine position. As a result, when the patient sleeps primarily in the supine position, symptoms of excessive fatigue increase; sleeping primarily in the lateral position may result in fewer daytime symptoms.[2,7,8]

Other daytime symptoms associated with OSA include memory loss, morning headache, decreased ability to concentrate, and personality changes.[1] Because of the decrease in mental function and increase in daytime sleepiness, patients with severe sleep apnea often have trouble performing routine daily functions. Patients with OSA often perform poorly at work and may even fall asleep while driving and have automobile accidents.

Loud snoring is a very common finding in patients with OSA. Typically, it is the bed partner who complains about the loud snoring. The snoring may be of such magnitude that the patient's spouse retreats to another room in the house to get some sleep. The bed partner often notices that the loud snoring is accompanied by pauses in breathing that end with a particular snorting gasp. In addition to the snoring, patients with sleep apnea may complain of other night-time symptoms such as enuresis (bedwetting), leg jerks, cardiac palpitations, and impotence.[1]

Physical Examination and Laboratory Data

Physical examination of the patient with OSA typically reveals an obese man with a short, thick neck. In those who are not obese, anatomic defects of the upper airway may be present. Such defects of the upper airway that predispose the patient to OSA include micrognathia, macroglossia, and adenotonsillar hypertrophy. If the sleep apnea is severe and has been occurring for many months or years, the signs of cor pulmonale (jugular venous distension [JVD], hepatomegaly, loud P_2) may be present. Otherwise, the physical examination is usually unremarkable.

Some patients with obstructive sleep apnea who are markedly obese may be labeled as having pickwickian syndrome, or obesity hypoventilation syndrome. In addition to the severe obesity, the patient with this syndrome usually has chronic hypoxemia and hypercapnia and signs of right heart failure. The term "pickwickian syndrome" is not popular today because it is not clinically useful.

Laboratory evaluation of the patient with sleep apnea is not usually helpful in making the diagnosis. Routine pulmonary function studies do not show specific abnormalities; however, flow volume loops may show variable extrathoracic airway obstruction.[9] The daytime blood gas studies are not helpful and often are normal unless an underlying lung disease is also present. Daytime ECG studies may be normal or demonstrate signs of cor pulmonale (e.g., large P waves and right-axis deviation) when a severe case occurs.

Clinical Polysomnography

The definitive diagnostic test for sleep apnea is the polysomnogram. This all-night recording of the patient's sleep is the "gold standard" for identifying the type, severity, and consequences of sleep apnea, when present. In addition, once the diagnosis is made and treatment implemented, the polysomnogram is helpful to identify the effects of treatment.

In patients with OSA the polysomnogram typically demonstrates frequent episodes of apnea in which the patient's effort of breathing continues while airflow through the nose and mouth stops. Each individual episode of apnea may last as long as 2 minutes but typically averages from 20 to 30 seconds.[2] Hypoxemia occurs during the period of apnea and is demonstrated on the pulse oximetry recording. Patients with coexisting lung disease typically start with some degree of hypoxemia before the onset of apnea and may experience severe hypoxemia as the result of even short episodes of apnea. The ECG monitoring typically reveals bradycardia during each apneic episode, with rebound tachycardia occurring immediately upon the end of the period of apnea. EEG monitoring shows sleep fragmentation with a reduced amount of delta sleep and delayed onset of REM sleep.

TREATMENT

The approach to treatment of patients with OSA depends on the severity of clinical symptoms (such as excessive daytime sleepiness) and severity of hypoxemia. Those with minimal daytime sleepiness and no signs of heart failure are considered to have mild disease. Those with moderate OSA often have more persistent sleepiness and may fall asleep performing many routine daytime functions. Severe OSA is present when daytime hypersomnolence results in potentially life-threatening events (such as automobile accidents) and is so severe that the patient cannot perform his or her job effectively. The patient with severe disease often has signs of heart failure.

For all patients with OSA, regardless of its severity, a few general rules apply. Avoiding alcohol, sleeping pills, and sedatives can be helpful, as their use can worsen OSA. Weight loss can result in significant reduction in the severity of the disease in those patients who are obese.[10-13] Although the exact amount of weight loss or percent of body fat needed for improvement is not known, a 20 percent decrease in weight often substantially improves the patient's symptoms. In addition, having the patient sleep on his or her side instead of supine can be effective in reducing daytime symptoms. This change in sleep position is a simple way to reduce the number of episodes of apneas and hypopneas in NREM sleep.[10]

For most patients with mild OSA the combination of weight loss and avoidance of alcohol and sedatives will be adequate. If the patient cannot lose weight, the attending physician may choose to initiate a low dose of protriptyline (10 to 30 mg) to be taken at bedtime.[10] Protriptyline is a nonsedating tricyclic antidepressant that may benefit patients with OSA.[14] Experts believe that protriptyline suppresses REM sleep and thereby reduces the period of time in which apneas are most severe. Other researchers have suggested that this medication increases the muscle tone of the upper airway.[15-16]

For patients with moderate to severe OSA, a trial of continuous positive airway pressure (CPAP) therapy may be indicated. CPAP acts by creating a "pneumatic splint" within the upper airway and thus maintains patency throughout the respiratory cycle. The level of pressure needed to prevent obstruction and apnea during sleep varies from patient to patient and must be determined by nocturnal oxygen saturation monitoring. CPAP is an effective therapy with few side effects, which can be administered by nasal mask. It has become one of the mainstays of therapy for the patient with moderate to severe OSA.[10]

In the surgical approach to OSA treatment the obstruction can be bypassed or the upper airway widened. Bypassing the obstruction, accomplished by tracheostomy, is very effective therapy. Tracheostomy is typically not popular with the patient but may be lifesaving in those with severe OSA when other treatments fail.[17] Nasal or oropharyngeal surgery may be indicated when these sites are identified as the location of obstruction and when removing excess tissue is feasible. In pediatric patients with OSA, removal of enlarged tonsils and adenoids increases airway size and is often effective.[10]

Case Study

HISTORY

Mr. L is a 47-year-old white man employed as a high school principal. Mr. L was seen in the outpatient clinic by his primary care physician because of excessive daytime sleepiness. He has had increasing problems over the past 6 months with daytime sleepiness, poor memory, and inability to concentrate. He often falls asleep while reading reports at work and while watching television at home. Within the past month he has been falling asleep while eating or during conferences with coworkers. Two weeks earlier, Mr. L was involved in a minor automobile accident in which he had fallen asleep while driving and ran off the road.

Mr. L's past medical history was noncontributory except for a tonsillectomy at age 6. He has no history of lung disease and denied problems with coughing, sputum, shortness of breath, orthopnea, or hemoptysis. Mr. L reported using alcohol two to three times per week and has smoked two packs of cigarettes per day for the past 25 years.

Questions

1. What could be causing the symptoms of daytime sleepiness, memory loss, and lack of concentration?
2. What other symptom should the physician explore during the initial interview?
3. What signs should the physician identify during the physical examination?
4. Is there a connection between Mr. L's use of alcohol and tobacco and his symptoms? If so, what is the connection and what should Mr. L be advised to do?
5. What simple techniques could the primary care physician suggest to Mr. L that might reduce his symptoms?
6. Does Mr. L require referral for objective evaluation of his condition?

Answers

1. Clinical depression or OSA could cause the symptoms of daytime sleepiness, lack of concentration, and memory loss. The automobile accident would be unusual as an event related to depression-related fatigue and is often seen in patients with OSA.[18] The physician should advise the patient to stop driving until the excessive daytime sleepiness resolves with treatment.[19]
2. The physician should ask the patient and his wife about Mr. L's snoring. Mr. L's wife would probably be the best source of information regarding the intensity of his snoring and the presence of pauses or snorts in breathing during sleep.
3. The physician should examine Mr. L for factors that may be contributing to upper airway obstruction (e.g., nasal polyps, obesity, neck size, large tongue) and for signs of heart failure. Evidence of heart failure would suggest that a more severe case of OSA is present if this tentative diagnosis proves accurate. The physical examination should also identify whether evidence of chronic lung disease is present in view of the patient's smoking history.
4. There probably is a connection between Mr. L's use of alcohol and his symptoms. Alcohol is known to worsen OSA and increases the patient's symptoms.

   There is no evidence that the use of tobacco increases the severity of symptoms in OSA; however, patients with chronic lung disease who also have OSA are prone to more severe hypoxemia during periods of apnea. The more severe hypoxemia relates to the fact that these patients have some hypoxemia before apnea occurs, and once breathing stops profound hypoxemia occurs more rapidly.

5. The primary care physician could recommend that Mr. L stop the consumption of alcohol, lose weight (if he is obese), sleep on his side or prone, and avoid the use of sleeping pills. Although these suggestions may not completely relieve Mr. L's symptoms, they may markedly improve his condition.

6. Mr. L's attending physician should refer him to a sleep center where a polysomnogram could be done to monitor his breathing during sleep.

PHYSICAL EXAMINATION

General — *Patient is alert and oriented but appears fatigued and sleepy. He is not in apparent distress. Mr. L is 5 feet 11 inches in height and weighs 225 lb.*

Vital Signs — *Temperature 36.9°C, pulse at rest 84/minute, respiratory rate 20/minute, and blood pressure 138/85 mm Hg*

HEENT — *No evidence of nasal obstruction, sinuses not tender or congested; pupils round, equal, and reactive to light*

Neck — *Supple, short, diameter of 19 inches; trachea midline; no stridor; carotid pulses ++ bilaterally with no bruits; no evidence of lymphadenopathy or thyromegaly; mild JVD with the head of the bed elevated to 20 degrees; no use of accessory muscles with breathing*

Chest — *Normal anteroposterior (AP) diameter with no use of accessory muscles at rest; no evidence of retractions or bulging with breathing*

Heart — *Regular rhythm with no evidence of murmurs or rubs; no heaves or abnormal pulsations noted over precordium*

Lungs — *Breath sounds slightly diminished bilaterally with no adventitious lung sounds; no abnormalities noted with percussion over the lungs*

Abdomen — *Soft, nontender, with marked obesity; normal bowel sounds present and no organomegaly identified*

Extremities — *No clubbing, edema, or cyanosis; capillary refill normal*

Questions

7. What is the most significant finding identified during the physical examination that may be contributing to Mr. L's problem?

8. Does the physical examination provide any evidence regarding the presence of lung disease?

9. What could explain the presence of mild JVD?

10. If OSA is causing Mr. L's problems, should the physical examination be more remarkable?

Answers

7. The most significant finding during the physical examination is the presence of obesity with a short, thick neck. Obesity appears to be the most common factor contributing to OSA.

8. The diminished breath sounds bilaterally may be the result of chronic obstructive pulmonary disease (COPD). It is also possible that obesity is making it more difficult to hear the breath sounds. Because Mr. L is a smoker, pulmonary function testing and a chest radiograph would be prudent to follow-up on the examination.

9. Some patients with OSA develop JVD because of the frequent episodes of hypoxemia that occur during sleep. The pulmonary hypertension causes the right ventricle to fail and leads to a backup of blood into the venous system, which is seen as JVD. Because Mr. L is a smoker, it is also possible that he has developed chronic lung disease with hypoxemia. This could lead to chronic right heart failure and JVD.

10. It is not uncommon for patients with OSA to have unremarkable findings during the physical examination. Only with very severe cases will complications such as heart failure cause significant findings during the examination.

At the conclusion of the physical examination the primary care physician referred Mr. L to a sleep laboratory for a polysomnogram. Fortunately for Mr. L, a nearby university hospital maintains a sleep disorders center.

At the sleep laboratory a pulmonologist interviewed and examined the patient. The pulmonologist agreed with the primary care physician's tentative diagnosis of sleep apnea and arranged for an all-night sleep study. During the interview it was identified that Mr. L has been a habitual snorer during sleep for many years. His wife stated that the snoring had gotten worse recently and she often slept in another room although she could hear her husband's snoring all over the house. She also had noted pauses in her husband's breathing but had never timed the pauses. She felt that the pauses were no more than 1 minute in length.

At the conclusion of the interview the purpose of and procedures for the sleep study were explained to Mr. L and his wife. They were given a brief tour of the facilities and advised to return later that evening for the sleep study. Mr. L returned to the sleep laboratory at 2110 hours and was put to bed at about 2300 hours. Mr. L had no trouble falling asleep in the laboratory and slept until 0530 the next day. The results of the sleep study follow:

Sleep Latency	*8 minutes*
Total Time in Bed	*381 minutes*
Sleep Efficiency	*85 percent*
Sleep Continuity	*23 awakenings; 56 minutes of wake time and 261 EEG arousals; which corresponded to an arousal index of 49*
Sleep Distribution	*Stage 1: 9 percent; stage 2: 69 percent; slow-wave sleep 2 percent; REM 5 percent; REM latency 213.5 minutes*
Apnea Indices	*Apnea plus hypopnea index 27; obstructive apnea index 19.5; central apnea index 9.9.*

Oxygen Parameters	*Baseline levels of Sao$_2$ 90 percent; minimal Sao$_2$ during test 69 percent; number of periods below 85 percent 33.*
Leg Movements	*Number of leg movements 148; 83 percent of leg movements resulting in EEG arousals; leg movement index 28.*
Cardiovascular Parameters	*The patient had 114 cardiac rhythm abnormalities during the recording including unifocal premature ventricular contractions (PVCs)*
Additional Findings	*Loud snoring throughout the night*

Questions

11. How do you interpret the following test results:
    (a) Sleep latency
    (b) Sleep efficiency
    (c) Sleep distribution
    (d) Apnea indexes
    (e) Oxygen parameters
    (f) Leg movements
    (g) Cardiovascular parameters
12. What is the probable cause of Mr. L's symptoms?
13. What recommendations should be made to the patient regarding treatment?

Answers

11. (a) The sleep latency is in the normal range. Normal values for nighttime sleep latency are less than 30 minutes.
    (b) Sleep efficiency is abnormally low. Normal is greater than 90 percent.
    (c) Sleep distribution is abnormal in this case. Normally stage 2 sleep represents 50 percent of sleep and slow-wave sleep 5 to 10 percent. REM latency is normally around 90 minutes. In this case the REM latency of 213.5 minutes represents a significant delay in the onset of REM sleep. This abnormal distribution of sleep is consistent with someone who has numerous interruptions in sleep during the night.
    (d) The apnea plus hypopnea index of 27 indicates that the patient averages 27 episodes per hour of abnormal ventilation during sleep. The obstructive apnea index of 19.5 suggests that of the 27 abnormal ventilation episodes each hour, about 20 of them are due to obstructive apnea. Figure 18–5 demonstrates an example of the patient's obstructive apnea. The remaining seven abnormal ventilatory periods each hour represent inadequate ventilation that may or may not be the result of upper airway obstruction. The central apnea index of 0.9 suggests that occasionally Mr. L experiences apnea resulting from a lack of ventilatory drive (Fig. 18–6). This is not uncommon in normal sleepers and often is present when obstructive sleep apnea is present.
    (e) The baseline Sao$_2$ of 90 percent represents a mild reduction in oxygenation while awake. The minimal Sao$_2$ value of 69 percent suggests that the patient experiences significant hypoxemia during sleep. An Sao$_2$ of 69 percent would correspond to a Pao$_2$ of less

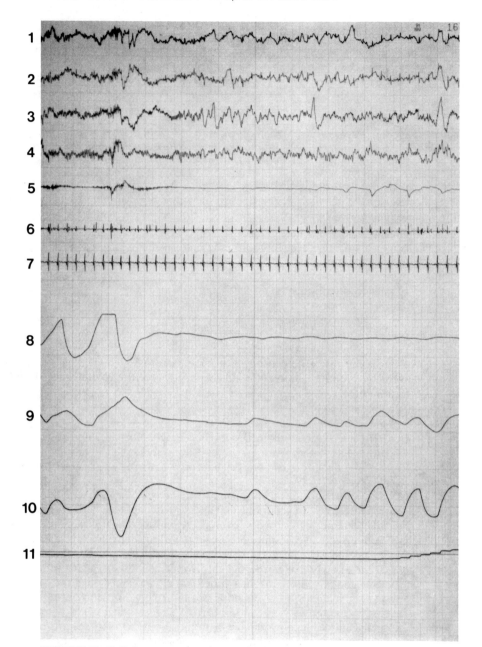

FIGURE 18–5 Polysomnogram demonstrating periods of apnea with persistent effort of breathing typical for OSA. Lines 1 and 2 = EOG of the left and right eyes; lines 3 and 4 = EEG tracings; line 5 = chin EMG; line 6 = leg EMG; line 7 = electrocardiogram (ECG); line 8 = flow at the nose or mouth; line 9 = upper chest; line 10 = lower chest; and line 11 = Sao_2. Note the onset of apnea seen as a lack of flow (line 8) with continued effort to breathe (lines 9 and 10).

than 40 mm Hg. The patient had 33 episodes of hypoxemia through-out the night.

(f) The leg movement monitoring demonstrates that the patient aver-aged 28 leg jerks per hour and experienced a total of 148 through-out the night. The majority (83 percent) of the leg jerks resulted

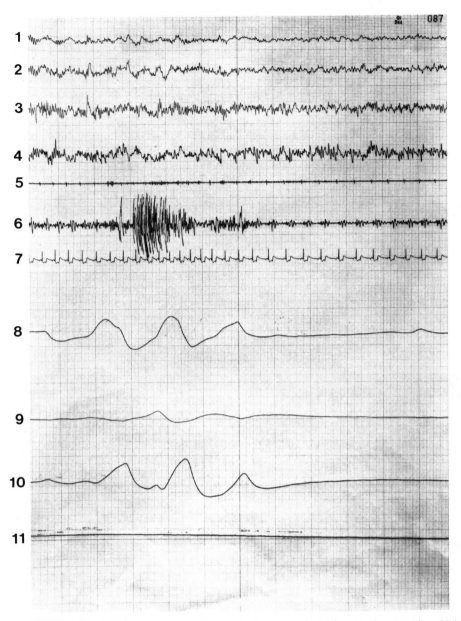

FIGURE 18–6 Polysomnogram demonstrating a period of central apnea in which the drive to breathe is temporarily absent. Note the lack of flow (line 8) and the lack of upper and lower chest movement (lines 9 and 10). Note leg jerks seen in line 6.

EEG arousal. This suggests that the leg jerks are contributing to Mr. L's sleep fragmentation and daytime sleepiness.

(g) The numerous episodes of hypoxemia are causing abnormal cardiac function during sleep. Changes in heart rate and unifocal PVCs are common when the patient is hypoxic.

12. Mr. L's symptoms of excessive daytime sleepiness are probably the result of sleep fragmentation, which in this case is caused by OSA and leg jerks. These two factors are combining to arouse Mr. L from a deeper stage of sleep to a lighter stage frequently throughout the night. As a result, Mr.

L has a delayed onset of REM sleep and very little slow-wave sleep. Because REM and slow-wave sleep promote refreshment and recovery, diminishing the time spent in these stages results in excessive daytime sleepiness and fatigue.

13. Treatment should include techniques for resolving the OSA and identifying the cause of the leg jerks. Mr. L should be put on a diet to lose weight and a trial of nasal CPAP during sleep would be reasonable. Mr. L should be advised to give up alcohol because this can contribute to the problem. The possible causes of leg jerks are not clear; however, diabetes has been shown to be a contributing factor in some patients. For this reason, Mr. L's attending physician should order tests to screen Mr. L for diabetes.

FOLLOW-UP

A diet plan was arranged for Mr. L. Nasal CPAP of 7 cm H_2O was successful in significantly reducing the number of apneas and hypopneas. Mr. L tolerated the nasal CPAP well and arrangements were made for Mr. L to use CPAP at home. The screening test for diabetes was positive and Mr. L responded well to the treatment, which included diet changes and daily insulin. When Mr. L visited his attending physician 1 month after the initiation of treatment, his symptoms were significantly improved.

REFERENCES

1. Romaker, AM and Ancoli-Israel, S: The diagnosis of sleep-related breathing disorders. Clin Chest Med 8:105, 1987.

2. Shepard, JW: Physiologic and clinical consequences of sleep apnea: In White, DP (ed): Disorders of Breathing During Sleep: Semin Respir Med 9:560, 1988.

3. White, DP: Disorders of breathing during sleep: Introduction, epidemiology, and incidence: In White, DP (ed): Disorders of Breathing During Sleep: Semin Respir Med 9:529, 1988.

4. Krieger, J: Breathing during sleep in normal subjects. Clin Chest Med 6:577, 1985.

5. Phillipson, EA: Sleep disorders: In Murray, JF and Nadel, JA: Textbook of Respiratory Medicine. WB Saunders, Philadelphia, 1988, pp 1841–1860.

6. Orr, WC: Sleep-related breathing disorders. Chest 84:475, 1983.

7. McEvoy, RD, Sharp, DJ, and Thronton, AT: The effects of posture on obstructive sleep apnea. Am Rev Respir Dis 133:662, 1986.

8. Phillips, BA, et al: Effect of sleep position on sleep apnea and parafunctional activity. Chest 90:424, 1986.

9. Smith, PL: Evaluation of patients with sleep disorders. Semin Respir Med 9:534, 1988.

10. George, C and Kryger, M: Management of sleep apnea. Semin Respir Med 9:569, 1988.

11. Browman, CP, Sampson, MG, and Yolles, SF: Obstructive sleep apnea and body weight. Chest 85:435, 1984.

12. Harman, EM, Wynne, JW, and Block, AJ: The effect of weight loss on sleep-disordered breathing and oxygen desaturation in morbidly obese men. Chest 82:291, 1982.

13. Smith, PL, et al: Weight loss in mildly to moderately obese patients with obstructive sleep apnea. Ann Intern Med 103:850, 1985.

14. Brownell, LG, West, P, and Sweatman, P: Protriptyline in obstructive sleep apnea. N Engl J Med 307:1037, 1982.

15.   Smith, PL, Haponik, EF, and Allen, RP: The effect of protriptyline on sleep disordered breathing. Am Rev Respir Dis 127:8, 1983.

16.   Bonora, M, St. John, WM, and Bledsoe, TA: Differential elevation by protriptyline and depression by diazepam of upper respiratory motor neuron activity. Am Rev Respir Dis 131:41, 1985.

17.   Partinen, M, Jamieson, A, and Guilleminault, C: Long term outcome for obstructive sleep apnea syndrome patients. Chest 94:1200, 1988.

18.   Findley, L, Unverzagt, M, and Surott, P: Automobile accidents in patients with obstructive sleep apnea. Am Rev Respir Dis 138:337, 1988.

19.   Findley, LJ and Bonnie, RJ: Sleep apnea and auto crashes; what is the doctor to do? Chest 94:225, 1988.

Robert L. Wilkins, MA, RRT
James R. Dexter, MD, FCCP

Chapter 19

CROUP and EPIGLOTTITIS

INTRODUCTION

The upper airway, which is made up of the nose, sinuses, pharynx, larynx, and trachea, is frequently exposed to a variety of irritants and infectious agents. It is not uncommon for these agents to cause inflammation and swelling of a portion of the upper airway. The inflammation may lead to significant narrowing of the airway and an increase in the work of breathing. Complete obstruction is possible if the airway inflammation affects a particularly vulnerable portion of the upper airway (e.g., epiglottis). As a result, diseases of the upper airway represent a potentially life-threatening medical problem that clinicians must recognize and treat promptly.

A large number of medical problems are associated with diseases of the upper airway, but this chapter focuses on croup and epiglottitis. Croup is a viral infection of the larynx, trachea, and/or bronchi that primarily affects infants and small children between 6 months and 3 years of age (Table 19–1). Epiglottitis, also called supra-glottitis, is a bacterial infection of the epiglottis. It most often affects children between the ages of 1 and 5 years but occurs occasionally in infants and adults.[1]

CROUP

Etiology

Croup is almost always caused by a virus, the most common of which are parainfluenza viruses 1 and 3, influenza viruses A and B, respiratory syncytial virus (RSV), and adenovirus.[2] Episodes of croup are much more common in the winter months.

Pathology and Pathophysiology

Croup causes inflammation and swelling of subglottic structures such as the larynx, trachea, and larger bronchi; thus, laryngotracheobronchitis (LTB) also refers to croup. Croup may result in intrathoracic airway involvement, which leads to ventilation-perfusion ratio ($\dot{V}/\dot{Q}$) mismatching and hypoxemia. Because croup may affect both upper and lower airways, the patient is at risk for ventilatory and oxygenation failure (see Chapter 1). If the upper airway obstruction becomes severe enough to jeopardize ventilation the patient's respiratory muscles eventually tire and the $Paco_2$ rises.

Table 19–1 Comparison of Croup and Epiglottitis

Parameter	Croup	Epiglottitis
Etiologic agent	Virus	Bacteria
Onset	Gradual	Acute
Most common age	6 months–3 years	1–5 years
Site of disease	Below the glottis	Above the glottis
CBC	Often normal	Shows leukocytosis
Fever	Mild	Moderate to severe
Admission criteria	Inspiratory and expiratory stridor at rest	Admit all patients
Treatment	Cool mist, oxygen, racemic epinephrine	Endotracheal tube, antibiotics

Clinical Features

Croup frequently has an insidious (slow) onset and commonly develops after 1 to 2 days of fever, nasal congestion, and coughing. The onset of croup is announced by an increasingly severe cough that takes on a brassy or barking quality. Hoarseness is common and indicates inflammation of the vocal cords and larynx. Symptoms of respiratory distress develop when the trachea and bronchi become inflamed and narrowed. The symptoms associated with croup typically worsen at night, perhaps because of the drop in absolute humidity at night which adds to the airway irritation.

Examination results of the croupy child may vary from nearly normal to markedly abnormal, with the degree of tachycardia and tachypnea identifying the severity. A diminished sensorium should alert bedside clinicians to the onset of respiratory failure.

Inspiratory stridor is common and may frequently be heard without the aid of a stethoscope in patients with croup. Stridor is more common on inspiration because narrowing of the upper (extrathoracic) airway is increased momentarily with each inspiratory effort. Stridor may occur on exhalation as well as on inhalation when the airway obstruction is severe. Retractions are seen when the inspiratory effort is severe enough to cause a large drop in pleural pressure. This draws the skin surrounding the rib cage inward with each inspiratory effort and suggests a more severe case. The retractions may be seen above or below the clavicles as well as in the intercostal spaces.

Treatment

The majority of patients with croup respond to cool mist and do not need hospitalization.[2] Keeping the child calm reduces stress on the respiratory system and may help minimize symptoms. Allowing the child to be held by a parent during examination and treatment may also be helpful.

Children with croup who have inspiratory and expiratory stridor at rest, severe retractions, and tachypnea usually need to be hospitalized. Respiratory care practitioners (RCPs) should administer cool mist and oxygen either by tent or face mask. Some infants and children do not tolerate a face mask and are more comfortable in a mist tent. A disadvantage of mist tents is that they make it difficult for clinicians to observe the patient and detect the onset of respiratory failure.

The use of racemic epinephrine may decrease airway edema and obstruction. Racemic epinephrine probably does not alter the overall course of illness but appears to offer temporary relief from upper airway edema and obstruction.[2] The typical dose for racemic epinephrine is 0.5 mL in 3 to 4 mL of saline given by medication nebulizer or intermittent positive airway pressure (IPPB) for 10 to 20 minutes. Repeat treatment may be needed in 1 to 2 hours. Tachyphylaxis is a common problem with racemic epinephrine and makes subsequent treatments less effective in some patients. Frequent use of racemic epinephrine may also lead to a rebound response that results in worsening of the airway obstruction.

Corticosteroids have been shown to reduce the severity and duration of illness in croup.[2] They are given if the patient appears severely ill and does not respond to initial therapy of cool mist and racemic epinephrine. A single dose of 0.3 to 0.5 mg/kg of dexamethasone or an equivalent dose of prednisone is frequently adequate.[3]

Most croupy children respond favorably to treatment, but close monitoring of the patient is very important to identify unexpected respiratory distress. Children with croup will sometimes develop respiratory muscle fatigue and proceed to respiratory failure. In such cases, the patient's sensorium, color, and arterial blood gases (ABG) deteriorate and endotracheal intubation is needed. In most cases the child can be extubated in 2 to 3 days after airway inflammation has subsided.

EPIGLOTTITIS

Etiology

Epiglottitis is most often caused by type B *Haemophilus influenzae*, although a small number of cases are caused by *Staphylococcus aureus*.[2] It occurs year-round and may follow a mild viral infection of the upper airway.

Pathology and Pathophysiology

Epiglottitis causes inflammation and swelling of the epiglottis, aryepiglottic folds, and arytenoids (Fig. 19–1). The epiglottis often turns a bright cherry color

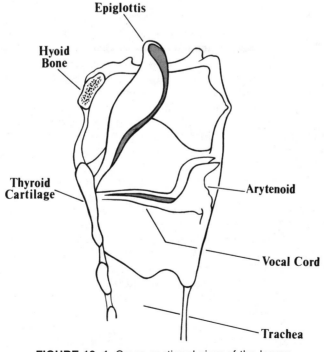

FIGURE 19–1 Cross-sectional view of the larynx.

with the onset of the infection. The structures below the glottis are usually not involved. Supraglottic inflammation leads to difficulty swallowing and airway narrowing that is more pronounced during inspiratory efforts.

Patients with a mild case of epiglottitis have normal ventilation and gas exchange as long as the upper airway remains patent. Ventilation will be impaired, however, when the obstruction is severe, and death from ventilatory failure and asphyxia may occur if clinicians do not initiate proper treatment.

Clinical Features

Patients with epiglottitis typically have an abrupt onset of symptoms and appear more acutely ill than do patients with croup. Older patients with epiglottitis may complain of fever, sore throat, and difficulty swallowing. Drooling is common because of the difficulty swallowing.

The patient with epiglottitis appears toxic and prefers sitting upright. Sitting upright and leaning forward may make it easier for the patient to maintain a patent airway, as this position can help keep the swollen epiglottitis out of the way. Inspiratory stridor and retractions are often present. Stridor varies with the position of the patient, level of activity, and degree of obstruction. Respiratory decompensation is associated with a diminished level of consciousness, and asphyxia may occur if treatment is not immediately implemented.

Although direct examination of the throat by depression of the tongue may reveal a bright red epiglottis and confirm the diagnosis, the procedure itself may result in a sudden complete obstruction of the upper airway. As a result, clinicians should perform the procedure only when equipment and personnel are available for intubation and tracheostomy.

Laboratory studies of the patient with epiglottitis will reveal an elevated white blood cell (WBC) count with a left shift. A lateral neck radiograph demonstrates a swollen epiglottis. A chest radiograph reveals a complicating pneumonia in about 25 percent of epiglottitis patients.[1]

Treatment

All patients with the diagnosis of epiglottitis should be hospitalized because intubation or tracheostomy are needed.[4,5] The risks associated with intubation or tracheostomy in patients with acute epiglottitis usually dictate placement of the artificial airway in the operating room. Initial airway management in the operating room is especially important because the upper airway will occasionally obstruct completely in response to attempts at intubation or even to simple inspection of the epiglottis. The physician and RCPs should stay with the patient at all times before successful placement of an artificial airway. Restraints may be needed in some cases to ensure against accidental extubation if paralysis and mechanical ventilation are not employed.

Sedation and mechanical ventilation are not routinely needed in uncomplicated cases of epiglottitis because the problem is upper airway patency and the lungs are normal.[6] Humidity therapy applied to the endotracheal tube may prevent further airway irritation and mobilize respiratory secretions. A small condenser humidifier attached to the endotracheal tube does not need tubing and may reduce the risk of accidental extubation.[6] Oxygen therapy is not typically needed following intubation unless a complicating pneumonia is present.

Culture specimens of the epiglottis should be obtained after the airway is in place.[7] The physician should order empiric intravenous (IV) antibiotic therapy to cover the most common organisms that cause acute epiglottitis (ampicillin 200 to 400 mg/kg per day and chloramphenicol 100 mg/kg per day in divided doses every 4 to 6 hours for 7 to 10 days). The chloramphenicol can be discontinued if the culture results demonstrate the *H. influenzae* strain is sensitive to ampicillin.

Extubation is often successful after 24 to 48 hours of treatment. Evidence that the patient is ready for extubation includes no fever within the past 12 hours, leak around the tube (which provides evidence that the inflammation has subsided), and improved general appearance of the patient. Extubation should be done with equipment and personnel available to replace the endotracheal tube should airway obstruction suddenly return.

Case Study No. 1

HISTORY

SR is a 6-year-old white girl brought to the emergency room by her parents at 3 AM. The parents stated that SR had been healthy until the afternoon of the previous day. At that time she had begun complaining of sore throat, difficulty swallowing, and fever. Her mother had obtained an oral temperature of 39.2°C and given her Tylenol. Later that evening she had become hoarse, her temperature had increased to 39.4°C, and her breathing had become rapid and labored. SR had refused solid foods but had been able to swallow small sips of juice. At 3 AM her parents had decided to take her to the emergency room.

Questions

1. What medical problems do the symptoms in this case suggest?
2. What is the significance of SR's age?
3. What is the significance of SR's rapid onset of symptoms?
4. What physical examination techniques are useful in this case and what purpose do they serve?

Answers

1. The medical history suggests croup, epiglottitis, tonsillitis, strep throat, or pneumonia.
2. SR's age suggests that croup is not likely, as it most often occurs in children 6 months to 3 years of age.
3. The rapid onset of symptoms suggests epiglottitis.
4. The initial examination should focus on the vital signs and sensorium. This will help determine the severity of the illness. Auscultation of the chest and neck will be useful to identify adventitious lung or airway sounds that might suggest the location and severity of respiratory abnormalities. Inspection of the patient's breathing pattern to identify the presence of retractions and use of accessory muscles will assist in evaluating the severity of the problem.

PHYSICAL EXAMINATION

General	*SR is alert and oriented. She is sitting upright and leaning forward, is drooling and appears anxious.*
Vital Signs	*Temperature 39.4°C, pulse 150/minute, respiratory rate 26/minute, blood pressure 110/75 mm Hg*
HEENT	*Unremarkable; throat not visualized at this time*
Neck	*Tracheal position normal; no lymphadenopathy; moderate use of accessory muscles with each inspiratory effort; inspiratory stridor noted with auscultation*

Chest	*Prolonged inspiratory time present; clear breath sounds noted bilaterally; intercostal retractions present*
Heart	*Tachycardia with regular rhythm; no murmurs*
Abdomen	*Grossly normal; patient refusal to lie down for abdominal examination*
Extremities	*No cyanosis or edema*

Questions

5. Should the examination include direct visualization of the epiglottis to assist in making a correct diagnosis? Why or why not?
6. What do the vital signs and sensorium tell you about the patient's condition?
7. Why is the patient drooling?
8. What pathophysiology accounts for the retractions?
9. Why is the stridor heard only on inspiration? What would be indicated by stridor heard on inhalation and exhalation?
10. What is the most likely reason for the patient not wanting to lie down for the abdominal examination?
11. What laboratory tests would help make the correct diagnosis in this case? What are the anticipated results for each potential diagnosis?

Answers

5. The attending physician should not attempt to visualize directly the patient's epiglottis until all the equipment and personnel are present to assist in emergency intubation and tracheostomy. This is important because the procedure of visualizing the back of the throat may initiate further inflammation of the epiglottis (if epiglottitis is the medical problem in this case) and result in sudden complete obstruction of the upper airway.
6. The rapid pulse and breathing rates suggest severe illness. The high fever is consistent with epiglottitis and is not common with croup. The normal sensorium indicates that respiratory failure is probably not present at this time.
7. The patient is drooling because of the painful swallowing. The pooling of secretions in the mouth and pharynx may promote aspiration.
8. The retractions are the result of changes in pleural pressure associated with strong contractions of the inspiratory muscles as the patient attempts to move air through a narrowed upper airway. This suggests that the patient's work of breathing is significantly increased.
9. Stridor is more common on inspiration because the extrathoracic airway tends to narrow as the inspiratory muscles pull gas through the airway into the thorax. Inflammation of the upper airway causes narrowing that becomes more pronounced as the patient attempts to inhale. If the stridor was present on inspiration and exhalation it would indicate a more severe case of upper airway obstruction.
10. Patients with a swollen epiglottis do not want to lie supine because this position makes breathing more difficult. The epiglottis is anterior to the tracheal opening and leaning forward allows gravity to hold it away from the larynx. The swollen epiglottis is more likely to obstruct the larynx

when the patient lays supine, which allows gravity to pull it back over the tracheal opening.

11. The complete blood count (CBC) helps to differentiate croup from epiglottitis. The WBC count, segmented neutrophils, and bands are usually elevated with epiglottitis. Lymphocytosis is more common with croup. A lateral neck radiograph may show narrowing below the glottis with croup and an enlarged epiglottis with epiglottitis.

LABORATORY DATA

CBC

WBC 15,500/mm³; segs 74 percent; bands 18 percent; lymphocytes 4 percent; hematocrit (Hct) 39 percent

LATERAL NECK RADIOGRAPH

Supraglottic narrowing consistent with epiglottitis (Fig. 19–2)

Questions

12. Is an ABG analysis important to obtain in this case? Why or why not?
13. Should the patient be hospitalized?
14. Should a throat culture be obtained?
15. What is the appropriate treatment?

Answers

12. An ABG analysis is not useful at this point. The procedure would probably add to the patient's anxiety and may worsen her condition.
13. All patients suspected of having epiglottitis should be hospitalized.
14. A throat culture should not be obtained until the integrity of the upper airway is ensured. The procedure could lead to more swelling of the epiglottis.
15. The most urgent treatment needed is placement of an endotracheal tube. This would ensure a patent airway and prevent sudden obstruction of the upper airway should the epiglottis continue to enlarge. The procedure should be performed in the operating room where an emergency tracheostomy can be performed if needed. IV antibiotics may be started as soon as an IV setup is available.

The patient was taken to the operating room, where an endotracheal tube was placed without complications. With the tube taped securely in place, a cool mist with a fraction of inspired oxygen (F_{IO_2}) of 0.35 was attached. The patient was taken to the pediatric intensive care unit (ICU) for further treatment. The vital signs were pulse rate 128/minute, respiratory rate 24/minute, blood pressure 115/70 mm Hg, and temperature 39.1°C. Pulse oximetry demonstrated a saturation of 97 percent upon arrival at the ICU. A throat culture specimen was obtained and IV ampicillin and chloramphenicol were given.

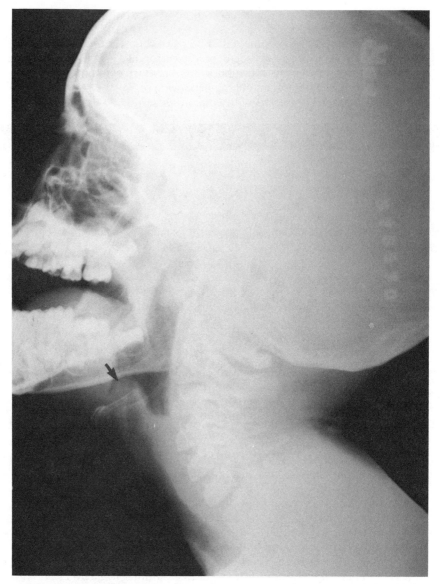

FIGURE 19–2 Lateral neck radiograph demonstrating an enlarged epiglottis *(arrow).* (Courtesy of Lionel Young, MD.)

Questions

16. What is the prognosis for this patient?
17. What is the most likely organism responsible for this infection?
18. When can the child be extubated?
19. How can accidental extubation be prevented?
20. Why apply humidity therapy to the endotracheal tube?

Answers

16. The prognosis for this patient is very good. A full recovery is expected.
17. The organism most likely responsible for this infection is *Haemophilus*

influenzae, which is a small gram-negative bacillus. It may be resistant to ampicillin.

18. The patient can be extubated once the fever has subsided for 12 hours and her general appearance has improved. This typically occurs 24 to 48 hours after intubation and the initiation of antibiotics.

19. Accidental extubation can be prevented by close observation of the patient, by careful explanation of the purpose of the tube to the child and parents, and by use of restraints and sedation.

20. Humidity therapy is given through the endotracheal tube to thin secretions and prevent obstruction of the tube with thick mucus. Because the upper airway is bypassed with an endotracheal tube, the inhalation of dry gas directly into the trachea could be irritating to the mucosa. The application of humidity therapy may reduce airway inflammation.

After 36 hours the patient's vital signs were normal and the patient was alert and oriented. At this point the patient was taken to the operating room where she was extubated without complications. She was returned to the pediatric ICU for observation and continued to receive IV antibiotics. Chloramphenicol was discontinued after the throat culture results demonstrated H. influenzae *sensitive to ampicillin. After she was stable on oral antibiotics for 24 hours the patient was discharged.*

Case Study No. 2

HISTORY

RD is a 23-month-old white boy brought to the emergency room by his mother at 10 PM. The patient's mother stated that RD had had a cold over the past 2 days and had developed a barking cough and respiratory distress earlier in the evening. The patient had been taking fluids poorly over the past 48 hours but refused to eat any solid food. He had been given pediatric Tylenol the day before and today. The mother stated that RD had "felt warm" but she had not actually taken his temperature.

Earlier this evening shortly after the barking cough started, RD began to have labored breathing. At this point he was taken into the bathroom with the shower turned on for humidity. Although this seemed to provide some relief initially, RD began to have increased difficulty with his breathing at about 9:30 PM. The patient's mother then brought him to the hospital for treatment.

Questions

1. What are the possible medical problems suggested by this history?
2. What is the significance of RD's age and sex?
3. What physical examination techniques are useful in this case?
4. Was it a good idea for the patient's mother to take RD into the bathroom to breathe in a steamy environment? Why or why not?

Answers

1. The differential diagnosis in this case would include laryngo-tracheobronchitis (croup), epiglottitis, tonsillitis, and pneumonia.
2. The patient's age and sex are typical for croup; however, they do not rule out pneumonia or tonsillitis.
3. Physical examination should identify the patient's general appearance,

vital signs, level of alertness, breathing pattern, breath sounds over the chest and upper airway, skin color, and presence of retractions.
4. Yes, it was a good idea for the mother to take RD into a steamy bathroom. The added moisture is often soothing to the irritated airways and may decrease respiratory distress.

PHYSICAL EXAMINATION

General   *RD is an alert child who appears anxious and is working hard to breathe.*

Vital Signs   *Temperature 37.3°C, pulse 144/minute, respiratory rate 36/minute, blood pressure 150/P*

HEENT   *Normocephalic; eyes equally reactive to light; ears normal; dried mucus discharge from nose, with flaring on inspiration; throat red upon brief inspection*

Neck   *Mild anterior cervical lymphadenopathy; loud inspiratory and expiratory stridor noted over the neck*

Chest   *Severe intercostal and subcostal retractions; expiratory low-pitched wheezing over both sides of chest, loudest on right*

Heart   *Regular rate and rhythm without murmur; no heaves or lifts*

Abdomen   *Normal*

Extremities   *Skin warm and pink with normal pulses bilaterally in the upper and lower extremities*

Questions

5. Based on the physical examination findings do you consider this a mild, moderate, or severe case of upper airway obstruction? Upon what do you base this assessment?
6. What is indicated by the nasal flaring?
7. What is suggested by the low-pitched wheezing heard over the chest?
8. What laboratory tests would be useful, and what are the expected findings for each potential diagnosis?

Answers

5. This appears to be a severe case of upper airway obstruction. This conclusion is based on the rapid pulse and respiratory rate, presence of inspiratory and expiratory stridor, and severe retractions.
6. The nasal flaring suggests that the patient's work of breathing is increased.
7. The low-pitched expiratory wheezing heard over the chest suggests that the intrathoracic airways are involved in addition to the upper airway.
8. A CBC would be useful to differentiate croup from epiglottitis. Epiglottitis generally increases the WBC count, with an increased percentage of segmented neutrophils and bands. The CBC may be normal with croup. If it is abnormal there is usually only a slight elevation in the lymphocyte count. The CBC may be markedly abnormal with either croup or epiglottitis if a complicating pneumonia is present.

A lateral neck radiograph would be useful. Narrowing below the glottis is typical for croup and narrowing above the glottis typical for epiglottitis.

A chest radiograph would be useful to evaluate the wheezing heard over the chest and to rule out pneumonia or atelectasis.

LABORATORY DATA

CBC

WBC 12,800; segs 50 percent; bands 3 percent; lymphocytes 45 percent, monocytes 2 percent

LATERAL NECK RADIOGRAPH

Subglottic narrowing (Fig. 19–3)

CHEST RADIOGRAPH

Patchy infiltrate in right middle lobe (Fig. 19–3B)

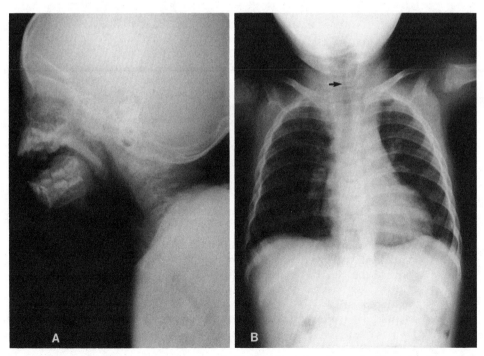

FIGURE 19–3 *A*) Lateral view and, *B*) *AP* view of radiograph demonstrating subglottic narrowing of the upper airway typical for croup *(arrow)*. (Courtesy of Lionel Young, MD.)

Questions

9. How do you interpret the CBC?
10. Should an ABG analysis be obtained?
11. Should the patient be admitted to the hospital? Upon what information do you base your answer?
12. What treatment is appropriate for this patient? State why each treatment modality is needed.

Answers

9. The CBC demonstrates a slight elevation in the WBC count. This appears to be primarily due to an elevation in the lymphocytes and is common with viral infections.
10. An ABG analysis is not needed at this point. The procedure would be traumatic for the patient and would probably increase the severity of the symptoms.
11. The patient should be admitted. Severe cases of croup can lead to respiratory failure and asphyxia.
12. Initial treatment should include oxygen, cool mist, and racemic epinephrine. Oxygen is needed because the chest radiograph abnormality and wheezing suggest that intrathoracic airways are involved. $\dot{V}/\dot{Q}$ mismatching is likely and would result in hypoxemia. Cool mist should thin secretions and soothe the irritated airways. Racemic epinephrine may temporarily reduce swelling and inflammation of the upper airway and reduce the child's dyspnea. Corticosteroids should be used if the child responds poorly to this treatment.

In the emergency room RD was given a cool mist by mask with an F_{IO_2} of 0.40. RCPs administered racemic epinephrine by face mask via IPPB. The patient's mother was present throughout the treatment and was helpful in obtaining the child's cooperation. RD was admitted because of the severity of his symptoms and the abnormal chest radiograph. He was taken to the pediatric ICU and placed in a mist tent with approximately 40 percent oxygen. A repeat treatment with racemic epinephrine was given 2 hours after the initial treatment. Following the second treatment the patient's vital signs were pulse 128/minute, respiratory rate 32/minute, and temperature 37.3°C. Pulse oximetry demonstrated a saturation of 95 percent in the mist tent. Stridor was present on inspiration and low-pitched wheezing continued to be heard over the chest. The retractions were less noticeable.

Questions

13. What dangers are associated with the use of mist tents?
14. Should RD be given corticosteroids?
15. Should the patient be given antibiotics?
16. What is a common problem associated with the use of racemic epinephrine?
17. Should the patient's mother be encouraged to remain at the bedside or to go home?

Answers

13. Mist tents can make it more difficult to observe the patient. This may delay treatment if respiratory decompensation occurs. A pulse oximeter

with an alarm may offer one useful monitoring tool for patients in a mist tent. Mist tents with oxygen represent a potential fire hazard and require appropriate posting of warning signs. The patient's mother should be advised of these concerns and should be told not to smoke or give the child any toys that may cause a spark.

14. Corticosteroids can be helpful in severe cases of croup. In this case the patient appears to be responding to more conservative treatment. Corticosteroids can be given if the patient does not continue to improve or if the upper airway obstruction worsens.

15. Antibiotics are not useful in the treatment of croup. This patient, however, has a suspicious infiltrate that may be pneumonia. It may be reasonable to administer a broad-spectrum antibiotic in this case while sputum specimens are obtained and analyzed.

16. Tachyphylaxis is a common problem with racemic epinephrine. This indicates that repeated treatments with racemic epinephrine may not be as effective as previous treatments. For this reason the medication should not be given in mild cases of croup or on an outpatient basis for more severe cases in an attempt to prevent hospitalization.[2]

17. RD's mother should be encouraged to remain at the bedside. This may help reduce the child's anxiety and assist the hospital staff. Provisions should be made for the mother to sleep at the bedside.

The next morning the patient awoke in the mist tent with minimal symptoms. Mild inspiratory stridor was noted over the upper airway, and some coarse crackles were present over the chest. Vital signs were nearly normal and the patient was transferred to the basic care area. The racemic epinephrine treatments were stopped but the mist tent continued. A repeat chest radiograph demonstrated improvement with partial resolution of the infiltrate. The patient continued to improve throughout the day and was discharged the following morning with normal vital signs and no symptoms.

Questions

17. Is the quick recovery in this case typical of most cases of croup?
18. Is this patient likely to experience repeated episodes of croup?

Answers

17. Yes, the quick recovery in this case is typical for croup.
18. Repeated episodes of croup are common in small children. As the child grows older the episodes are likely to decrease in severity and frequency.

REFERENCES

1. Robotham, JL: Obstructive airways disease in infants and children. In Kirby, RR and Taylor, RW (eds): Respiratory Failure. Year Book Medical, Chicago, 1986, pp 169–190.

2. Bass, JW and Wehrie, PF: Croup and epiglottitis. In Nussbaum, E and Galant, SP (eds): Pediatric Respiratory Disorders. Grune & Stratton, Orlando, 1984, pp 109–127.

3. Super, DM, et al: A prospective randomized double-blind study to evaluate the effect of dexamethasone in acute laryngotracheitis. J Pediatr 115:323, 1989.

4. Winn, RE: Other important ICU infections. In Civetta, JM, Taylor, RW, and Kirby, RR (eds): Critical Care. JB Lippincott, Philadelphia, 1988, p 876.

5. Kimmons, HC and Peterson BM: Management of acute epiglottitis in pediatric patients. Crit Care Med 14:278, 1986.

6. Butt, W, et al: Acute epiglottitis: A different approach to management. Crit Care Med 16:43, 1988.

7. Letourneau, MA: Respiratory disorders. In Berkin, RM, et al (eds): Pediatric Emergency Medicine. Mosby–Year Book St. Louis, 1992, pp. 969–1007.

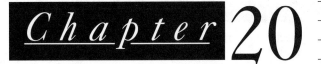

Victoria C. Sciacqua, BS, RRT

RESPIRATORY SYNCYTIAL VIRUS

INTRODUCTION

Respiratory syncytial virus (RSV) was initially isolated in 1956 by Morris, Blount, and Savage,[1] and continues to be a major cause of morbidity and mortality worldwide. It is recognized as the most common viral respiratory pathogen in infancy and early childhood. It is a leading cause of bronchiolitis (43 percent of patients) and pneumonia (25 percent of patients).[3]

Syncytium, as defined by Dorland's[4] is a "multinucleate mass of protoplasm produced by the merging of cells." At the level of the bronchioles, the virus causes neighboring cells to fuse together to form a syncytium; hence, the name respiratory syncytial virus.

By the age of 2 years, nearly 100 percent of children have been exposed to the virus. Although infection occurs throughout one's life, children less than 1 year old tend to have the most severe disease. This appears to be due to their decreased immune response, smaller airway size, and lack of collateral ventilation. Because of protection from maternal antibodies, it is very rare for RSV to infect infants during the first 4 weeks after birth.[5]

RSV outbreaks occur throughout the world every year and typically last from 2 to 5 months. The virus is extremely common during the midwinter and early spring months. These epidemics tend to occur at regular, predictive intervals. During each epidemic the number of infants and small children with lower respiratory tract infections who are admitted to hospitals increases significantly.

ETIOLOGY

The virus is usually introduced into the family by an older sibling or parent who is exhibiting coldlike symptoms. This infection poses a more serious threat to the younger siblings in the family. While reinfections are common in both adults and children, the severity of illness usually decreases with reinfection.

Incubation period for the virus is from 2 to 8 days, with an average of 4 days.[2,6] The two most common modes of transmission are (1) large particle aerosols that are transmitted during close personal contact, and (2) physical contact with contaminated secretions. The latter type of transmission can occur with hand-to-hand contact or touching of infected material. Infection usually occurs when the virus comes in contact with the victim's conjunctiva or mucous membranes via airborne particles or direct contact.[2] Although the virus is very labile (fragile), it remains infective on cloth and paper for more than 30 minutes and is still contagious in nasal secretions after 6 hours.[7]

PATHOLOGY AND PATHOPHYSIOLOGY

Once infection has occurred, the virus is spread along the respiratory tract by cell-to-cell transfer. Involvement of the lower respiratory tract may be a result of aspiration of secretions from the infected upper respiratory tract. Replication of the virus is limited to the respiratory tract mucosa but may involve the entire respiratory tract, thus increasing the severity of illness.

The pathologic findings associated with RSV infection include peribronchiolar mononuclear infiltration and necrosis of the epithelium of the small airways.[2] Peribronchiolar mononuclear infiltration leads to edema of the bronchiole walls, submucosa, and adventitial tissue. Proliferation of the epithelium into the airway lumen owing to necrosis leads to sloughing of the necrotic tissue into the airway. This sloughing, along with edema and the accumulation of mucus, leads to a decrease in airway lumen size. The airway may actually become completely occluded. The virus causes an increase in mucus production, which enhances the severity of the plugging.

Once plugging of the airway occurs, the patient is likely to develop hyperinflation in some areas of the lungs and atelectasis in other regions. Inspiration increases airway diameter and air enters the lung around the obstructions. During expiration the airways become narrower and inhibit the gas from escaping around the plug, which results in air trapping. Atelectasis may occur in regions of the lung where the mucus plugging is more severe, resulting in minimal or no ventilation of the affected regions.

The combination of hyperinflation and atelectasis leads to abnormalities in ventilation-perfusion ($\dot{V}/\dot{Q}$) matching, resulting in hypoxemia. Reduced lung compliance and increased airways resistance result in increased work of breathing.

CLINICAL FEATURES

The clinical manifestations associated with RSV vary with both the age of the patient and the severity of the illness. Infants most often present with serious clinical manifestations. Certain groups of children are also at an increased risk for having severe illness: children less than 3 months old; children with congenital heart disease, bronchopulmonary dysplasia (BPD) (see Chapter 22), cystic fibrosis, or immunodeficiencies; and premature infants (Table 20–1).

History of Present Illness

The infant who presents with RSV infection often has a history of being exposed to an older sibling or parent who has cold symptoms. Exposure to other children with RSV often occurs in daycare centers or as a result of nosocomial transmission while hospitalized. Often signs and symptoms of an upper respiratory tract infection (mild rhinorrhea, pharyngitis, cough, and a low-grade fever) precede the onset of more severe symptoms. As the disease progresses into the lower respiratory tract, the symptoms increase in severity.

Table 20–1 Risk Factors for Severe RSV Infection

Infants with any of the following:
1. Congenital heart disease
2. Bronchopulmonary dysplasia
3. Prematurity
4. Immunodeficiency or immunosuppression
5. Undergoing chemotherapy

Physical Examination

The patient with RSV infection of the lower airways may exhibit several signs indicating an increased work of breathing. An increase in respiratory rate is typically present. Tachypnea is the best clinical sign correlating with hypoxemia.[2] The patient typically has intercostal or subcostal retractions (or both) and uses his or her accessory muscles to breathe. Other signs of increased work of breathing include nasal flaring, grunting, and the appearance of being "air hungry." As a result of an increased respiratory rate, the patient is likely to feed poorly. The increased respiratory rate also puts the patient at risk for aspiration if vomiting occurs.

Apneic episodes may occur during RSV infection and are a sign of severe illness. The cause of these episodes is uncertain; however, the immaturity of the central respiratory control mechanisms of very young children is thought to be a contributor.[8] As the disease becomes more severe, frequency and severity of apneic episodes also increase. Patients who are at highest risk for apneic episodes are those of young postnatal age, premature infants, and infants with a history of apnea.[8]

Breath sounds may help assess the severity of pulmonary involvement. Expiratory wheezing, diminished breath sounds, and crackles are most common. Wheezing is a result of the narrowed airways caused by inflammation and edema. Because the patient's lungs are often hyperexpanded, there is less airflow moving with each respiratory cycle and breath sounds are diminished. The cause of the crackles can be inferred from their pitch and timing during the respiratory cycle. If crackles are fine and occur at late inspiration, the most likely source is atelectasis due to plugging of the airways. On the other hand, if the crackles are coarse and occur throughout the respiratory cycle, pneumonia or retained bronchial secretions, or both, may be the cause. The extent to which the adventitious lung sounds occur over the chest indicates the amount of lung involved. Stridor may be heard over the upper airway if the trachea or larynx is affected.

Laboratory Data

The complete blood count (CBC) with RSV infection is typically normal. An increase in white blood cell (WBC) count with a left shift (increase in the proportion of immature WBCs) may be seen when a superimposed bacterial infection is present.

Assessment of arterial blood gases (ABGs) confirms the degree of hypoxemia and the ventilatory status of the patient. The Pao_2 is usually decreased due to $\dot{V}/\dot{Q}$ mismatching. Hypoxemia due to RSV infection may last for weeks after recovery.[9] The arterial carbon dioxide level may be decreased owing to hyperventilation. An increase in $Paco_2$ indicates fatigue of the respiratory muscles from an increased work of breathing. Progression to metabolic acidosis may occur if hypoxemia is severe and increases in circulation are compromised. Serial ABGs may help identify a worsening trend in time to avert problems.

Chest radiographs commonly demonstrate at least one of two findings: hyperinflation or interstitial pneumonitis or both.[2] The signs of hyperinflation and air trapping include flattened diaphragms, widened intercostal spaces, and an increase in anteroposterior (AP) diameter. If a lateral radiograph is available, a prominence of the retrosternal space will also be noted when hyperinflation is present. Interstitial pneumonitis is commonly present in several lobes and is seen as areas of increased density. Atelectasis may also be seen on the radiograph.

Diagnosis

RSV should be suspected as the cause of illness based on the time of year, presence of a local outbreak, age of the patient, the history of present illness, and the clinical picture. A definite diagnosis of RSV infection can be made by isolation of the virus or its antigens from the patient's respiratory secretions.[2] A good sputum specimen must be obtained and rapidly analyzed to ensure accurate results.

The bedside clinician can obtain a specimen by several different techniques; the most common are nasal washing (aspirate) and nasal swabs. Although both techniques can be effective, some studies have shown that nasal washing is a more sensitive test than nasal swabs,[2,6] whereas others have found nasal swabs to be nearly as effective as nasal washing.[10]

Once the specimen is obtained, rapid detection of the virus is found using immunofluorescent techniques. One of these techniques is the enzyme-linked immunosorbent assay (ELISA). Results from immunofluorescent types of tests can usually be obtained within 2 to 4 hours. It is very important to be able to diagnose the virus rapidly so that specific therapy can be initiated as soon as possible (see farther on).

TREATMENT

The treatment of RSV, like many diseases, varies with the degree of severity. Most children require only supportive care for their illness. Some will require supplemental oxygen to treat hypoxemia, especially if lower respiratory tract infection is present. The patient with RSV should be adequately hydrated with intravenous (IV) fluids until normal feeding can be resumed. Pulse oximetry can be useful to watch for hypoxemia and ABGs help to evaluate the degree of hypercapnia.

Bronchodilators may be helpful if the patient demonstrates wheezing or an increased work of breathing. Racemic epinephrine may be useful to decrease upper airway swelling when inflammation is severe enough to cause stridor. Mechanical ventilation may be necessary if the patient demonstrates increasing $Paco_2$ with therapy, excessive work of breathing, or episodes of apnea.

Since January 1986, ribavirin has been commonly used for those patients who are extremely ill or at high risk for severe illness. Ribavirin is a virostatic agent whose exact mechanism of action is uncertain.[11,12] In some viruses, it prevents cap formation on the viral messenger RNA, which may preclude translation of the virus. Another mechanism may be inhibition of viral nucleic acid polymerases and prevention of RNA replication. Ribavirin is different from most other antiviral drugs in both its spectrum of activity and its mode of administration.

Ribavirin is administered in aerosol form via a small particle aerosol generator (SPAG-2; Fig. 20–1). The SPAG-2 delivers particles in the size range of 1.1 to 5.0 μm. These small particles remain suspended in air until they reach the distal airways, where they are deposited. The drug is administered to the patient via a hood, tent, or mechanical ventilation. Ribavirin is typically given 12 to 18 hours per day for 3 to 7 days. The cost in 1991 for 3 days of treatment was approximately $700. Because of the cost involved, this drug is usually given only after a sputum sample has been found to be positive for RSV. Exceptions to this include patients who have a high probability of having RSV and are severely ill. The use of ribavirin in the treatment of RSV leads to more rapid clinical improvement with an increase in Pao_2 and oxygen percent saturation (Sao_2) and a decrease in both hospital stay and time of viral shedding.[13,14]

Because ribavirin is very sticky, it may precipitate in either the ventilator circuit or the endotracheal tube. This precipitation can lead to malfunction of the expiratory valve in the circuit. The precipitate may also narrow the patient's endotracheal tube and increase expiratory resistance. The increase in resistance may inadvertently cause positive end-expiratory pressure (PEEP), also known as auto PEEP. The risks associated with ribavirin and mechanical ventilation may be reduced by:

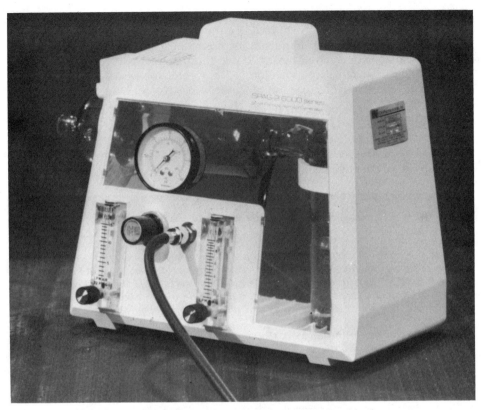

FIGURE 20–1 SPAG-2 unit used to administer ribavirin therapy.

1. Frequent ventilator circuit changes (every 8 hours)
2. Modifications to the circuit such as filters and one-way valves
3. Frequent suctioning of the endotracheal tube
4. Close and constant monitoring of the patient[15,16]

Concern to Health Care Workers

Because safety reports are based primarily on animal studies, the toxic effects of ribavirin in humans are unknown; however, the drug has teratogenic effects in animals. A teratogen is "an agent or factor that causes the production of physical defects in the developing embryo of a pregnant woman."[4] Pregnant women and those trying to become pregnant should avoid exposure to ribavirin and should not provide care for people receiving ribavirin treatments.[18] This recommendation is based primarily on animal research, and no cases of human toxicity have been reported.[19] The most common human side effects have been rash, mild bronchospasm, and reversible skin irritation.[20] Health care workers may also complain of eye irritation and headache associated with ribavirin exposure.[20] Caregiver exposure can be limited by a tight-fitting mask that filters out particles with a diameter of 0.5 μm or greater. The use of a containment system has been shown to be effective in decreasing the level of exposure to ribavirin.[19,21]

Prevention of Nosocomial Infection

Because hospital-acquired RSV infection remains a major problem, many studies have evaluated techniques to decrease the spreading of the infection. One study showed that handwashing and isolating patients reduced the incidence of nosocomial infection.[22] Another study showed that the use of gloves and gowns was found beneficial in decreasing the frequency of nosocomial infection.[23] Screening and isolating patients suspected of having RSV at the time of admission are also useful in decreasing nosocomial transmission.[24] The Center for Disease Control (CDC) recommends the following:

1. Use of masks if close to the patient
2. Use of gowns if soiling is likely
3. Use of gloves to prevent touching infected material
4. Use of disposable material or isolation of material prior to reprocessing
5. Use of effective handwashing.[17]

Case Study

HISTORY

NJ is a 2-month-old white girl born to a 25-year-old gravida 4, para 3 (four pregnancies, three live births) woman via normal vaginal delivery. NJ had been in her usual state of health until February, when she had developed slight nasal congestion. The patient had been seen by her primary physician and sent home with a regimen of amoxicillin for symptoms associated with an upper respiratory tract infection (URI).

Two days after the initial visit, the mother had noticed that NJ had progressively worsening respiratory distress. She had also noted that the patient had increased congestion, decreased appetite, vomiting, and diarrhea. The mother reported that the patient's three older siblings had recently had a URI. The patient was brought to the emergency room for repeat evaluation.

Questions

1. What risk factors indicate that RSV is the likely source of infection?
2. What suggests that this patient is at risk for a more severe case?

Answers

1. A number of factors may point to RSV as the source of infection. First, the child's age puts her in a high-risk group. Second, RSV is common in February. Most outbreaks appear to peak in January, February, or March.[8] Third, the patient was treated a few days earlier for symptoms associated with a URI. Fourth, the patient was exposed to older siblings with symptoms of URI. This is a very common clinical scenario for RSV infection.
2. The patient's age puts her more at risk for severe RSV infection.

PHYSICAL EXAMINATION

General   *NJ is awake and grunting and is in moderate to severe respiratory distress. She was connected to a pulse oximeter, which revealed saturations of 80 to 85 percent on room air. She experienced frequent coughing spells, during which her saturation fell into the 60 percent range.*

Vital Signs   *Temperature 38.7°C; respiratory rate 50/minute; pulse 180/minute; blood pressure 80/60 mm Hg, with a mean of 63 mm Hg*

HEENT	Reveals normal anterior fontanelle; pupils equal, round, and reactive to light and accommodation (PERRLA); tympanic membranes were erythematous bilaterally; nasal flaring with small amount of yellow nasal discharge and crusting noted in nostrils; throat clear
Neck	Trachea midline and mobile; inspiratory stridor noted
Chest	Costal and substernal retractions present with each inspiration; chest hyperexpanded
Heart	Regular rhythm with a rate of 180/minute; no murmurs
Lungs	Diffuse inspiratory and expiratory coarse crackles and expiratory wheezes throughout all lung fields
Abdomen	Soft, nontender, nondistended; normoactive bowel sounds
Skin	Pale, cool, dry; no rashes; no evidence of cyanosis
Musculoskeletal	Slightly decreased tone
Neurologic	Deep tendon reflexes + + and equal bilaterally; no ankle clonus elicited; equivocal Babinski's signs
Measurements	Weight 4.3 kg (in 20th percentile for age); length 57 cm (in 50th percentile); head circumference 37 cm (in 10th percentile)

Questions

3. What effect does the elevated body temperature have on the patient's work of breathing?
4. What is the likely cause of the inspiratory stridor?
5. What are the likely causes of the crackles and wheezes heard upon auscultation?
6. Why is the patient's chest hyperexpanded? How does this hyperexpansion affect the patient's work of breathing?
7. What clinical signs indicate that the patient's work of breathing is increased?

Answers

3. Elevated body temperature increases metabolic rate and oxygen consumption. The patient's heart and respiratory rates will increase to accommodate the increased demand on both the pulmonary and cardiovascular systems.
4. Stridor is a high-pitched inspiratory sound often described as a "crowing" sound. It is usually caused by partial obstruction of the upper airway, which in this case is most likely due to inflammation from the viral infection.
5. Retained secretions are the most likely cause of the crackles because they are heard upon inspiration and expiration and are coarse. Viral infections often cause an increase in the production of mucus. The expiratory wheezing may be produced by edema, bronchospasm, or secretions in the airways.
6. The patient's chest is hyperexpanded because of the air trapping that is the result of intrathoracic airway obstruction. When the intrathoracic

airways are obstructed, air enters the lung more easily than it exits the lung. This is because airways dilate slightly during inspiration and narrow with exhalation. As a result of air trapping, hyperexpansion of the chest occurs. Air trapping also leads to an increase in the patient's functional residual capacity (FRC). As the FRC increases, the patient breathes at a higher lung volume. At high lung volumes, the elastic force of both lung and chest wall make chest expansion very difficult. The patient must exert her respiratory muscles to inhale in order to overcome these two forces opposing inhalation.

7. The patient is exhibiting many signs of an increased work of breathing including increased respiratory rate, retractions, expiratory grunting, and nasal flaring.

LABORATORY FINDINGS

CHEST RADIOGRAPH

(Fig. 20–2)

ABG (ON ROOM AIR)

	Patient Value	Normal Values
pH	7.37	7.35–7.45
$Paco_2$	48 mm Hg	35–45 mm Hg
Pao_2	52 mm Hg	85–100 mm Hg
HCO_3^-	25 mEq/liter	22–26 mEq/liter
Base excess (BE)	−1 mEq/liter	(−2)–(+2) mEq/liter

CBC

	Observed	Normal
WBCs	12,200	4000–11,000/mm³
Red blood cells (RBCs)	3.9	4.1–5.5 million/mm³
Hemoglobin	11.1	11.5–15.5 g/dL
Hematocrit	37.2	30–40%
Platelets	583,000	175–415,000
WBC morphology		
Segs	35%	38–79%
Bands	9%	0–7%
Lymphocytes	52%	12–30%
Monocytes	4%	0–10%

CHEMISTRY

All within normal limits except for sodium (Na^+), which is slightly decreased at 132 mEq/liter.

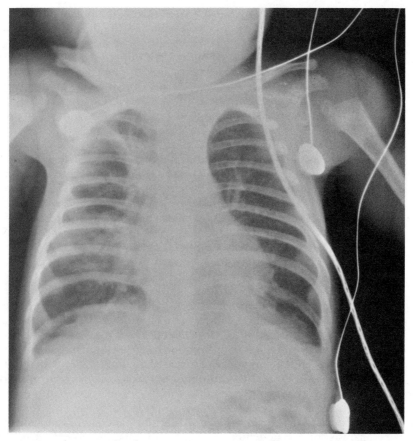

FIGURE 20–2 Chest radiograph demonstrating presence of diffuse opacities. (See text for complete description.)

Questions

8. What findings on the chest radiograph (Fig. 20–2) are consistent with the diagnosis of RSV? How do the findings on the chest radiograph relate to the patient's symptoms?
9. Interpret the ABG and describe possible causes of the findings.
10. Interpret the CBC. What is the likely cause of the increase in the WBCs? Of what significance is the decreased hemoglobin?
11. What further diagnostic procedures should be done at this time?
12. What therapeutic interventions should be instituted in the emergency room?
13. Should this patient be mechanically ventilated?

Answers

8. Hyperinflation and the presence of diffuse opacities are consistent with RSV infection. This chest radiograph demonstrates both of these features. Flattened diaphragms, increased intercostal spaces, and increased radiolucency are consistent with hyperinflation.

    The presence of diffuse opacities is common with RSV infection. Infiltrates are present in the right middle lobe (RML) and right lower lobe (RLL), as shown by the increased opacity of the radiograph in those areas. These densities are consistent with the diagnosis of RSV pneumonia.

The linear density seen in the right upper lobe (RUL) is consistent with subsegmental atelectasis secondary to plugging of the airway.

The patient's symptoms correlate with the chest radiograph findings. Pulmonary hyperinflation leads to an increased work of breathing as the infant is forced to breathe at a higher lung volume. The presence of infection can account for the air hunger, increased congestion, and elevated body temperature.

9. The ABG analysis reveals a mild respiratory acidosis. The decreased Pao_2 indicates moderate hypoxemia on room air. The increase in respiratory rate with an elevated $Paco_2$ suggests that the child's effectiveness of ventilation is impaired. Respiratory muscle fatigue is the most likely cause for the elevated $Paco_2$. $\dot{V}/\dot{Q}$ mismatching and shunt from excessive airway secretions and atelectasis are probable sources of the hypoxemia.

10. The CBC reveals a slightly elevated WBC count as well as a slightly reduced RBC count. The increase in WBC (leukocytosis) is most likely a response to the stress of the infection. WBCs are an integral part of the body's immune system and increase in response to the stress of infection. Acute bacterial infection or stress is noted by the increase in the number of bands. An increase in the percent of lymphocytes and WBC is consistent with viral infection. A decrease in hemoglobin reduces the oxygen-carrying capacity of the blood. This patient's oxygen content is low because of the decreased amount of circulating RBCs and the decreased PaO_2. This will stimulate cardiovascular compensation but a decreased oxygen delivered to the tissues may occur if the compensation is inadequate.

11. Appropriate diagnostic procedures at this time should include sputum analysis for the detection of RSV by an immunofluorescent technique. Either a nasal swab or a nasal aspirate should be done to detect the virus or its antigens in the nasal secretions of the patient.

12. Oxygen therapy is a mainstay in the treatment of RSV and should be instituted at this time to relieve the patient's hypoxemia. The amount of oxygen delivered to the patient should be titrated to maintain saturations between 90 and 95 percent.

The stridor present in this patient requires immediate intervention because upper airway obstruction is potentially life threatening. The drug of choice to treat stridor is racemic epinephrine (Micronephrine or Vaponefrin), which can be useful to reduce the amount of upper airway swelling. It should be continued if found to benefit the patient (decreased work of breathing and stridor) and discontinued if no relief is noted. Broad-spectrum antibiotics should be given until a specific infectious agent is identified.

13. Although the patient's $Paco_2$ is elevated, the respiratory acidosis dictates careful observation but is not yet life threatening. Mechanical ventilation will be needed if the patient does not respond to therapy or if the respiratory acidosis becomes more severe.

The patient was admitted to the pediatric intensive care unit (ICU). Physician orders include:

1. Nothing by mouth (NPO)

 2. *IV dextrose 5%/normal saline 0.2%, with 10 mEq KCl/liter at 15 mL/hour*
 3. *Aminophylline 1:1 at 4.5 mL/hour*
 4. *Theophylline level checked every morning (Q_{AM})*
 5. *Medication nebulizer 0.25 mL Micronephrine (Q_{AM}) every 3 hours as needed for stridor (Q3 prn)*
 6. *Medication nebulizer 0.3 mL albuterol in 2.5 mL normal saline every 3 hours (Q3)*
 7. *Chest physiotherapy every 3 hours after medication nebulizer*
 8. *O₂ via hood to keep saturation at 90 to 95 percent*
 9. *Continuous pulse oximeter and respiratory monitor*

Questions

14. Why did the physician make the patient NPO and start administering IV fluids?
15. What level of blood theophylline is considered therapeutic?
16. Are medication nebulizers and chest physiotherapy indicated in this patient?
17. Is ribavirin indicated in this case? If so, how should it be given and what precautions should be taken by the respiratory care practitioner to minimize his/her exposure to the drug?
18. What precautions should be taken by all health care workers caring for this patient to prevent the spread of RSV to other patients?
19. What change in breathing pattern might occur in this patient that would indicate a more severe case of RSV infection?

Answers

14. The physician ordered nothing by mouth for the patient because the patient is experiencing moderate to severe respiratory distress. The patient not only would have difficulty eating but also is at risk for aspiration. IV fluids are necessary in this patient to maintain adequate hydration.
15. The patient's aminophylline drip should be titrated to a level of 10 to 20 μg/mL to ensure maximum benefits of bronchodilatation with minimum risk for toxicity.
16. Chest physiotherapy and medication nebulizer treatments are indicated for the treatment of bronchospasm. The presence of bronchospasm is suspected when wheezing is identified. Chest physiotherapy is indicated for patients having difficulty raising secretions. The child's age and condition suggest that she will need assistance with secretion removal.
17. Ribavirin is indicated in this case because the patient is experiencing a relatively severe illness. The respiratory care practitioner (RCP) should administer ribavirin in aerosol via a SPAG-2, which delivers particles in the range of 1.0 to 5.0 μm that are needed to reach the peripheral lung units.

    The RCP should wear a mask that will filter all particles with a mass median aerodynamic diameter of 0.5 μm or larger. Additionally, a containment system (e.g., vacuum system) should be used whenever possible. This will minimize the RCP's exposure to the drug. Any RCP who may be pregnant should not administer the ribavirin treatments.
18. All health care workers associated with this patient should wash their hands thoroughly before and after each patient contact. The use of gown and gloves with each contact is also important to prevent the spread of infection to other patients. The patient should be isolated from other patients who do not have RSV.

19. Apneic episodes, increased respiratory rate, and increased use of accessory muscles would indicate a more severe case of RSV infection.

NJ was placed in isolation and started on ribavirin 6 g in 300 mL sterile water via mist hood. With the exception of an increased respiratory rate, vital signs remained stable throughout her hospitalization. The patient improved daily and was afebrile by day 3. On day 4, her medication nebulizers and chest physiotherapy were decreased to every 4 hours. They were decreased further as the patient improved, until they were no longer required after day 6. Hypoxemia also decreased during that time, and her F_{IO_2} was titrated by pulse oximeter until by day 7. Room air saturations were 90 to 95 percent. The aminophylline drip was eventually discontinued and she was started on oral Somophyllin with the dose titrated to maintain a therapeutic level. At the time of discharge, NJ was feeding without difficulty, breath sounds were clear and no signs of respiratory distress were noted. NJ was discharged 8 days after admission and was sent home on a regimen of oral theophylline syrup. NJ's mother was advised to bring her in for a follow-up visit with her private physician in 1 week.

REFERENCES

1. Morris, JA, Blount, RE, and Savage, RE: Recovery of cytopathogenic agent from chimpanzees with coryza. Proc Soc Exp Biol Med 92:544, 1956.

2. Hall, CB: Respiratory syncytial virus. In Fergin, RD and Cherry, JD (eds): Textbook of Pediatric Infectious Diseases, ed 2. WB Saunders, Philadelphia, 1987, pp 1247–1267.

3. Kim HW, et al: Epidemiology of respiratory syncytial virus infection in Washington, DC. Am J Epidemiol 98:216, 1973.

4. Dorland's Illustrated Medical Dictionary. WB Saunders, Philadelphia, 1988, p 1628.

5. Heierholzer, JC and Tannock, GA: Respiratory syncytial virus: A review of the virus, its epidemiology, immune response and laboratory diagnosis. Aust Paediatr J 22:77, 1986.

6. McIntosh, K: Respiratory syncytial virus infections in infants and children. Pediatr Rev 9:191, 1987.

7. Hall, CB, Geiman, JM, and Douglas, RG: Possible transmission by fomites of respiratory syncytial virus. J Infect Dis 141:98, 1980.

8. Hayden, FG and Gwaltney, JM: Viral infections. In Murray, JF and Nadel, JA: Textbook of Respiratory Medicine. WB Saunders, Philadelphia, 1988, pp 782–785.

9. Hall CB, Hall WG, and Speers, DM: Clinical and physiological manifestations of bronchiolitis and pneumonia. Am J Dis Child 133:798, 1979.

10. Barnes, SD, et al: Comparison of nasal brush and nasopharyngeal aspirate techniques in obtaining specimens for detection of respiratory syncytial viral antigen by immunofluorescence. Pediatr Infect Dis J 8:598, 1989.

11. Boruchoff, SE and Cheeseman, SH: Antiviral chemotherapy. In Kass, EH and Platt, R: Current Therapy in Infectious Disease, ed 3. BC Decker, Toronto, 1990, pp 3–4.

12. Patterson, JL and Fernandez-Larsson, R: Molecular mechanisms of action of ribavirin. Rev Infect Dis 12:1139, 1990.

13. Rodriquez, WJ, et al: Aerosolized ribavirin in the treatment of patients with respiratory syncytial virus disease. Pediatr Infect Dis J 6:159, 1987.

14. McBride, JT: Study design considerations for ribavirin: Efficacy studies. Pediatr Infect Dis J 9:574, 1990.

15. Adderley, RJ: Safety of ribavirin with mechanical ventilation. Pediatr Infect Dis J 9:5112, 1990.

16. Outwater, KM, Meissner, HC, and Peterson, MB: Ribavirin administration to infants receiving mechanical ventilation. Am J Dis Child 142:512, 1988.

17. Peter, G (ed): Report of the Committee on Infectious Diseases, ed 21. American Academy of Pediatrics, Elk Grove Village, IL, 1988.

18. Assessin, G: Exposures of health-care personnel to aerosols of ribavirin—California. MMWR 37:560, 1988.

19. Torres, A, et al: Reduced environmental exposure to aerosolized ribavirin using a simple containment system. Pediatr Infect Dis J 10:217, 1991.

20. Janai, HK, et al: Ribavirin: Adverse drug reactions, 1986 to 1988. Pediatr Infect Dis J 9:209, 1990.

21. Bradley, J: Environmental exposure to ribavirin aerosol. Pediatr Infect Dis J 9:595, 1990.

22. Isaacs, D, et al: Handwashing and cohorting in prevention of hospital acquired infections with respiratory syncytial virus. Arch Dis Child 66:227, 1991.

23. LeClair, JM, et al: Prevention of nosocomial respiratory syncytial virus infections through compliance with glove and gown isolation precautions. N Engl J Med 317:329, 1987.

24. Krasinski, K, et al: Screening for respiratory syncytial virus and assignment to a cohort at admission to reduce nosocomial transmission. J Pediatr 116:894, 1990.

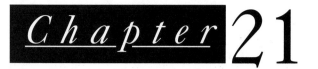

Chapter 21

Patrice A. Johnson, BS, RRT
Cynthia Malinowski, MA, RRT

RESPIRATORY DISTRESS SYNDROME in the NEWBORN

INTRODUCTION

Respiratory distress syndrome (RDS) of the infant is characterized by progressive atelectasis and respiratory failure and is found primarily in the premature newborn. Although many forms of respiratory failure can occur in the newborn, RDS is the most prevalent among premature infants. Advances in the prevention of premature delivery and treatment of RDS have reduced the number of deaths; however, RDS continues to be a significant cause of morbidity and mortality.[1] All neonatal intensive care unit (ICU) clinicians should be able to recognize and treat this common cause of respiratory failure.

ETIOLOGY

The infant with RDS suffers from a surfactant deficiency. Surfactant must be produced in sufficient quantity and quality at birth to prevent collapse of the infant's alveoli at end exhalation. Functionally intact type II alveolar cells are responsible for producing this surface-active material so important for postnatal pulmonary function. The premature infant, however, often does not have a sufficient amount of type II cells at birth and therefore lacks adequate surfactant production. Therefore, the incidence of RDS is inversely related to gestational age and any newborn born prematurely (less than 38 weeks' gestation) is at risk. RDS is most prevalent in the very premature (less than 29 weeks' gestational age) and very low birth weight (less than 1500 g) newborn.[2]

Initially experts thought the sole problem focused on the decreased amount of surfactant produced in the immature lung of premature infants. However, recent research points to more complex problems.[3] The premature newborn not only has a decreased quantity of surfactant but the surfactant that is present is immature and lacks the effectiveness of mature surfactant. It is not clear how well the premature newborn can reuse the existing surfactant.[4] Additionally, the infant with RDS has immature lung parenchyma with decreased alveolar surface area for gas exchange, increased alveolar-capillary membrane thickness, a reduced lung defense system, immature chest wall, and increased capillary permeability.[5,6] A left-to-right shunt through the patent ductus arteriosus is often present with RDS. This shunting pattern leads to increased pulmonary blood flow and pulmonary edema (Fig. 21–1).

353

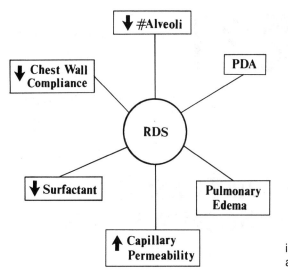

FIGURE 21–1 Diagram showing the abnormalities often associated with RDS.

Any acute episode of asphyxia or reduction in pulmonary perfusion can interfere with appropriate surfactant production and contribute to the onset of RDS. Numerous maternal risk factors such as diabetes, cesarean section without labor, and previous delivery of a newborn with RDS increase the incidence of RDS.[7,8]

PATHOPHYSIOLOGY

The surfactant abnormality leads to alveolar collapse and irregular distribution of ventilation. As more and more alveoli collapse, the newborn must generate greater negative intrapleural pressures during inspiration in order to ventilate. The compliant chest wall of the newborn is an advantage during delivery when the fetus must pass through the birth canal. The compliant chest can be a disadvantage, however, when the infant with RDS inhales and attempts to expand noncompliant lungs. As greater negative intrapleural pressures are generated in an attempt to expand the stiff lungs, the compliant chest wall is pulled inward. This limits lung expansion. The progressive atelectasis causes a reduced functional residual volume, which impairs gas exchange in the lungs.

Hyaline membranes, a proteinaceous substance caused by lung injury, are formed and further reduce the lung compliance; thus, the name hyaline membrane disease is also used to describe this syndrome. Proteinaceous fluid, leaking from areas of epithelial disruption into alveoli, further inactivates any surfactant that may be present.[9] This fluid and worsening hypoxemia resulting from large areas of intrapulmonary shunt lead to further inhibition of surfactant function. A vicious cycle is produced by the continuing pattern of atelectasis, decreased compliance, ventilation-perfusion ($\dot{V}/\dot{Q}$) mismatching, and hypoxemia, which causes further decreases in surfactant production and worsening atelectasis (Fig. 21–2).

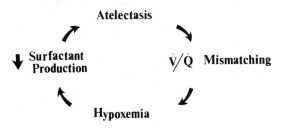

FIGURE 21–2 The vicious cycle contributing to the deteriorating clinical condition of the infant with RDS.

MATERNAL HISTORY

A thorough maternal history is necessary in order to rule out other causes of respiratory distress such as sepsis or congenital cardiac defects. β-streptococcal pneumonia, transmitted prenatally, can mimic RDS.[10] A maternal history of prolonged rupture of the membranes or fever should cause suspicion of sepsis. A maternal history that includes alcohol ingestion, exposure to rubella virus, and maternal diabetes or a previous child with a congenital cardiac defect should lead to investigation for a cardiac defect.[11]

Maternal history also helps to confirm the diagnosis of RDS if risk factors for RDS are present. Those factors include maternal diabetes, history of RDS in siblings, second-born twin, cesarean section with labor, and perinatal asphyxia.[1,12]

CLINICAL FEATURES

The newborn with RDS has signs of distress soon after delivery.[4,12] Retractions are present early in the disease. Grunting, the sound of expiration against a closed glottis, is a mechanism used by the newborn to increase functional residual capacity (FRC). Tachypnea is a common early finding, whereas bradypnea or periods of apnea are late signs of respiratory failure. Nasal flaring and central cyanosis on room air are also typically present.[13] Auscultation may reveal either fine crackles from distal lung units abruptly opening or diminished breath sounds because of shallow tidal volumes.[14]

The chest radiograph will show bilaterally decreased lung volumes, alveolar consolidation, and a ground-glass appearance with air bronchograms. Increased pulmonary vascularity will be seen on the chest radiograph if a patent ductus arteriosus is present.

Pulmonary function testing will show moderate to severe reductions in lung compliance and FRC, but these tests are not regularly done in unstable, critically ill infants. Some newborns will have elevated airway resistance, which, when present, indicates the infant is likely to develop bronchopulmonary dysplasia (see Chapter 22).[15]

The most common abnormality present on arterial blood gas (ABG) analysis in the infant with RDS is hypoxemia. Respiratory acidosis is also common in newborns with moderate to severe disease when the increased work of breathing leads to fatigue.[5,8,9] If a left-to-right shunt through the patent ductus arteriosus is a complicating factor, there may be a metabolic acidosis from the decreased perfusion to the lower body.

The clinical course of the newborn with RDS progresses through a predictable sequence. Typically there is a worsening of symptoms from delivery through the second or third day of life.[16] Respiratory function then generally improves within 72 hours when type II alveolar cell regeneration occurs and surfactant production reappears. Without complications, the newborn recovers within 5 to 7 days. The severely ill infant, who is usually of very low birth weight, often does not respond as quickly to treatment and frequently needs some type of ventilatory assistance.

TREATMENT

The initial resuscitation of the newborn suspected of having RDS should include careful thermoregulation to avoid increased oxygen consumption and metabolic acidosis.[4,17] Oxygen therapy should be instituted to treat hypoxemia and monitored with the use of a continuous noninvasive device such as a transcutaneous monitor or pulse oximeter.

If the infant requires a fraction of inspired oxygen (FIO_2) greater than 0.60 to achieve adequate oxygenation, continuous positive airway pressure (CPAP) is needed. The use of CPAP greatly improves outcome for newborns with RDS when the patient population is of a larger birthweight and older gestational age.[18] The obvious advantage of CPAP in these patients is that it increases FRC and keeps alveoli open throughout exhalation. This increases lung compliance and decreases the work of breathing and usually leads to improved arterial oxygenation at a lower FIO_2.

Currently, a larger population of patients is being treated for RDS in the very low birthweight category (less than 1500 g). CPAP has not been as widely accepted as the most effective treatment in these smaller, more immature newborns who appear to benefit from early intubation and mechanical ventilation rather than a trial of CPAP.[4,19]

Continuous mechanical ventilation is needed when the infant fatigues and cannot maintain adequate ventilation as evidenced by a $PaCO_2$ that exceeds 60 to 70 mm Hg or when sustained apnea is present. If mechanical ventilation is required, high peak inspiratory pressures and positive end-expiratory pressures (PEEP) may be necessary initially because of poor lung compliance.[4,20] Mechanical respiratory rates of up to 60/minute may be needed. The general goals of mechanical ventilation in the infant with RDS are to keep the PaO_2 in the range of 60 to 70 mm Hg, $PaCO_2$ less than 50 to 60 mm Hg, and pH greater than 7.3 while minimizing peak inspiratory pressures and FIO_2. Minimizing peak inspiratory pressures and FIO_2 may reduce the risk of oxygen toxicity, barotrauma, cardiovascular compromise, and bronchopulmonary dysplasia (see Chapter 22).

As mentioned, many premature newborns with RDS have a patent ductus arteriosus (PDA) with a left-to-right shunt complicating their clinical course. Left-to-right shunting through the PDA causes blood to be shunted from the aorta into the pulmonary artery, leading to "flooding" of the pulmonary circulation with blood, which increases pulmonary capillary hydrostatic pressure and leakage of fluid into the alveolar space. The shunting also leads to a decreased perfusion to the descending aorta, which may cause a metabolic acidosis. Clinicians should rapidly identify the presence of a PDA and employ pharmacologic or surgical interventions to close the PDA. Indomethacin, a prostaglandin inhibitor, is often given to help close the PDA (Chapter 23).

Treatment for RDS can include the administration of exogenous surfactant through the endotracheal tube. Improvements in lung compliance and ABGs are likely after the administration of artificial surfactant.[21] The appropriate clinical criteria for the use of surfactant are still under investigation.

Case Study

MATERNAL HISTORY

A 24-year-old, gravida 2, para 1, white woman, approximately 31 weeks pregnant, was admitted with a complaint of lower back pain. She had received prenatal care with regular visits. Medications taken during her pregnancy included only prenatal vitamins. She had been in a car accident 2 weeks earlier; she had been seen by her obstetrician after the accident but had had no difficulty until an hour before admission. Upon arrival to the hospital, she had been determined to be in premature labor and had spontaneous rupture of membranes. The amniotic fluid was clear. Delivery occurred 8 hours after the onset of labor via normal vaginal delivery.

DELIVERY HISTORY

A 31-week estimated gestational age boy was born who weighed 1750 g. The weight was appropriate for the gestational age of the infant. The Apgar scores were 6 and 8 for 1 minute and 5 minutes, respectively. The mother received no Demerol before the delivery. Forceps aided the delivery of the infant, whose presentation was cephalic. No complications were documented by the delivery team.

Questions

1. Why is it important to know the color of the amniotic fluid?
2. Does the fact that there was a normal vaginal delivery have any bearing on the respiratory status of the infant?
3. What significance is there in knowing that the mother did not receive Demerol before the infant's delivery?
4. Is 31 weeks' gestational age considered to be premature?

Answers

1. The amniotic fluid is typically clear. Yellow or green amniotic fluid or green particles in the fluid usually indicates release of meconium (newborn's initial stool), which may occur for different reasons. Most often the release takes place when the infant has had periods of asphyxia. Through the resulting hypoxia, vasoconstriction, peristalsis, and ultimately anal sphincter relaxation, the meconium is emitted to the amniotic fluid.[22] Meconium can cause severe lung damage if drawn into the lungs before or during delivery. If blood is present, the amniotic fluid appears red. Other discolorations can be caused by infection that may develop when there is a prolonged period of time following rupture of the membranes.
2. Yes, the type of delivery can influence the respiratory status of the infant. A vaginal delivery assists with the "squeeze" of the thoracic cavity, which helps to expel amniotic fluid from the lungs. When the chest has not been squeezed, as with cesarean section deliveries, the infant is prone to transient tachypnea of the newborn.[23]
3. Demerol can cross the placental barrier and affect the infant. If a mother received Demerol within a few hours before delivery, the infant has the potential of being lethargic and apneic, requiring more advanced resuscitation.[24] The resuscitation may need to include Narcan to reverse the effects of the Demerol.[17]
4. The gestational age of 31 weeks is considered premature. Term (mature) infants are from 38 to 42 weeks gestational age, with any age less than 38 weeks considered preterm or premature.[11,25]

PHYSICAL EXAMINATION

Vital Signs	*Temperature 36.8°C; pulse 168/minute; respiratory rate 64/minute; blood pressure 53/31 mm Hg; mean arterial pressure 42 mm Hg; and pulse oximeter oxygen saturation 93 percent*
Measurements	*Weight 1750 g (near 50th percentile); head circumference 28 cm (50th percentile); length 42 cm (greater than 50th percentile)*
HEENT	*Head round with some mild molding and mild bruising; anterior fontanelle flat and soft, sutures overlapping; external auditory canals patent; pupils equal, round, and reactive to light and accommodation (PERRLA); nares patent*
Lungs	*Subcostal and intercostal retractions; breathing irregular and fine, with inspiratory crackles (rales) in both lungs*

Heart	*Regular rate and rhythm with no murmur auscultated; pulses equal but diminished bilaterally, brachial, and femoral*
Skin	*Acrocyanosis present; multiple bruising on extremities; initial capillary refill 3 seconds*
Extremities	*Creases on hands and feet; fingers and toes intact bilaterally*
Neurologic	*Good muscle tone; good activity*
Abdomen	*Soft, no bowel sounds heard; no distension; liver down 1.5 cm; umbilical cord containing three vessels*
Genitalia	*Normal male; has voided once, loose meconium stool*

Questions

5. How do you interpret the vital signs?
6. What is indicated by the retractions and inspiratory crackles?
7. What is the differential diagnosis of this infant and what is the most likely diagnosis?
8. What diagnostic tools can be helpful in confirming the diagnosis?

Answers

5. The infant has tachycardia and tachypnea. The normal heart rate for a newborn is 120 to 160/minute, and the normal respiratory rate varies between 35 and 60/minute.[4,17] The infant should be observed closely because these signs could indicate hypoxemia. The blood pressure is within normal range.
6. Retractions indicate a significant increase in the work of breathing. Infants have a very compliant thoracic cage in contrast to adults, who have a very rigid thoracic cage. Retractions occur when the infant generates a more negative intrathoracic pressure to overcome low lung compliance. Because the lungs of the infant with RDS are often less compliant than is the chest wall, the forces of negative intrathoracic pressure collapse the chest wall inward instead of expanding the lungs. The fine crackles indicate either fluid or atelectasis and are consistent with RDS.
7. The differential diagnosis for this patient would include sepsis, pneumonia, and RDS. The history does not indicate a long period of time with ruptured membranes or any maternal fever or infection, so sepsis is not the most likely diagnosis. RDS is the likely diagnosis, but further analysis is necessary to confirm this.
8. A complete blood count (CBC) with white blood cell (WBC) count and differential may help identify the presence of infection. A chest radiograph could help confirm the diagnosis of RDS or pneumonia.

The patient's clinical status began to deteriorate over the next hour with substernal (xiphoid) retractions in addition to the subcostal and intercostal retractions that were observed initially. A chest radiograph was obtained (Fig. 21–3). The infant exhibited nasal flaring and audible grunting. The pulse oximeter saturation was 86 percent on room air. The infant became cyanotic and required a 30 percent oxygen hood in order to improve his color.

The infant's current vital signs were as follows: a heart rate of 160/minute, a

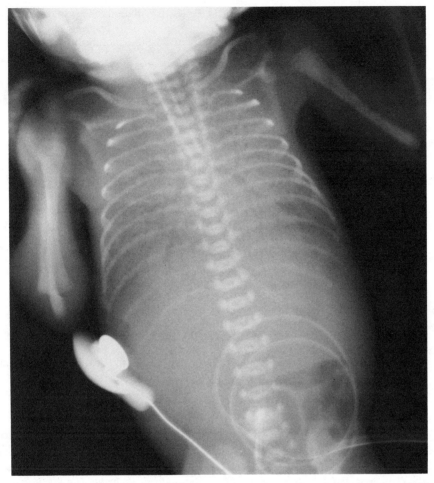

FIGURE 21–3 Chest radiograph obtained in the neonatal intensive care unit (ICU).

respiratory rate of 72/minute, and blood pressure 52/29 mm Hg with a mean arterial pressure of 40 mm Hg. An ABG sample was drawn after the placement of an umbilical artery catheter. The results were as follows: pH 7.31, $Paco_2$ 37, Pao_2 47, HCO_3^- 18 mEq/liter, base excess (BE) −7 mEq/liter.

Questions

9. What is your interpretation of the chest radiograph?
10. What is the cause of the nasal flaring and the audible grunting?
11. Interpret the ABG results.

Answers

9. The chest radiograph demonstrates consolidation throughout both lungs with decreased lung volumes and bilateral air bronchograms.
10. Nasal flaring is an infant's response to an increase in the work of breathing. In an attempt to decrease resistance to airflow into the lungs, the infant increases the diameter of the nostrils upon inspiration. This enables the infant to increase the inspiratory airflow. The audible grunting occurs during exhalation when the exhaled volume is pushed

through a partially closed glottis. With this maneuver an infant may be able to increase FRC.

11. The ABG assessment shows an uncompensated metabolic acidosis with hypoxemia.

The infant's oxygen requirements continued to increase. He was breathing an FI_{O_2} of 0.60 by oxygen hood with the pulse oximeter reading a saturation of 88 percent. The ABG results are: pH 7.26, PaCO_2 50 mm Hg, PaO_2 40 mm Hg. The patient was placed on four (4) cm H_2O CPAP via nasal prongs with an FI_{O_2} of 0.65. The saturation continued to be below acceptable levels and the FI_{O_2} was increased to 0.80.

After increasing the CPAP to 6 cm H_2O and the FI_{O_2} to 0.80, the ABG results were as follows: pH 7.25, PaCO_2 53 mm Hg, PaO_2 39 mm Hg, HCO_3^- 21 mEq/liter, BE −3 mEq/liter.

Questions

12. Interpret the most recent ABG.
13. What treatment is indicated at this time?

Answers

12. The most recent ABG reveals respiratory and metabolic acidosis with severe hypoxemia.
13. Intubation and mechanical ventilation are indicated at this time. Mechanical ventilation is needed because the infant appears to be tiring as evidenced by an increasing PaCO_2. Additionally, the CPAP is not correcting the hypoxemia.

The physician intubated the infant with a 3.5-mm endotracheal tube. Auscultation of the chest and abdomen suggested proper placement of the tube. The infant was manually ventilated to determine the optimal pressures for chest expansion. The mechanical ventilator was set at a peak inspiratory pressure of 22 cm H_2O, a PEEP of 4 cm H_2O, an intermittent mandatory ventilation (IMV) rate of 40/minute, and an FI_{O_2} of 0.80. Within 1 hour of mechanical ventilation the pulse oximeter reading was 96 percent saturation. The infant was pink and had increased activity. The heart rate was 145/minute, respiratory rate 50/minute, mean arterial pressure 48 mm Hg, and skin temperature 37.2°C.

Questions

14. Is this patient a candidate for exogenous surfactant therapy?
15. Why was the infant given CPAP and not directly placed on pressure limit ventilation?
16. What is the cause of the metabolic and respiratory acidosis and the hypoxemia in this patient?

Answers

14. Exogenous surfactants are used as a prophylactic treatment or rescue treatment in infants with RDS. As long as the diagnosis of RDS has been established through clinical and laboratory assessments and all other differential diagnoses have been ruled out, the infant would be consid-

ered a candidate for surfactant therapy.[24,26] Some experts suggest specific criteria be met before rescue treatment with surfactant therapy is implemented. For example, the patient should be mechanically ventilated with peak inspiratory pressures of greater than 18 cm H_2O, an FIO_2 greater than 0.80 to achieve a PaO_2 of greater than 50 mm Hg, and should have an arterial-to-alveolar (a–A) ratio of less than 0.22.[24,27] Additional research needs to be done in order to provide a standard for inclusion criteria.

15. In some premature infants the use of nasal CPAP alone can maintain the patency of the alveoli and avoid the possible trauma of an endotracheal tube and the barotrauma of mechanical ventilation. If the patient does not respond well to CPAP and continues to deteriorate, mechanical ventilation should be considered as in this case.

16. Alveolar collapse throughout the lungs leads to severe problems with gas exchange. With RDS, large areas of the lungs are perfused but not ventilated (shunt), which explains the refractory hypoxemia. The respiratory acidosis is probably the result of inspiratory muscle fatigue from the increased work of breathing. The metabolic acidosis may be caused by tissue hypoxia and the resulting lactic acidosis. Maintaining the infant in a neutral thermal environment will help minimize the tissue hypoxia and lactic acidosis.

The patient improved and by day 4 was extubated and given an FIO_2 of 0.30 by oxygen hood. By the end of the fourth day of life, the FIO_2 was increased to 0.40 because of low SaO_2 values. Upon examination, the patient had mild intercostal retractions and an increase in respiratory rate from 40/minute to 52/minute compared with that of the previous examination. The patient had inspiratory crackles bilaterally and a systolic murmur upon auscultation. It was noted that the patient had bounding pulses and an active precordium. The chest radiograph revealed pulmonary edema and cardiomegaly. Umbilical line ABG measurements were pH 7.30, $PaCO_2$ 37 mm Hg, PaO_2 52 mm Hg, HCO_3^- 18 mEq/liter, and BE −8 mEq/liter.

Questions

17. What is the most likely cause of this patient's respiratory distress?
18. Would the absence of a murmur change the suspected diagnosis?
19. What is the most likely cause of the metabolic acidosis as seen by the ABG?
20. What is the suggested treatment for this patient?

Answers

17. This patient is exhibiting symptoms of a PDA, which is associated with respiratory disease in newborn infants.[28] The ductus arteriosus is the fetal vascular connection between the pulmonary artery and aorta. During the acute stages of respiratory disease, pulmonary vascular resistance can remain high. If the ductus arteriosus remains patent, a small amount of shunting will occur, but not enough to be clinically significant. When the pulmonary vascular resistance drops, with resolving RDS, a PDA will allow for a large amount of blood to shunt from the aorta through the ductus into the pulmonary artery (left-to-right shunt). The increase in pulmonary blood flow leads to pulmonary edema and symptoms of respiratory distress.[4,25] Symptoms of a PDA include bounding pulses, mur-

mur, active precordium, and respiratory distress including retractions, tachypnea, and crackles. The incidence of PDA is highest in low birth-weight infants.[29]

18. Even in the presence of a large PDA, a murmur may be absent. In the absence of a murmur, findings of bounding pulses, active precordium, pulmonary edema, and cardiomegaly should make one suspicious of a PDA.[4,25]

19. The metabolic acidosis is caused by decreased blood flow to the descending aorta and lower extremities. There is a shunting of blood into the pulmonary artery instead of to the descending aorta. The reduction of blood flow leads to the buildup of lactic acids and a metabolic acidosis.

20. A PDA can be treated with indomethacin, which is a prostaglandin synthetase inhibitor. The ductus arteriosus is stimulated to remain open by prostaglandins. Reducing the production of prostaglandins may lead to the closure of the ductus arteriosus. A second method to close the ductus arteriosus is surgical ligation.

After administration of indomethacin, the systolic murmur and pulmonary edema resolved. The patient was weaned to room air within 24 hours. He remained hospitalized for three more weeks until he gained an appropriate amount of weight. There were no other respiratory complications and he was discharged at a weight of 2510 g.

REFERENCES

1. Bryan, H, et al: Perinatal factors associated with the respiratory distress syndrome. Am J Obstet Gynecol 162:476, 1990.

2. Robertson, B: Background to neonatal respiratory distress syndrome and treatment with exogenous surfactant. Dev Pharmacol Ther 13:159, 1989.

3. Morton, N: Pulmonary surfactant: Physiology, pharmacology and clinical uses. Br J Hosp Med 42:52, 1989.

4. Thibeault, D and Gregory, G: Neonatal Pulmonary Care, ed 2. Appleton-Century-Crofts, Norwalk, CT, 1986.

5. Hallman, M and Gluck, L: Respiratory distress syndrome—update 1982. Pediatr Clin North Am 29:1057, 1982.

6. O'Brodovich, H and Mellins, R: Bronchopulmonary dysplasia: Unresolved neonatal acute lung injury. Am Rev Respir Dis 132:694, 1985.

7. Kjos, S, et al: Prevalence and etiology of respiratory distress in infants of diabetic mothers: Predictive values of fetal lung maturation tests. Am J Obstet Gynecol 163:898, 1990.

8. Hodson, W: Hyaline membrane disease—remaining challenges. Semin Respir Med 6:111, 1984.

9. Ikegami, M. et al: A protein from airways of premature lambs that inhibits surfactant function. J Appl Physiol 57:1134, 1984.

10. Ablow, R and Driscoll, S: A comparison of early-onset group B streptococcal neonatal infection and the respiratory distress syndrome of the newborn. N Engl J Med 294:65, 1976.

11. Streeter, N: High Risk Neonatal Care, Aspen Publishers, Rockville, MD, 1986.

12. Lapido, M: Respiratory distress revisited. Neonatal Network 8:9, 1989.

13. Walti, H, et al: Neonatal diagnosis of respiratory distress syndrome. Eur Respir J (Suppl) 3:22s, 1989.

14. Downes, J: Respiratory distress syndrome of newborn infants: New clinical scoring system (RDS score) with acid-base and blood-gas correlations. Clin Pediatr 9:325, 1970.

15. Kraybill, E, et al: Risk factors for chronic lung disease in infants with birth weights of 751 to 1,000 grams. J Pediatr 115:115, 1989.

16. Chatburn, R: Similarities and differences in the management of acute lung injury in neonates (IRDS) and in adults (ARDS). Respir Care 33:539, 1988.

17. Bloom, RS and Cropley, C: Textbook of Neonatal Resuscitation. American Heart Association, American Academy of Pediatrics, Los Angeles, 1988.

18. Gregory, G, et al: Treatment of the idiopathic respiratory-distress syndrome with continuous positive airway pressure. N Engl J Med 284:1333, 1971.

19. Drew, J: Immediate intubation at birth of the very-low birthweight infant. J Dis Child 136:207, 1982.

20. Goldsmith, J and Karotkin, E: Assisted Ventilation of the Neonate, ed 2. WB Saunders, Philadelphia, 1988, p 161.

21. Morton, N: Pulmonary surfactant: Physiology, pharmacology and clinical uses. Br J Hosp Med 42:52, 1989.

22. Rossi, EM, et al: Meconium aspiration syndrome: Intrapartum and neonatal attributes. Am J Obstet Gynecol 161:1106, 1989.

23. Taeusch, HW, Ballard, RA and Avery, ME: Schaffer and Avery's Diseases of the Newborn, ed 6, WB Saunders, Philadelphia, 1988, p 505.

24. Yeh, TF: Neonatal Therapeutics, ed 2. Mosby Year Book, St Louis, 1991.

25. Avery, G: Neonatology, ed 3. JB Lippincott, Philadelphia, 1987.

26. Kwong, M and Egan, E: Reduced incidence of hyaline membrane disease in extremely premature infants following delay of delivery in mother with preterm labor: Use of ritodrine and betamethasone. Pediatrics 78:767, 1986.

27. Exosurf Neonatal: Guidelines for use: 1990. Burroughs Wellcome, Research Triangle Park, NC.

28. Hubbard, C: Ligation of the patent ductus arteriosus in newborn respiratory failure. J Pediatr Surg 21:3, 1986.

29. Cunningham, M, et al: Perinatal risk assessment for patent ductus arteriosus in premature infants. Obstet Gynecol 68:41, 1986

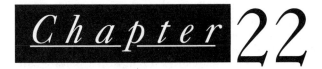

Cynthia Malinowski, MA, RRT

BRONCHOPULMONARY DYSPLASIA

INTRODUCTION

Bronchopulmonary dysplasia (BPD) is a chronic lung disease that occurs in infants who have received mechanical ventilation. The newborns most at risk for developing this disease are those who are born prematurely and are ventilated with high peak inspiratory pressures and/or an increased fraction of oxygen inspired (FIO_2) during mechanical ventilation.[1] Although occurring less often, BPD has been reported in full-term newborns who have also received mechanical ventilation.[2] The reported incidence of BPD varies widely and is inversely related to gestational age. Up to 85 percent of newborns who weigh 500 to 699 g will develop the disease, with the incidence dropping as low as 5 percent in newborns weighing more than 1300 g.[3] The definition of BPD is not standardized and this contributes to the wide variance in the reported incidence.

There is little agreement on the criteria for diagnosis of BPD or for the definition of the disease, and suggestions range from a liberal view, which would include all infants with respiratory sequelae who required an increased FIO_2 for more than 28 days after birth,[4] to more specific criteria involving radiographic and clinical findings. The presence of specific radiographic findings, discussed later in this chapter, helps to confirm the diagnosis. Chest radiographic changes that indicate BPD may not be clearly seen for several weeks after the newborn has developed clinical symptoms of the disease. In the absence of radiographic findings, infants may be diagnosed with BPD if they received mechanical ventilation for more than 7 days, have persistent respiratory distress, and require an FIO_2 higher than room air after 28 days of age.[5] These criteria are usually associated with ruling out other causes of continued respiratory distress such as pneumonia, pulmonary edema, and apnea of prematurity.

Infants treated for BPD can range in age from 3 weeks to a few years. The 3-week-old premature neonate presents different challenges in management than the 1-year-old with home care needs and repeated hospitalizations.

ETIOLOGY

BPD is caused primarily by trauma to the lungs associated with mechanical ventilation.[6,7] The high incidence found in infants with lower gestational ages and birth weights is due to the increased risk of that population to lung injury.[8] The majority of babies with BPD have first been diagnosed with respiratory distress syndrome (RDS) and may have required high inflating pressures and oxygen concentrations because of the poor lung compliance associated with their initial disease process.[9] The fragile immature lung may not tolerate the stretching forces likely to be present with mechanical ventilation. Efforts have been made to single out the factor associated with mechanical ventilation that causes the most harm; for example, is it high peak inspiratory pressures or high mean airway pressures? The evidence is inconclusive as to the exact factor, although most clinicians agree that the use of minimal peak inspiratory pressures may lessen the risk.[10,11]

In addition to delicate airways and alveoli, the premature newborn has immature antioxidant systems. Without antioxidant systems to neutralize oxygen radicals, even a low FIO_2 (0.25 to 0.50) may predispose the lung to damage.[12] The infant with BPD has an increased number of inflammatory cells in the airway. The inflammatory response may be abnormal with an imbalance of protective cells versus destructive cells.[13] This imbalance promotes hydrolysis of the connective tissue matrix. The presence of an endotracheal tube or infection, or both, may also contribute to the injury.[14]

Many infants with BPD have had a patent ductus arteriosus (PDA) at some point in their clinical course, which leads to left-to-right shunting of blood, flooding the pulmonary vasculature.[15,16] The resulting pulmonary edema may contribute to the lung injury in several ways. The presence of pulmonary edema results in greater oxygen requirements (an increased FIO_2), which may worsen the oxygen toxicity problem. Pulmonary edema can render surfactant inactive, resulting in atelectasis, decreased compliance, and the need for higher ventilator pressures.[17] Destruction of the alveolar-capillary membrane also predisposes the infant with BPD to pulmonary edema.

A link between BPD and family history has been suggested owing to the discovery of a high association between a familial history of asthma and reactive airway disease and an increased risk of development of BPD.[4] The etiology of BPD is more likely a combination of factors rather than one single mechanism. Although mechanical ventilation obviously plays a role, disadvantages in premature lung anatomy and physiology contribute to the development of the disease.

PATHOPHYSIOLOGY

In 1967, when BPD was first described by Northway, Rosan, and Porter,[7] it was described as a disease that occurred in stages, associated with specific radiographic changes. Since that time, other clinical investigators, including Northway himself, have reported that many patients with this chronic disease do not clearly follow these specific chest radiographic stages.[18] It is helpful to examine the pathologic changes in the lung that were associated with the originally described radiographic stages.

Stage I is characterized by the presence of hyaline membranes and is often indistinguishable from RDS. Atelectasis is present and necrosis of bronchiolar mucosa has begun. Radiographic findings are similar to those of RDS (Chapter 21).[19]

In stage II there is repair of bronchiolar and alveolar epithelium but also areas of widespread necrosis. Areas of emphysema become evident, and cellular debris may block airways. Atelectatic areas remain a problem, and the radiographic findings may show opacification.[5,20]

Stage III is associated with transition to the classic chronic findings in the lungs of the newborn with severe BPD. There is extensive bronchial and bronchiolar metaplasia and hyperplasia. Thickening of basement membranes occurs, and the alveolar emphysema that has been developing now leads to larger, spherically circumscribed groups of alveoli, often surrounded by continuing atelectatic areas. Increased mucus secretion and interstitial edema are present.[21]

Stage IV is characterized by the presence of fibrosis. Smooth muscle hypertrophy is present. Progressive destruction of alveoli, airways, and vasculature can be seen. Lymphatic and mucous glands are deformed.[5,20]

The results of the lung changes cause ventilation to perfusion defects with areas of atelectasis having less ventilation than perfusion and areas of emphysema having high ventilation and little perfusion. The overall ventilation-perfusion ($\dot{V}/\dot{Q}$) mismatch results in hypoxemia.[9] Thickening membranes and pulmonary edema lead to diffusion defects and decreased gas exchange. Air trapping from alveolar destruction causes elevated Pa_{CO_2}. The infant with severe BPD (stage IV) has an increased FRC because of the air trapping.[2] The airways lose their structural integrity and become floppy, leading to scattered expiratory wheezing.

Mechanical characteristics of the lungs of newborns with BPD include decreased lung compliance and increased airway resistance. Increased airway resistance, possibly due to bronchospasm, may also be related to the development of BPD. Newborns who have subsequently developed BPD have had elevated airway resistance on the first day of life.[22] The infant with BPD may also have an increased amount of secretions and thickening of secretions, contributing to the elevated airway resistance.

CLINICAL FEATURES

The clinical feature first noticed in the infant with BPD may be an inability to wean from mechanical ventilation. Later, there can exist a sensitivity to changes in F_{IO_2} of such a magnitude that there may be large drops in saturation with small decreases in F_{IO_2}.

The infant's general appearance will demonstrate an increased work of breathing, tracheal tugging, chest wall retractions, and tachypnea.[2] The infant in respiratory failure or impending respiratory failure will often remain pink, even in the presence of moderate hypoxemia, because fetal hemoglobin shifts the oxygen-dissociation curve to the left, allowing a higher saturation of hemoglobin for a lower Pa_{O_2}.

Auscultation reveals diffuse fine crackles and expiratory wheezes. The crackles are heard because of the presence of pulmonary edema, which is associated with BPD, or the opening of atelectatic areas on inspiration that have closed during expiration. Wheezes result from bronchospasm, anatomic narrowing of airways, or narrowing due to secretions.

The chest radiograph may not be definitive for BPD until later in the disease when various degrees of irregular densities (from atelectasis and the formation of fibrosis), and areas of hyperlucency can be seen.[23] The overexpansion is caused by air trapping similar to that occurring in adult chronic obstructive pulmonary disease (COPD) patients. The radiographic pattern in advanced BPD is often described as "bubbly" or cystic in appearance.[24] Complications such as pulmonary edema or pneumonia may obscure the radiographic chronic changes of BPD.

Pulmonary function studies typically reveal elevated total airway resistance, decreased lung compliance, and increased work of breathing.[25] In most cases pulmonary function testing is not done.

Arterial blood gas (ABG) measurements are similar to those seen in adults with COPD. Hypoxemia and a compensated to partially compensated respiratory acidosis are common findings. The hypoxemia usually responds to oxygen therapy.

An important part of the assessment of the newborn suspected of having BPD is to rule out other causes of continuing respiratory compromise such as sepsis, aspiration, seizure disorders, apnea, immature chest wall, the presence of PDA, or intraventricular hemorrhage (IVH). In the newborn with respiratory distress and oxygen dependency lasting for longer than 28 days, a complete blood count (CBC), blood cultures, and ultrasound for PDA and IVH may be needed to rule out other causes of the respiratory compromise.

TREATMENT

Treatment of BPD is supportive, emphasizing adequate nutrition and oxygenation to provide an environment for healthy lung growth. Although areas of lung damage may be permanent, the newborn has the ability to continue generating alveolar tissue. If the ratio of healthy alveoli to damaged alveoli improves, the newborn has a better opportunity to be weaned from the damaging effects of the mechanical ventilator.

Pharmacologic agents used in treatment of BPD include bronchodilators, diuretics, and steroids.[26] Bronchodilators decrease the high airway resistance that is often seen in these infants.[27] Treatment with bronchodilators is warranted if wheezing, retractions, and gas trapping are noted. Isoproterenol, terbutaline, metaproterenol, albuterol, and isoetharine are the bronchodilators most commonly used in the treatment of BPD.[28] There does not appear to be a superiority of one bronchodilator over another.

Theophylline may be beneficial in reducing airway resistance and improving compliance in infants who are difficult to wean from mechanical ventilation.[4,28,29]

Diuretics are often necessary in infants with increased oxygenation requirements associated with pulmonary edema.[30] Excessive weight gain from the retention of fluid may precede pulmonary edema and identify the patient in whom diuretics may be necessary.

Steroid administration leads to short-term improvements in pulmonary function in infants with BPD.[24] There is no clear evidence that the use of steroids leads to a decreased hospital stay, decreased duration of oxygen therapy, or decreased mortality. Steroids are also associated with side effects such as infection, hyperglycemia, and hypertension. Immunosuppression associated with the use of steroids is also a concern in the newborn who may already have an underdeveloped immune system.[6] Even with the potential hazards and lack of evidence of long-term efficacy, steroids occasionally are used in the infant with BPD who has become ventilator dependent and is difficult to wean.

The spontaneously breathing newborn suspected of having BPD may need intubation and mechanical ventilation. ABG criteria for respiratory failure in the newborn vary but generally are considered as pH less than 7.25, $Paco_2$ greater than 60 mm Hg, and/or Pao_2 less than 50 mm Hg on an Fio_2 greater than 0.60 to 0.80.[19,26]

Mechanical ventilation may be necessary for weeks or even months in some infants with BPD. Although there is no conclusive evidence that one strategy for mechanical ventilation is superior to another in these infants, it is generally agreed that the lowest peak inspiratory pressure and Fio_2 necessary to achieve acceptable ABG levels should be employed.[4,11] Inspiratory times should be long enough to provide even distribution of gases but allow adequate expiratory times to ensure emptying of the lung and prevention of gas trapping. Low levels of positive end-expiratory pressure (PEEP) (2 to 4 cm H_2O) are helpful in preventing atelectasis. Higher levels may be necessary in the presence of complicating pulmonary edema but should be used with caution as the infant with BPD is prone to air trapping and overexpansion.

The acceptable arterial blood gas values are often different for the infant with BPD. For example, the newborn with BPD may be allowed to have a $Paco_2$ within a range of 50 to 70 mm Hg as long as the pH remains greater than 7.28. Although the infant with BPD often requires an increased Fio_2 and is difficult to oxygenate, it appears beneficial for their growth to maintain an adequate Pao_2.[31] In addition, hypoxemia leads to pulmonary vasoconstriction and pulmonary hypertension in infants with BPD.[32] A Pao_2 range of 55 to 65 mm Hg is considered acceptable in these patients.[11]

If mechanical ventilation is an important etiologic factor, then weaning as soon as possible may reduce lung damage. Aggressive weaning from the ventilator in the newborn not yet diagnosed with BPD or showing very mild symptoms of BPD can prevent a severe chronic pattern from developing. The early use of continuous positive airway pressure (CPAP) in premature newborns with RDS has been advocated to avoid the need for mechanical ventilation, also possibly preventing BPD.[33] Intravenous (IV) aminophylline can be used in conjunction with weaning from mechanical ventilation to facilitate the success of the weaning procedure.

Monitoring of the infant during mechanical ventilation usually includes the use of pulse oximetry. Transcutaneous monitoring has been less popular than oximetry in these infants because their transcutaneous Po_2 and Pco_2 values do not correlate well with their arterial values.[34]

Vitamins A and E are being investigated for use as a prophylactic treatment for BPD, to reduce oxygen induced lung damage and promote normal lung healing.[2,11] Controlled trials with the use of these vitamins are necessary before conclusions can be made.

The infant with BPD needing long-term mechanical ventilation may benefit from tracheotomy.[35] A tracheotomy can allow greater movement of the infant's head and improvement in feeding, both contributing to better overall development. However, because the complication rate and mortality from tracheotomies in pediatric patients is higher than those in adults, many clinicians leave the infant with chronic lung disease intubated for long periods of time, even several months, before considering tracheotomy.[36]

The infant may be discharged while still receiving oxygen therapy, and home care must be provided. The home care of infants and children requiring respiratory therapy is evolving into a subspecialty that requires special education.

OUTCOME

Mortality rates associated with BPD have been reported between 11 and 29 percent.[37,38] Northway[39] had reported that 34 percent of infants with BPD had handicaps that included cerebral palsy, neurologic deficit, deafness, and blindness. Others[4] have reported similar adverse outcomes, although if placed in a favorable home environment with proper attention to nutrition, the patient has improved neurologic development.

An increased incidence of infections and repeated hospitalizations are frequently found in this population of infants. Pulmonary function studies may remain abnormal, demonstrating reactive airway disease. The infant with BPD may become a child with respiratory problems such as wheezing and airway obstruction.[40]

Case Study

HISTORY

Baby N is a 33-day-old prematurely born boy who weighs 1420 g. At birth his estimated gestational age was 28 weeks. His initial diagnosis was RDS and PDA. He received mechanical ventilation for 3 weeks with peak inspiratory pressure recorded as high as 38 cm H_2O with an Fio_2 between 0.60 and 0.80 for more than 1 week. Initial radiographic findings were low lung volumes, ground-glass appearance, and air bronchograms. The patient received indomethacin therapy to close his ductus arteriosus at 1 week of age. He was extubated and was on a 35 percent oxygen hood. An examination revealed a respiratory rate of 78/minute; moderate substernal, subcostal and intercostal chest wall retractions; and crackles bilaterally. ABG findings show pH 7.28, $Paco_2$ 62 mm Hg, Pao_2 40 mm Hg, base excess (BE) +4, HCO_3^- 30 mEq/liter.

Questions

1. What are the indications of respiratory distress and what further information should be gathered?
2. What is the differential diagnosis of this patient's problem and what is the most likely diagnosis?
3. What is your interpretation of the ABG and what is the most likely cause of the decreased Pao_2?

Answers

1. The indications of respiratory distress include tachypnea (respiratory rate 78/minute) and chest wall retractions. Additionally, an ABG analysis reveals hypoxemia on an Fio_2 of 0.35. Average respiratory rates for newborns are between 30 and 60/minute, with rates in the higher range typical for infants of this patient's gestational age group. More importantly, the infant's current respiratory rate should be compared with rates counted in the past 48 hours to see if there has been an increase. Further information to gather includes a chest radiograph and CBC.
2. Differential diagnosis includes sepsis, aspiration, pulmonary edema from fluid overload, and BPD. There is not enough evidence at this point to identify which of the suggested problems is causing the respiratory distress. The history of mechanical ventilation strongly suggests BPD. In sepsis, there are more likely findings of apnea and bradycardia episodes,[41] which are not a part of this patient's clinical findings. Blood cultures and a CBC would be important to rule out sepsis as a cause of the infant's respiratory distress. If the patient had aspirated, the clinical findings would likely be more acute.
3. The ABG reveals partially compensated respiratory acidosis with moderate hypoxemia. The decreased Pao_2 is caused by $\dot{V}/\dot{Q}$ mismatching and alveolar hypoventilation. The hypoxemia could also be caused by pulmonary edema, occurring as a result of injury to the aveolar capillary membranes.

PHYSICAL EXAMINATION

General   *Patient is alert and agitated, under an oxygen hood. He is pink but appears to be in moderate respiratory distress.*

Vital Signs   *Temperature 36.3°C, respiratory rate 78/minute, pulse 166/minute, blood pressure 64/48 mm Hg*

HEENT   *Patient normocephalic with anterior fontanelle 2 × 2 cm soft and normotensive; pupils equally round and reactive to light; mild nasal flaring present; throat clear*

Neck   *Supple, without lymphadenopathy, but slightly increased tracheal tugging noted; no stridor*

Chest   *Normal anteroposterior (AP) diameter with symmetric expansion; moderate substernal, subcostal, and intercostal retractions present*

Lungs   *Rapid respiratory rate with fine inspiratory crackles throughout anterior lung fields bilaterally; wheezes heard on expiration*

Heart   *Regular rate and rhythm without murmur*

Abdomen	*Soft, nontender, nondistended with active bowel sounds and no hepatosplenomegaly*
Extremities	*Strong pulses in the upper and lower extremities bilaterally; no evidence of clubbing, cyanosis, or edema*

Questions

4. What is the cause of the chest wall retractions?
5. Does the absence of a fever indicate no infectious process is occurring?
6. Does the fact that the infant's color is pink ensure adequate oxygenation?
7. Why does tracheal tugging occur and what is the cause of it?
8. What is the cause of the expiratory wheezes?
9. What is the significance of the presence of crackles?

Answers

4. Chest wall retractions are present because of a high chest wall compliance and low lung compliance. When a large intrapleural subatmospheric pressure is generated by the diaphragm, the compliant chest wall collapses inward at the points of least resistance. As the infant's lung compliance worsens and greater diaphragmatic contractions are generated, the retractions will worsen.

5. The absence of fever does not necessarily indicate that the patient is free of infection. Sepsis can be associated with transient temperature imbalances that include hyperthermia or hypothermia.[4] An additional complicating factor with regard to assessment of body temperature is that the premature newborn's body temperature is often regulated by an incubator. The incubator temperature must be assessed as well as the infant's body temperature to help with the interpretation of changes in body temperature.[41] For example, if the newborn has a normal core temperature but the incubator temperature has been increased several degrees to maintain the normal core temperature, this may indicate thermal instability.

6. The term newborn has only 25 percent adult hemoglobin and the premature newborn may have 0 percent adult hemoglobin.[42] Pink color in an infant does not ensure adequate oxygenation because fetal hemoglobin shifts the oxygen-hemoglobin dissociation curve to the left. The left-shifted curve means that the infant has a higher saturation at a lower Pao_2. The higher saturation of hemoglobin makes the detection of cyanosis difficult. The newborn may remain pink until the Pao_2 drops very low — as low as 40 mm Hg in some premature newborns.[6,42] Fetal hemoglobin can be present in infants until 6 months of age. Although this patient is 33 days old, it is likely that he has significant amounts of fetal hemoglobin. The amount may vary as a result of the amount and frequency of transfusions of adult hemoglobin blood that this infant may have received. Therefore, adequate oxygenation cannot be assumed based on the patient's pink color.

7. Tracheal tugging is an indication of respiratory distress. The infant with BPD has a low, flat diaphragm, similar to that of an adult with emphysema. When this low, flat diaphragm moves downward, the central diaphragmatic tendon pulls the trachea downward also, causing a tracheal tug.[43]

8. Wheezing can be caused by narrowing of the airways, viscous airway secretions, and floppy airway walls. Bronchospasm with increased airway resistance is associated with BPD.

9. Crackles are often present in infants with BPD complicated by pulmonary

edema. Pulmonary edema can be present in BPD owing to increased capillary permeability, fluid overload, or the presence of an open ductus arteriosus. Left-to-right shunting through the ductus arteriosus causes blood to be shunted away from the aorta and into the pulmonary vasculature, leading to high hydrostatic pressure and leaking of fluid into the lung. This patient is 33 days old and the presence of a PDA is usually diagnosed earlier in the clinical course.

LABORATORY EVALUATION

CHEST RADIOGRAPH

(Fig. 22–1)

ABGs

pH 7.30; $Paco_2$ 71 mm Hg; Pao_2 49 mm Hg; BE^+ 6, HCO_3^- 35 mEq/liter; oxygen by hood at Fio_2 0.6

CBC (See Appendix for normal values.)

White blood cells (WBCs) 13,000/mm³; red blood cells (RBC) 3.7 million/mm³, segs 58 percent, bands 1 percent, lymphocytes 37 percent, monocytes 1 percent, eosinophils 1 percent, hemoglobin (Hb) 12.9 g/100 mL, hematocrit (Hct) 38 percent.

During the time of this laboratory evaluation, the infant required the Fio_2 to be increased to 0.70 based on pulse oximetry saturation values below 88 percent. The respiratory rate increased to 82/minute, and chest wall retractions became severe.

Questions

10. How would you interpret the ABG results?
11. What abnormalities are present on the chest radiograph and what pathophysiology is causing the chest radiograph results?
12. What is significant about the CBC results?
13. What is your suggestion for therapy for this patient?
14. At what point would you consider intubation?
15. What range would you like to have the Pao_2 in?

Answers

10. These ABGs reflect a partially compensated respiratory acidosis and hypoxemia. The pH is lower than normally acceptable; however, infants with BPD may not have the ability to compensate completely for a respiratory acidosis because of a decreased ability for renal retention of bicarbonate.[44]

    In order to make decisions for care of this patient, the ABG results would best be interpreted by examining the trend of the patient's ABGs. If the acid-base status is typical for this patient, there may be a different recommendation for therapy than if this represents a significant change. Interpreted alone, these ABGs represent typical values for infants with BPD. The Pao_2 is below the acceptable range and represents significant hypoxemia.

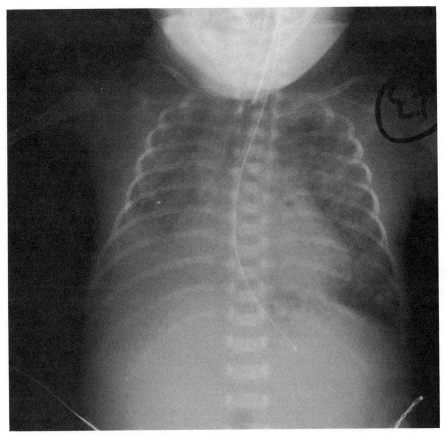

FIGURE 22–1 Chest radiograph of the infant.

11. The chest radiograph shows hyperexpanded lungs with irregular bilateral perihilar streaky densities. The hyperinflation is typical of infants with BPD. Grossly, the lungs of infants with BPD have been described as having areas of emphysematous alveoli caused by cystic dilation of distal airways interspersed with dense fibrotic areas.[45] The air trapping from the emphysematous component leads to the hyperinflation, and the fibrotic areas are represented by the irregular streaky densities.

12. The significance of the CBC results is the absence of findings consistent with sepsis. There is no left shift or abnormally low or high WBC value. A newborn can have an abnormally low or high number of WBCs during an active infection.[41] A WBC value of 13,000 is considered normal for an infant this age.

13. The presence of wheezing is an indication for bronchodilator therapy. Aerosolized sympathomimetic agents such as metaproterenol, terbutaline, or isoetharine may provide relief for bronchoconstriction. The use of theophylline in infants with BPD has appeared beneficial in some cases, but because of potential relaxation of the cardiac esophageal junction allowing reflux, these agents are used with caution. Additional therapy for this patient would include an increase in the F_{IO_2} to alleviate the hypoxemia.

14. There are two factors to consider in a decision to intubate this patient: The work of breathing and the evidence of respiratory failure by ABGs. This patient does not meet the ABG criteria for respiratory failure

because the pH is greater than 7.28, but he may be considered to be in impending respiratory failure as evidenced by an increase in respiratory rate, increased respiratory retractions, and increasing F_{IO_2} requirements. This may be cause for intubation even before the stated ABG criteria are met.

15. The Pa_{O_2} should be maintained in the range of 55 to 65 mm Hg. If values greater than 55 mm Hg can be achieved it is better to use the lowest F_{IO_2} necessary to be within the stated range. It is important to understand that these desired Pa_{O_2} values are ABG values and not those obtained from the heel (capillary blood gas values). Heel-stick P_{O_2} values do not reflect arterial values. Because of the difficulty in acquiring accurate arterial Pa_{O_2} values in the chronically ill newborn, pulse oximetry is used to monitor oxygenation. Values in the 90 to 95 percent saturation range are commonly the goal of oxygen therapy. It is necessary to maintain adequate oxygenation in patients with BPD because their growth rate and right ventricular function improve when chronic hypoxemia is avoided.[31]

The patient's F_{IO_2} was increased to 0.80 over the course of an hour while monitoring the infant with a pulse oximeter, to keep the saturation between 90 and 95 percent. He continued to have evidence of respiratory distress with retractions and tachypnea. Aerosolized medication treatments were ordered with terbutaline 0.25 mL in 2.75 mL saline. The patient's wheezing decreased after treatment. Oxygen requirement fluctuated but was eventually reduced to 0.45. Two days later it was noted that a weight gain in excess of 60 g/day (normal weight gain should be less than 50 g/day in a newborn this size) had been measured for two consecutive days. Crackles continued to be heard bilaterally and a repeat chest radiograph revealed pulmonary edema superimposed on changes consistent with BPD. Respiratory rate increased to 90/minute, and heart rate was 150/minute. ABG results on a 1-liter/minute nasal cannula were pH 7.27, Pa_{CO_2} 85 mm Hg, Pa_{O_2} 40 mm Hg, HCO_3^- 37 mEq/L, BE^+ 8. Because of evidence of impending respiratory failure, the patient was intubated and given pressure-limited ventilation.

Questions

16. What is the cause of this patient's pulmonary edema?
17. Can any bronchodilator therapy changes be made?
18. Can the low Pa_{O_2} be treated with a higher F_{IO_2} instead of intubation and mechanical ventilation?
19. What is the F_{IO_2} for this patient on 1 liter/minute?
20. Is there any additional pharmacologic therapy that can be used in this patient?
21. What initial ventilator settings would you suggest for this patient?

Answers

16. This patient had a previous history of PDA, which was treated with indomethacin. It is unlikely at the age of 33 days, the ductus would reopen and cause pulmonary edema. Because a PDA seems unlikely, the probable cause of pulmonary edema is the combination of increased capillary permeability and high pulmonary vascular pressures. Because pulmonary edema can be caused by fluid overload, the intake and output on this patient should be examined.

17. The findings do not indicate that the cause of his increasing respiratory distress is bronchoconstriction. This pattern of pulmonary edema and increased respiratory distress may be repeated during the course of his disease. As there is no evidence that one bronchodilator agent is superior to another in treatment of BPD, changing the medication probably will not have any effect on the patient's course.

18. Even though the patient shows evidence of continuing compensation for the respiratory acidosis, other signs indicate that he is in impending respiratory failure. His continued low Pao_2, increase in respiratory rate, increase in heart rate, crackles, and weight gain all indicate a clinical picture of decompensation. Increasing his Fio_2 may improve his Pao_2 and is indicated as an immediate step, but will probably be only a temporary solution to his continued low Pao_2.

19. The Fio_2 of an infant on a 1-liter/minute cannula is not known. As in adults, the Fio_2 is variable and influenced by the patient's ventilatory pattern. It is more likely that the infant will have a high Fio_2 associated with low flows because of their small peak inspiratory flows and shallow breathing patterns. This patient may be receiving an Fio_2 as high as 0.60 on 1-liter/minute nasal cannula. In this case it can be deceptive to consider the patient stable because he is on only a 1-liter/minute cannula.

20. Because he has had excessive weight gain, crackles, and chest radiograph indicative of pulmonary edema, diuretics should be considered. Conservative management of this patient may include the use of diuretics before intubation to see if there is improvement in his respiratory distress. It may still be considered appropriate to intubate him before or during the administration of diuretics because of his continued deterioration and hypoxemia.

21. In order to determine ventilator settings, an assessment can be made after the patient is intubated and is being manually ventilated. Chest excursion is observed and a peak inspiratory pressure chosen that causes chest movement. The lowest possible peak inspiratory pressure should be used to avoid further lung damage. PEEP should be applied to all newborns on mechanical ventilation, and in this case levels of 2 to 4 cm H_2O should be used.[46] A typical respiratory rate to start out with is 40 to 50 breaths/minute. Inspiratory to expiratory (I:E) ratios should favor longer expiratory times to avoid air trapping. A common order for settings on a infant with this diagnosis would be intermittent mandatory ventilation (IMV) 40/minute, peak inspiratory pressure (PIP) 24 cm H_2O, PEEP 2 cm H_2O, Fio_2 0.60, I:E ratio 1:2.5.

Over the next 3 weeks the patient was extubated twice and reintubated twice for respiratory failure. In each instance of extubation, he required an increased Fio_2 and demonstrated worsening respiratory distress. He has had one more episode of pulmonary edema treated with diuretics. His ventilator settings were 20 to 30 cm H_2O, IMV 40 to 50/minute, PEEP 2 to 5, Fio_2 0.50 to 0.80. The patient became very sensitive to small Fio_2 and PIP changes.

Questions

22. What are the possibilities for treatment of this patient at this point?
23. What is the prognosis for this patient based on his current course?

Answers

22. A trial of aminophylline may decrease airway resistance, improve diaphragmatic function, and allow the infant to be weaned from mechanical ventilation. Tracheotomy may be considered if the patient continues to be ventilator dependent. Advantages of tracheotomy in this patient include better opportunities for environmental stimulation, better range of motion, and more normal feeding habits.

    The use of steroids could also be considered at this point, although, as previously mentioned, there is no evidence that steroid administration in infants with BPD alters long-term outcome.

23. Mortality rates from 11 to 29 percent have been reported for BPD. It is not possible to predict if this patient will survive at this time.[47] The patients who die of BPD often have histories of weeks of mechanical ventilation, difficulty weaning, and high F_{IO_2} requirements. If this patient does survive his chronic lung disease, his future outcome may involve ongoing health problems, neurologic developmental problems, abnormalities of language development, and hearing difficulties.

The hospital course of this patient included another 3 months in the newborn intensive care unit, repeated attempts at extubation, pneumonia, and nutritional difficulties. He was eventually successfully extubated 6 months after admission and went home on oxygen therapy. Three months later he was weaned from oxygen therapy. He was followed and treated for reactive airway problems, which led to his home use of bronchodilator therapy.

REFERENCES

1. Palta, M, et al: Development and validation of an index for scoring baseline respiratory disease in the very low birth weight neonate. Pediatrics 86:714, 1990.

2. O'Brodovich, H: Bronchopulmonary dysplasia. Unsolved neonatal acute lung injury. Am Rev Respir Dis 132:694, 1985.

3. Bancalari, E: Pathogenesis of bronchopulmonary dysplasia: An overview. In Bancalari, E and Stocker, JT (eds): Bronchopulmonary Dysplasia. Hemisphere Publishing, Cambridge, 1988, pp 3–15.

4. Taeusch, H, Ballard, R, and Avery, M: Schaffer and Avery's Diseases of the Newborn, ed 6. WB Saunders, Philadelphia, 1991, p 519.

5. Bailey, P and Giltman, L: Bronchopulmonary dysplasia: An update. Respir Care 30:771, 1985.

6. Avery, G: Neonatology, ed 3. JB Lippincott, Philadelphia, 1987, p 451.

7. Northway, WH, Rosan, RC, and Porter, DY: Pulmonary disease following respirator therapy of hyaline membrane disease—bronchopulmonary dysplasia. N Engl J Med 276:357, 1967.

8. Murphy, J: The human lung at 24 to 26 weeks gestation: Watershed of survival. Semin Respir Med 6:103, 1984.

9. Jackson, J: Bronchopulmonary dysplasia: Challenges for research. Semin Respir Med 6:119, 1984.

10. Kraybill, E and Runyan, D: Risk factors for chronic lung disease in infants with birth weights of 751 to 1000 grams. J Pediatr 115:115, 1989.

11. Goldberg, R and Bancalari, E: Therapeutic approaches to the infant with bronchopulmonary dysplasia. Respir Care 36:613, 1991.

12. Frank, L and Groseclose, EE: Preparation for birth into an O_2 rich environment: The antioxidant enzymes in the developing rabbit lung. Pediatr Res 18:240, 1984.

13. Ogden, B, et al: Neonatal lung neutrophils and elastase/proteinase inhibitor imbalance. Am Rev Respir Dis 130:817, 1984.

14. Stern, L, et al: Negative pressure artificial respiration: Use and treatment of respiratory failure of the newborn. Can Med Assoc J 102:595, 1970.

15. Dudell, GG and Gersony, WM: Patent ductus arteriosus in neonates with severe respiratory disease. J Pediatr 104:915, 1984.

16. Brown, ER, et al: Bronchopulmonary dysplasia: Possible relationship to pulmonary edema. J Pediatr 92:982, 1978.

17. Kobayashi, T, Nitta, K, and Ganzuka, M: Inactivation of exogenous surfactant by pulmonary edema fluid. Pediatr Res 29:353, 1991.

18. Bancalari, E, Abdenour, G, and Feller, R: Bronchopulmonary dysplasia: Clinical presentation. J Pediatr 95:819, 1979.

19. Thibeault, D and Gregory, G: Neonatal Pulmonary Care, ed 2. Appleton-Century-Crofts, Norwalk, CT, 1986, p 698.

20. Kirkpatrick, B and Mueller, D: Bronchopulmonary dysplasia. In Kendig, E (ed): Disorders of the Respiratory Tract in Children, ed 4. WB Saunders, Philadelphia, 1983, p 819.

21. Taghizadeh, A and Reynolds, E: Pathogenesis of bronchopulmonary dysplasia following hyaline membrane disease. Am J Pathol 82:241, 1976.

22. Oliphant, M, et al: Pulmonary parenchymal patterns at one month as a prognostic indicator in neonatal chronic lung disease. Perinatol Neonatol Sept/Oct:21, 1987.

23. Fitzgerald, P, et al: Bronchopulmonary dysplasia: A radiographic and clinical review of 20 patients. Br J Radiol 63:444, 1990.

24. Greenough, A: Bronchopulmonary dysplasia: early diagnosis, prophylaxis, and treatment. Arch Dis Child 65:1082, 1990.

25. Gerhardt, T, et al: Serial determination of pulmonary function in infants with chronic disease. J Pediatr 110:448, 1987.

26. Koff, P, et al: Neonatal and Pediatric Respiratory Care. CV Mosby, St Louis, 1988, p 75.

27. Kao, L, et al: Effect of isoproterenol inhalation on airway resistance in chronic bronchopulmonary dysplasia. Pediatrics 73:509, 1984.

28. Davis, J, Sinkin, R, and Aranda, J: Drug therapy for bronchopulmonary dysplasia. Pediatr Pulm 8:117, 1990.

29. Northway, W: Bronchopulmonary dysplasia: Then and now. Arch Dis Child 65:1076, 1990.

30. Southall, D and Samuels, M: Bronchopulmonary dysplasia: A new look at management. Arch Dis Child 65:1089, 1990.

31. Cox, M, et al: Improved growth in infants with bronchopulmonary dysplasia treated with nasal cannula oxygen (abstract). Pediatr Res 13:492, 1979.

32. Southall, DP, Samuels, MP, and Talbert, DG: Recurrent cyanotic episodes with severe arterial hypoxaemia and intrapulmonary shunting: A mechanism for sudden death. Arch Dis Child 65:953, 1990.

33. Avery, ME, Tooley, WH, and Keller, JB: Is chronic lung disease in low birthweight infants preventable? A survey of 8 centres. Pediatrics 79:26, 1987.

34. Hamilton, PA, Whitehead, MD, and Reynolds, EOR: Underestimation of arterial oxygen tension by transcutaneous electrode with increasing age in infants. Arch Dis Child 60:1162, 1985.

35. Carlo, W and Chatburn, R: Neonatal Respiratory Care, ed 2. Year Book Publishers, Chicago, 1988, p 360.

36. Handler, S: Pediatric tracheostomy: Experience during the past decade. Ann Otol Rhinol Laryngol 91:628, 1982.

37. Sauve, R and Singhal, N: Long-term morbidity of infants with bronchopulmonary dysplasia. Pediatrics 76:725, 1985.

38. Yip, Y and Tan, K: Bronchopulmonary dysplasia in very low birthweight infants. J Paediatr Child Health 27:34, 1991.

39. Northway, WH: Observations on bronchopulmonary dysplasia. J Pediatr 95:815, 1979.

40. Smyth, JA, et al: Pulmonary function and bronchial hyperreactivity in long term survivors of bronchopulmonary dysplasia. Pediatrics 68:336, 1981.

41. Streeter, N: High Risk Neonatal Care. Aspen Publishers, Rockville, MD, 1986, p 389.

42. Bancalari, E and Flynn, J: Respiratory physiology, oxygen therapy, and monitoring. Birth Defects 24:41, 1988.

43. Glauser, F: Signs and symptoms in pulmonary medicine. JB Lippincott, Philadelphia, 1983, p 113.

44. Farnaroff, A and Martin, R: Neonatal-Perinatal Medicine: Diseases of the Fetus and Infant, ed 5. St Louis, CV Mosby, 1987, p 1296.

45. Taghizadeh, A and Reynolds, E: Pathogenesis of bronchopulmonary dysplasia following hyaline membrane disease. Am J Pathol 82:241, 1976.

46. Carlo, W and Martin, R: Principles of neonatal assisted ventilation. Pediatric Clin North Am 33:221, 1986.

47. Markestad, T and Fitzharding, P: Growth and development in children recovering from BPD. J Pediatr 98:597, 1981.

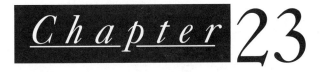

Cynthia Malinowski, MA, RRT

PERSISTENT PULMONARY HYPERTENSION of the NEWBORN

INTRODUCTION

The lungs do not participate in gas exchange before birth, as this is the function of the placenta. The lack of oxygen in the lungs causes the pulmonary vasculature to constrict, resulting in a marked elevation of the pulmonary vascular resistance (PVR). The elevated PVR inhibits blood flow through the lungs and causes blood to bypass the lungs via two normal fetal circulatory shunts known as the **ductus arteriosus** and the **foramen ovale.** The ductus arteriosus is a connection between the pulmonary artery and the aorta. The foramen ovale is an opening between the right and left atria (Fig. 23–1). Blood flow through these two fetal shunts allows most of the oxygenated blood returning from the placenta to bypass the lungs by shunting from right to left into the systemic circulation.

After birth, the pulmonary vasculature dilates as oxygen enters the lungs. The associated drop in PVR and simultaneous increase in systemic blood pressure cause the fetal shunts to close and pulmonary blood flow to increase significantly. If the PVR does not decrease after birth, the fetal shunts will remain patent and blood flow to the lungs will remain low. This syndrome, which consists of a high PVR, low pulmonary blood flow, and a fetal state of circulation, is known as persistent pulmonary hypertension of the newborn (PPHN).[1] Although this condition may be treatable, the newborn with persistent pulmonary hypertension has a high mortality risk.[2]

ETIOLOGY

PPHN is a syndrome with a variety of clinical causes. Any pulmonary or cardiac disease that causes reactive pulmonary capillary constriction, an increase in pulmonary arterial musculature, or hypoplasia of the pulmonary vascular bed (with decreased total vascular area) may cause PPHN (Table 23–1).[1,3–5] After birth these babies maintain an elevated PVR that leads to persistent pulmonary hypertension (PPH).

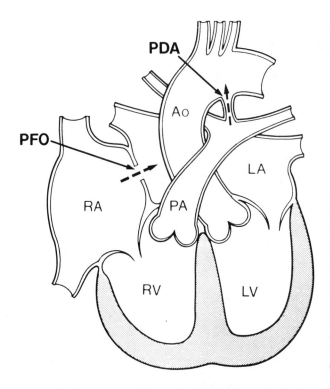

FIGURE 23–1 Fetal circulation is illustrated, showing right-to-left shunting *(dashed arrows)* through patent ductus arteriosus (PDA), pulmonary artery (PA) to aorta (AO), and patent foramen ovale (PFO), right atrium (RA) to left atrium (LA). (Modified from Graves, E, et al: Persistent pulmonary hypertension in the neonate. Chest 93:638, 1988, with permission.) RV = Right ventricle; LV = left ventricle.

PATHOPHYSIOLOGY

Diminished pulmonary blood flow associated with PPHN results in areas of the lung where ventilation exceeds perfusion (high ventilation-perfusion ratio [$\dot{V}/\dot{Q}$]). Although the blood returning to the heart from the lung is well oxygenated (unless respiratory disease is the cause of the PPH), a significant portion of the venous return is shunted through the ductus arteriosus and the foramen ovale into the arterial system. As a result the arterial blood is a mixture of desaturated venous blood and oxygenated arterial blood. Tissue oxygenation is often inadequate and

Table 23–1 Causes of PPHN

Reactive pulmonary vasoconstriction
Hypoxia/acidosis
Pneumonia
Atelectasis
Meconium aspiration
Hypoventilation
Increased pulmonary vascular musculature
Chronic fetal hypoxia
Prenatal pulmonary hypertension
Decreased cross-sectional area of pulmonary vasculature
Hypoplasia of the lung
Space-occupying lesions
Diaphragmatic hernia
Lung cysts

(Adapted from Rudolph, AM: High pulmonary resistance after birth. Clin Pediat 19, (9):588, 1980.

lactic acidosis occurs as tissue hypoxia develops. The combination of acidosis and hypoxemia results in a more profound increase in PVR and promotion of a vicious cycle that leads to respiratory failure and death if not reversed.[4]

CLINICAL FEATURES

The infant with PPH may not exhibit signs of respiratory distress at birth. This is especially true if respiratory disease is not the cause of the PPHN. Cyanosis is often intense and responds poorly to oxygen therapy.[6] A prominent right ventricular heave is visible or easily palpable during examination of the precordium. A loud second heart sound or a narrowly split second heart sound with a loud pulmonic component is often found during auscultation of the heart. A murmur is usually present as blood squirts through the ductus arteriosus or foramen ovale.[2,7] The lack of a murmur does not rule out PPHN because a large opening through the foramen ovale or ductus arteriosus may not result in turbulent blood flow. Examination of the respiratory system may reveal retractions and nasal flaring if lung disease is the cause of the PPHN. Otherwise, the lung examination is normal.

The infant with PPH may demonstrate signs and symptoms of neurologic impairment when intrauterine asphyxia has been present. Neurologic impairment may be seen as seizures and abnormalities in the level of consciousness, muscle tone, posture, reflexes, and pattern of breathing (e.g., periods of apnea).[8] Neurologic impairment is an important finding, as it often determines the ultimate outcome.[9]

The chest radiograph will reveal clear lung fields and reduced pulmonary blood flow in the absence of lung disease. Although the chest radiograph is not diagnostic for PPH, it is useful to assess sudden clinical deterioration caused by pneumothorax, bronchial intubation, or pneumonia.

The arterial blood gas (ABG) findings vary with the severity of the shunting, with the presence of underlying lung disease (e.g., meconium aspiration pneumonia), and with the site at which the arterial sample is drawn. Postductal arterial blood (blood in the arterial system that represents a mixture of shunted and non-shunted blood) will demonstrate severe hypoxemia. Preductal arterial blood (blood from the aorta before the opening of the ductus arteriosus) will often have good oxygenation because it has passed through the lung. (This issue is explained in greater detail farther on, under Diagnosis.) The arterial P_{CO_2} value of postductal blood is often found to be normal or elevated and is typically higher than expected for the level of ventilation. This is related to the large amount of dead space ventilation occurring while the lungs are inadequately perfused.

DIAGNOSIS

Neonates with PPH may appear clinically similar to those with a cyanotic heart defect or any number of respiratory disorders. Bedside diagnostic tests such as the hyperoxia test, comparison of preductal to postductal arterial P_{O_2}, and hyperoxia-hyperventilation test are often useful in the differential diagnosis.

The hyperoxia test identifies whether the patient's Pa_{O_2} is responsive to the administration of oxygen. The newborn with a Pa_{O_2} of 100 mm Hg or greater while breathing a fraction of inspired oxygen (FI_{O_2}) of 1.0 probably has a $\dot{V}/\dot{Q}$ problem from an intrapulmonary source (e.g., meconium aspiration) and not a fixed right-to-left cardiac shunt as in PPHN.[2] If the patient's Pa_{O_2} remains below 100 mm Hg while breathing an FI_{O_2} of 1.0, it is assumed that the hypoxemia is due to true shunting.[10] In such cases PPHN or a cardiac lesion is the more likely diagnosis.

Comparing preductal to postductal Pa_{O_2} can reveal a right-to-left shunt through the ductus arteriosus. Blood that enters the root of the aorta from the left ventricle is considered preductal blood because it has not reached the point at which the ductus arteriosus empties into the aorta. Preductal blood represents oxygenated blood that has returned from the lung to the left side of the heart and exits the left ventricle into the aorta according to normal mechanisms. Postductal blood is blood distal to the ductus arteriosus in the arch of the aorta. This represents blood that is a mixture of venous blood that shunted through the ductus arteriosus and oxygenated blood from the left ventricle (Fig. 23–2).

The assessment of preductal or postductal blood can be done with either ABGs or transcutaneous monitors. If ABGs are to be used, the right radial artery is the common source of obtaining preductal blood. The right radial artery represents preductal blood because the right subclavian artery, which feeds blood into the right arm, branches from the brachiocephalic trunk of the aorta before the site at which the ductus arteriosus empties venous blood into the arch of the aorta (Fig. 23-2). The left radial artery is avoided because of the anatomic proximity of the left subclavian artery to the ductus arteriosus. Postductal blood can be obtained from the umbilical artery. Transcutaneous (Tc) monitors can be used on the right upper body for preductal $TcPO_2$ and on the lower body for postductal $TcPO_2$. If simultaneous sampling reveals a difference of more than 15 mm Hg, then right-to-left shunting through the ductus arteriosus is probably present. A negative test result, however, does not rule out PPHN because shunting through the foramen ovale could be occurring and would not cause a significant difference between preductal and postductal PaO_2.[1,2]

The hyperoxia-hyperventilation test is accomplished by giving the newborn a high oxygen concentration (FIO_2 greater than 0.70) while a ventilator or manual resuscitator hyperventilates the patient. If the hypoxemia is due to PPHN, the respiratory alkalosis should decrease PVR, lessen the right-to-left shunting pattern, and improve oxygenation. A newborn with a fixed congenital heart lesion will not usually improve during this test.

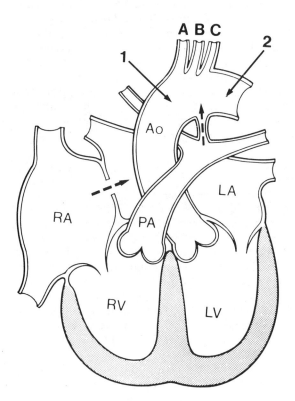

FIGURE 23–2 Preductal and postductal blood illustrated. 1 = Preductal blood in the ascending aorta; 2 = postductal blood in the arch of the aorta; A = brachiocephalic trunk; B = left common carotid artery; C = left subclavian artery. (Modified from Graves, E, et al: Persistent pulmonary hypertension in the neonate. Chest 93:638, 1988.) Abbreviations as in Figure 23–1.

Echocardiography can also confirm the presence of a right-to-left shunt through the ductus arteriosus. This noninvasive procedure represents little risk to the patient.

TREATMENT

Treatment for PPHN focuses on lowering PVR and increasing systemic vascular resistance (SVR). This should result in a reduction of the right-to-left shunting and increase pulmonary blood flow.

Some infants may respond favorably to supplemental oxygen, but most require assisted ventilation. The principal goal of mechanical ventilation in the treatment of PPHN is respiratory alkalosis. Respiratory alkalosis from hyperventilation should cause pulmonary vascular dilatation when the pH exceeds 7.50.[11] Hydrogen ion concentration rather than $Paco_2$ appears to be the mediating factor in the reduction of PVR.[12,13] As PVR decreases, blood flow through the PDA decreases and blood flow to the lung increases.

The newborn who is agitated and breathing out of synchrony with the ventilator may have periods of hypoxemia that may worsen the right-to-left shunting pattern. In such cases paralysis and sedation can be used. The use of neuromuscular blockers is not universally accepted and some physicians manage PPHN without paralysis.[1,7]

Pharmacologic treatment of PPHN may include tolazoline (Priscoline) because of its potential ability to cause pulmonary vasodilatation. Tolazoline is an α-adrenergic blockade with histaminelike action that has direct vasodilating effects. Unfortunately the use of tolazoline in infants with persistent pulmonary hypertension has had mixed results.[4,11] Tolazoline is not a selective pulmonary vasodilator and can lower both systemic as well as pulmonary vascular pressures. If systemic pressures are lowered more than pulmonary pressures, the right-to-left shunting can increase. The use of tolazoline is also limited by complications, which include hypotension and gastrointestinal bleeding.[14] It may cause the infant to have a flushed appearance as systemic vasodilatation occurs.

Severe systemic hypotension in patients with PPHN must be treated promptly because it increases the pressure gradient between the pulmonary artery and the aorta leading to increased blood flow through the ductus arteriosus. Pharmacologic agents such as dopamine may be needed to correct hypotension when it occurs.

Extracorporeal membrane oxygenation (ECMO) has been an important option in the treatment of patients with PPHN when conventional methods have failed.[15] Arteriovenous ECMO is a method in which the infant's blood is withdrawn through a venous catheter and then perfuses a membrane oxygenator. After the blood is oxygenated, it is warmed and replaced into the infant's arterial system. This may be a lifesaving technique in severe PPHN because it allows adequate oxygenation and a reduction of the PVR. Poor prognostic signs such as a $P(A-a)o_2$ greater than 600 mm Hg for 12 hours suggest that ECMO may be of value.

High-frequency ventilation has also been used to treat PPHN. It is most commonly used for newborns with a pulmonary air-leak problem resulting in pulmonary interstitial emphysema. The role of high-frequency ventilation in the treatment of PPHN has not been clearly identified.

Case Study

HISTORY

Baby C is a full-term newborn girl who weighs 3250 g. She was delivered from an uncomplicated pregnancy to a 34-year-old mother with two healthy children at *home. One hour before delivery, the presence of fetal heart rate decelerations was noted. At delivery there was meconium in the amniotic fluid. After delivery, the patient's airway was suctioned to remove any meconium that may be present in the trachea. The patient had APGARs of 7 at 1 minute (owing to poor color and respiratory effort) and 8 at 5 minutes (the patient had a more vigorous spontaneous respiratory effort). It was noted that the patient's color was cyanotic immediately after delivery and she did not respond to an F_{IO_2} of 0.40 by oxygen hood. Examination revealed a respiratory rate of 40/minute, heart rate of 130/minute, clear breath sounds, and the absence of grunting or respiratory retractions. The F_{IO_2} was increased to 0.50, with no change in the patient's color. The infant was intubated and placed on a time-cycled, pressure-limited, continuous-flow infant ventilator.*

Questions

1. What are pertinent factors in the delivery history of this patient?
2. What is the differential diagnosis of this patient's problem and what is the most likely diagnosis?
3. What diagnostic tests should be suggested to assess this patient further?
4. What could explain why the cyanosis did not respond to oxygen therapy?

Answers

1. Pertinent factors related to this patient's delivery history include the presence of meconium in the amniotic fluid, which indicates that the patient may have suffered an asphyxia episode in utero or during delivery. The most common cause for asphyxia is a reduction in placental blood flow which impairs the transfer of oxygen from the mother to the fetus.[16] Symptoms of respiratory distress shortly after the delivery of a newborn through meconium-stained amniotic fluid are typically due to inhalation of meconium particles. The inhalation of meconium can cause pneumonitis, atelectasis, or pulmonary hyperinflation resulting from airway plugging.

   An additional factor of importance in the patient's history is the presence of fetal heart rate decelerations. A normal fetal heart rate is between 120/minute and 160/minute. When bradycardia occurs, it is referred to as a deceleration. A common cause of heart rate decelerations in the fetus is asphyxia. A history of perinatal asphyxia can be an important finding in establishing the differential diagnosis.
2. Differential diagnosis includes meconium aspiration syndrome, PPHN, or congenital heart disease. It is necessary to have additional information before choosing the most likely cause of this patient's cyanosis. Because an increase in F_{IO_2} did not improve the patient's color, true shunting is likely to be the cause of the hypoxemia.
3. Diagnostic tests that would further identify the cause of the infant's cyanosis are ABG analysis, chest radiograph, and echocardiography. Bedside tests such as the use of preductal and postductal Pa_{O_2} comparison may also be helpful.
4. The cyanosis may not have improved because of the shunting of blood past the lungs. This is common in congenital heart disease and PPHN.

PHYSICAL EXAMINATION ————————

General   *Patient is alert and active, intubated with a 3.5-mm endotracheal tube, and receiving mechanical ventilation.*

Vital Signs	*Temperature 36.5°C; respiratory rate 50/minute by mechanical ventilator and 20/minute spontaneously; pulse 140/minute, blood pressure 60/45 mm Hg with a mean arterial pressure 50 mm Hg*
HEENT	*Normocephalic, with soft anterior fontanelle; eye motion normal, pupils equally round and reactive to light; nasal shape normal with no flaring; pinnae well formed; intubation precluding throat examination*
Neck	*No masses, glands, or redundant tissue folds*
Chest	*Symmetric with no retractions*
Heart	*Regular rate and rhythm without murmur or gallops*
Lungs	*Inspiratory crackles present bilaterally*
Abdomen	*Nondistended; no masses or organomegaly on palpation; no bowel sounds heard on auscultation; umbilical cord with clean stump, umbilical arterial line and umbilical venous catheter lines in place*
Extremities	*Strong pulses in the upper and lower extremities bilaterally, no evidence of edema; normal muscle tone demonstrated; cyanosis noted*

Questions

5. Why are both a mechanical respiratory rate and a spontaneous respiratory rate given?
6. What is the significance of the patient's active alert state, reactive pupils, and normal muscle tone?
7. What does the finding of clear equal breath sounds indicate?
8. Does the lack of a murmur rule out a patent ductus arteriosus (PDA) in this patient?
9. Why would the monitoring of the blood pressure or arterial mean be important in this patient?
10. Is it significant that no chest wall retractions are present in this patient? If so, what is the significance?

Answers

5. The patient is reported to be receiving mechanical ventilation at a respiratory rate of 50/minute, with a spontaneous rate of 20/minute. It is important to document both spontaneous and mechanical respiratory rates to identify whether the patient is exhibiting any spontaneous effort and how much of the total minute ventilation the infant is providing. The presence of spontaneous respirations is a positive neurologic sign.
6. A normal sensorium, reactive pupils, and normal muscle tone represent significant positive findings in a patient with this kind of history (perinatal asphyxia and meconium-stained amniotic fluid) and indicate an intact neurologic system. Meconium in the amniotic fluid can be considered a risk factor for the presence of an asphyxial episode in utero.[17] Although the normal neurologic findings do not completely rule out future neurologic abnormalities, it is unlikely that this infant has suffered more than minimal asphyxia.[18] If the patient were suspected of sustaining a moderate to severe brain injury, preparations should be made for the treatment of apnea episodes and seizures.

7. The findings of equal breath sounds could be important in ruling out pneumothorax or right mainstem intubation. A newborn with a history of meconium in the trachea is at risk for meconium aspiration syndrome (MAS), which is associated with a higher than normal incidence of pneumothorax. Unequal breath sounds may indicate pneumothorax. The presence of clear breath sounds does not rule out a lung parenchymal disease, although it makes it less likely.

8. The absence of a murmur does not rule out PDA. A newborn with PDA may not have a murmur if the opening is wide and blood flow through the ductus arteriosus is not turbulent.[1]

9. Patients with suspected PPHN syndrome should have their blood pressure monitored because changes in blood pressure may lead to changes in right-to-left shunting. The amount of blood bypassing the lungs and emptying directly into the aorta depends on both systemic and pulmonary pressures in addition to the size of the shunt. Systemic hypotension can facilitate a greater pressure gradient between the pulmonary artery and the aorta and more shunting of blood from the pulmonary artery into the aorta through the PDA, worsening the right-to-left shunt.

10. The absence of chest wall retractions is significant because it is a pertinent negative sign when trying to distinguish between a lung parenchymal problem and a right-to-left shunt such as occurs with PPHN. Chest wall retractions are usually associated with the reduced lung compliance typical of lung parenchymal diseases. The presence of chest wall retractions is possible with lung disease or PPHN, but the absence of retractions would be more common in PPHN than in lung disease.

LABORATORY EVALUATION

CHEST RADIOGRAPH

Right lung somewhat hyperexpanded; irregular bilateral perihilar streaky densities; an endotracheal tube terminating approximately 1 cm above the carina (Fig. 23–3).

ABGs

pH 7.26, $Paco_2$ 44 mm Hg, Pao_2 46 mm Hg, base excess (BE) −10 mEq/liter, HCO_3^- 18 mEq/liter, Fio_2 0.50, intermittent mandatory ventilation (IMV) 40/minute, peak inspiratory pressure (PIP) 20 cm H_2O, positive end-expiratory pressure (PEEP) 4 cm H_2O

COMPLETE BLOOD COUNT (CBC)

White blood cells (WBC) 13,000, segs 52 percent, bands 8 percent, lymphocytes 27 percent, monocytes 6 percent, Eosinophils 2 percent, hemoglobin (Hb) 18.2 g/dL

OXIMETER

Pulse oximeter on the left foot reading 85 percent saturation

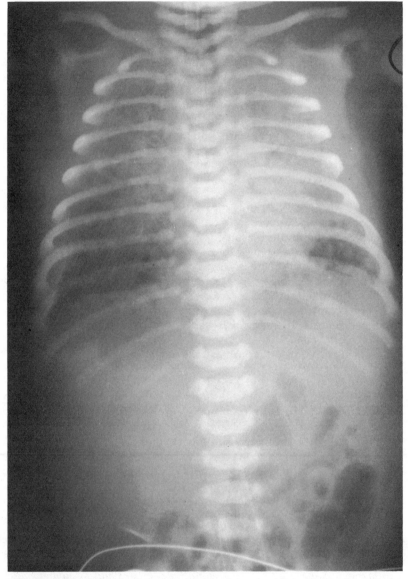

FIGURE 23–3 Chest radiograph showing irregular bilateral densities. Endotracheal tube is in good position.

Questions

11. What is the pathophysiology causing the chest radiographic results?
12. Are these radiographic findings typical for PPHN?
13. How would you interpret the ABG results?
14. What is the cause of the hypoxemia?
15. What are the desired ABG values?
16. What is the significance of the anatomic location on the baby from which the pulse oximeter reading was taken?
17. What is the significance of the CBC findings?
18. What other diagnostic tests could be performed on this patient to confirm the presence of a right-to-left shunt?

Answers

11. The radiographic findings are consistent with the patient's history of meconium in the amniotic fluid and with meconium aspiration syndrome.[19] Aspiration of meconium causes pneumonitis and can lead to atelectasis. Particulate meconium particles can lead to plugging of the airways and a pattern of hyperinflation, diffuse infiltrates, and areas of atelectasis. It is not clear if this patient's ABG abnormalities are caused by the meconium aspiration or by PPHN.

12. The radiologic findings are not unusual in a patient with suspected PPHN, caused by MAS. The radiographic findings suggest only that the meconium found in the amniotic fluid has been inhaled. They do not confirm or rule out PPHN and a right-to-left shunt as the cause of cyanosis.

13. These ABGs show an uncompensated metabolic acidosis and moderate hypoxemia on 50 percent oxygen. The cause of the metabolic acidosis could be the in utero asphyxia the patient may have suffered, reduced perfusion, or severe hypoxemia from PPHN.

14. The cause for this patient's hypoxemia could be atelectasis, small airway obstruction leading to $\dot{V}/\dot{Q}$ abnormalities, or a right-to-left shunting of blood through the ductus arteriosus.

15. The therapeutic range for ABG values in this patient would depend on the diagnosis. If the patient has PPH, a pH greater than 7.50, Pa_{CO_2} between 20 and 30 mm Hg, and Pa_{O_2} greater than 100 mm Hg may lead to a lowering of pulmonary vascular resistance.[2,6,7,11] The patient with MAS without PPHN may be managed more conservatively, with lower ventilator rates and a lower F_{IO_2}.

16. The pulse oximeter reading is to be interpreted as a postductal (left foot) sample. To help confirm a right-to-left shunt through the ductus arteriosus, both preductal and postductal samples of blood should be obtained (described earlier in this chapter).

17. This is a normal CBC for a newborn. PPHN can be caused by sepsis; therefore, a normal CBC is helpful in evaluating for sepsis as the etiology of the persistent hypertension.

18. A diagnostic test that could confirm the presence of a right-to-left shunt through the ductus arteriosus is echocardiography.

Echocardiography confirmed the presence of a right-to-left shunt through the ductus arteriosus and the absence of any other structural heart disease. With the patient receiving 100 percent oxygen, the Pa_{O_2} remained in the 40s. On an IMV of 40/minute, PIP 20 cm H_2O, PEEP 4 cm H_2O, and F_{IO_2} of 1.0, the umbilical artery blood gas results were a pH 7.29, Pa_{CO_2} 48 mm Hg, Pa_{O_2} 40 mm Hg, BE −8, HCO_3^- 19 mEq/L. The patient had episodes of decreased Sa_{O_2} by pulse oximeter during suctioning or other procedures. During these procedures, the patient became agitated, respiratory efforts became uncoordinated with the ventilator, and saturation readings from the pulse oximeter dropped as low as 70 percent.

Questions

19. Would you suggest any ventilator parameter changes for this patient?

20. What probably happens to this patient's delivered tidal volumes when her respiratory efforts are not coordinated with the ventilator breaths?

21. What is the approach needed to decrease the patient's episodes of low Sao_2 values?

Answers

19. This patient is hypoventilating and may benefit from hyperventilation in order to improve her Pao_2 and pH, which should decrease PVR. Increasing the IMV rate to between 60 and 80/minute may result in a higher pH and a lower $Paco_2$. These ABG changes may facilitate a decrease of the right-to-left shunting and improve the Pao_2. A Pao_2 of between 80 and 100 mm Hg is a reasonable goal. This patient is much below that Pao_2. An alternative may be to increase the PIP, which will also have the effect of decreasing $Paco_2$ and increasing pH. The disadvantage of using an increased peak pressure to achieve a higher pH is that excessive pressures can lead to barotrauma.[6,20]

20. The newborn receiving pressure-limited, time-cycled, continuous-flow ventilation may have a reduction in volume delivered to the lung when fighting the ventilator. If the patient exhales during an inspiratory phase of the ventilator, the expiratory effort results in an increased resistance to the gas entering the lung through the ventilator. This increased resistance will cause a buildup of pressure in the circuit until the pressure limit of the ventilator is reached and no more gas enters the lung. On any given breath, it is difficult to determine how much volume actually reached the lungs of a patient who is not breathing in synchrony with the ventilator. Because the pressure developed in the lungs with pressure-limited ventilation determines the tidal volume (VT), breathing out of synchrony with the ventilator is associated with a reduced VT and minute ventilation. Decreases in minute ventilation can cause an increased $Paco_2$ and decreased pH, worsening the PVR and decreasing pulmonary blood flow in patients with PPH.

21. Most clinicians would agree with the use of minimal stimulation, including a quiet environment, infrequent suctioning, and restrictions on handling the patient to reduce the patient's episodes of low Sao_2. Paralysis of the patient with PPHN is controversial and is usually reserved for patients like the one in this case, in which breathing out of synchrony with the ventilator is leading to impairment of oxygenation. Sedation can be attempted and if the patient improves, paralysis may not be necessary.

Baby C was managed with hyperventilation (PIP increased to 30 and an IMV rate of 60) and responded with an increase in Pao_2 to 60 mm Hg. She remained unstable, having several episodes of cyanosis despite sedation. The episodes of cyanosis became longer and lasted up to 3 minutes. Her blood pressure was unstable (hypotensive). She showed no evidence of sepsis and had improved breath sounds. Her chest radiograph demonstrated improvement with reduced pulmonary vascular markings. At 36 hours of age the following two ABG values were recorded, a half an hour apart:

1. *pH 7.23, $Paco_2$ 49 mm Hg, Pao_2 45 mm Hg, BE −8 mEq/liter, HCO_3^-, 20 mEq/liter*
2. *pH 7.12, $Paco_2$ 68 mm Hg, Pao_2 40 mm Hg, BE −9 mEq/liter, HCO_3^- 22 mEq/liter.*

These ABGs were obtained with the patient receiving IMV 65/minute, PIP 35cm H_2O, PEEP 4 cm H_2O, Fio_2 1.0.

Questions

22. What physical assessment information would you now gather?
23. What is the effect of the hypotension on the pathophysiology of PPHN in this patient?
24. Is this patient a candidate for ECMO?

Answers

22. The physical assessment of this patient should include auscultation to determine if breath sounds are bilateral. There has been a deterioration in the patient's ABGs and two abnormalities that should be considered are pneumothorax and a right mainstem bronchus intubation. If breath sounds and chest radiograph confirm the absence of pneumothorax or right mainstem intubation, these ABG values could be indicative of intractable respiratory failure, which can occur in the course of PPHN.

23. Systemic hypotension associated with PPHN can increase the right-to-left shunt through the ductus arteriosus. Hypotension often leads to lower systemic vascular pressures but not lower pulmonary vascular pressures and increases blood flow across the ductus arteriosus.

24. Several criteria that have been suggested for ECMO are based on historic mortality predictions.[21] A $P(A\text{-}a)O_2$ greater than 600 mm Hg for 12 hours is a poor prognostic sign and means that ECMO may be warranted.[22] In this patient, calculations for the first ABG (assuming 760 mm Hg barometric pressure) reveals a $P(A\text{-}a)O_2$ of 607 and for the second, 588. Another criteria for ECMO is acute deterioration associated with PaO_2 less than 40 mm Hg for 2 hours or pH less than 7.15 for 2 hours; PaO_2 less than 55 mm Hg and pH less than 7.40 for 3 hours; *or* evidence of barotrauma defined as four of the following seven: (1) pulmonary interstitial emphysema, (2) pneumothorax or pneumomediastinum, (3) pneumoperitoneum, (4) pneumopericardium, (5) subcutaneous emphysema, (6) persistent air leak for greater than 24 hours, and (7) mean airway pressure greater than 15 cm H_2O.[23] Even though there is an acute deterioration in this patient, many physicians would manage this patient with conventional therapy (stabilize blood pressure, optimize ventilator settings), at least temporarily, unless she continued to deteriorate.

The hospital course of this patient included a few more hours of instability in which dopamine was used to control her blood pressure and neuromuscular blockers and sedation were administered in an attempt to reduce her cyanotic episodes. Her pH, $PaCO_2$, and PaO_2 improved and after 24 hours of hyperventilation, she was gradually weaned from mechanical ventilation. She was discharged from the hospital 10 days later in good health.

REFERENCES

1. Thibeault, D and Gregory, G: Neonatal Pulmonary Care, ed 2. Norwalk, CT, Appleton-Century-Crofts, 1986, p 462.

2. Duara, S and Gewitz, M: Use of mechanical ventilation for clinical management of persistent pulmonary hypertension of the newborn. Clin Perinatol 11:641, 1984.

3. Haworth, S and Reid, L: Persistent fetal circulation: Newly recognized structural features. J Pediatr 88:614, 1976.

4. Peckham, GJ and Fox, WW: Physiologic factors affecting pulmonary artery pressure in infants with persistent pulmonary hypertension. J Pediatr 93:1005, 1978.

5. Geggel, R and Redi, L: The structural basis of PPHN. Clin Perinatol 11:525, 1984.

6. Graves, E, et al: Persistent pulmonary hypertension in the neonate. Chest 93:638, 1988.

7. Taeusch, H, Ballard, R, and Avery, M: Schaffer and Avery's Diseases of the Newborn, ed 6, Philadelphia, WB Saunders, 1991.

8. Brann, A: Hypoxic ischemic encephalopathy. Pediatr Clin North Am 33:451, 1986.

9. Sexson, et al: The multisystem involvement of the asphyxiated newborn. Pediatr Res 10:432, 1976.

10. Lawson, M: Persistent pulmonary hypertension of the newborn: Current trends in classification and diagnosis. Neonatal Network 27–35, August 1987.

11. Drummond, W, et al: The independent effects of hyperventilation, tolazoline, and dopamine on infants with persistent pulmonary hypertension. J Pediatr 98:603, 1981.

12. Morray, J, et al: Effect of pH and PCO2 on pulmonary and systemic hemodynamics after surgery in children with congenital heart disease and pulmonary hypertension. J Pediatr 113:474, 1988.

13. Schreiber, M, et al: Increased arterial pH, not decreased PaCO2, attenuates hypoxia-induced pulmonary vasoconstriction in newborn lambs. Pediatr Res 20:113, 1986.

14. Ward, R: Pharmacology of tolazoline. Clin Perinatol 11:703, 1984.

15. Beck, R, et al: Criteria for extracorporeal membrane oxygenation in a population of infants with persistent pulmonary hypertension of the newborn. J Pediatr Surg 21:297, 1986.

16. Abramovici, H, et al: Meconium during delivery: A sign of compensated fetal distress. Am J Obstet Gynecol 118:251, 1974.

17. Jacobsa, M and Phibbs, R: Prevention, recognition, and treatment of perinatal asphyxia. Clin Perinatol 16:785, 1989.

18. Amiel-Tison, C and Ellison, P: Birth asphyxia in the fullterm newborn: Early assessment and outcome. Dev Med Child Neurol 28:671, 1986.

19. Yeh, T, et al: Roentgenographic findings in infants with meconium aspiration syndrome. JAMA 242:60, 1979.

20. Dworetz, A, et al: Survival of infants with persistent pulmonary hypertension without extracorporeal membrane oxygenation. Pediatrics 84:1, 1989.

21. Nading, J: Historical controls for extracorporeal membrane oxygenation in neonates. Crit Care Med 17:423, 1989.

22. Loe, W, Graves, E, and Ochsner, J: Extracorporeal membrane oxygenation in newborn respiratory failure. J Pediatr Surg 20:684, 1985.

23. Bartlett, RH, et al: Extracorporeal circulation in neonatal respiratory failure: A prospective randomized study. Pediatrics 76:479, 1985.

Glossary

A₂: Aortic component of the second heart sound

ABG: Arterial blood gas

Abdominal Paradox: Abnormal inward movement of the abdomen with inspiratory effort; occurs with diaphragm fatigue or paralysis

Acrocyanosis: Cyanosis of the extremities

Afterload: Resistance to blood flow out of the ventricle during ventricular contraction

Amniotic Fluid: Liquid produced by the fetal membranes that surrounds the fetus throughout pregnancy

Anabolic Metabolism: Constructive process by which the body converts simple substances into more complex compounds

Anaerobic: Usually used in reference to metabolism in the body that occurs without oxygen

Anemia: Condition in which there is an abnormal reduction in number of circulating red blood cells

Angina: Severe chest pain associated with coronary artery disease

Angiography: Visualization of coronary arteries by radiograph after injection of radiopaque contrast medium

Anion Gap: Mathematic difference between the positive and negative ions of the blood

Apgar Score: Evaluation system used to assess the newborn immediately after birth, based on a scale of 1 to 10, with 10 indicating the best physical condition of the infant

Apnea: Cessation of spontaneous breathing for more than 10 seconds

ARDS: Adult respiratory distress syndrome

Arrhythmia: Abnormal rhythm of the heartbeat

Asbestosis: Condition of pulmonary fibrosis related to the chronic inhalation of asbestos fibers

Ascites: Accumulation of serous fluid in the peritoneal cavity of the abdomen

Asphyxia: Apparent or actual cessation of life caused by the lack of effective gas exchange in the lungs

Aspiration: Drawing in or out by the application of suction; in respiratory care patients, often used to indicate the abnormal inhalation of vomit into the trachea and lungs

Asthma: Pulmonary disease characterized by reversible airways obstruction

Atelectasis: Collapsed or airless condition of the lung

Atopy: Clinically applies to a group of diseases of an allergic nature that differ from most allergies in that (1) they are inherited; (2) the antibody produced, called atopic reagin or skin-sensitizing antibody, is deposited in cutaneous tissues and may enter the bloodstream; and (3) the primary reaction that appears is edema, as occurs in hayfever or rhinitis; with principal atopic manifestations being bronchial asthma, vasomotor rhinitis, and chronic urticaria

Atrophy: Reduction in the size of a body part because of disease

Auto PEEP: Inadvertent buildup of positive end-expiratory pressure (PEEP) in the lung during mechanical ventilation as a result of inadequate expiratory time

Bands: Immature neutrophils that are recognized by the lack of nucleus segmentation

Bronchiolitis: Inflammation of the bronchioles, most often occurring in infants and children

Bronchitis: Inflammation of the bronchi usually because of infection

Bronchospasm: Abnormal contraction of the smooth muscles lining the intrathoracic airways

Bruit: Adventitious sound of venous or arterial origin heard on auscultation and produced by turbulent blood flow

Cachexia: State of ill health, malnutrition, and wasting; may occur in many chronic diseases such as certain malignancies, advanced chronic pulmonary disease, and the like

Carboxyhemoglobin: Hemoglobin bound with carbon monoxide

Cardiac Index: Cardiac output divided by the patient's body surface area in m^2; normal cardiac index, 2.5 to 4.0 liters/minute/m^2

Cardiac Output: Quantity of blood pumped out of the left ventricle per minute; normal values in the adult, 4 to 8 liters/minute

Cardiomegaly: Hypertrophy (enlargement) of the heart

Cardiomyopathy: Disease of the heart muscle

Catabolic Metabolism: Destructive process by which the body breaks down more complex compounds into more simple substances

CBC: Complete blood count; a laboratory test reporting the red blood cell and white blood cell counts in the circulating blood

Cheyne-Stokes Breathing: Abnormal pattern of breathing characterized by periods of apnea lasting 10 to 60 seconds followed by gradually increasing depth and frequency of breathing

CHF: Congestive heart failure

Clubbing: Abnormal enlargement of the distal phalanges

Consolidation: Process of becoming more dense or consolidated; often used in reference to the lung tissue when pneumonia is present

Contractility: Having the ability to contract or shorten

Contusion: Injury to the body in which the skin is not broken; a bruise

COPD: Chronic obstructive pulmonary disease

Cor Pulmonale: Right heart failure due to chronic lung disease

Coryza: Profuse discharge from the mucous membranes of the nose

CPAP: Continuous positive airway pressure

Crackles: Discontinuous adventitious lung sounds produced by the sudden opening of collapsed airways or by the movement of excessive airway secretions

Crepitus: Dry, crackling sound or sensation

CVP: Central venous pressure

Cyanosis: Slightly bluish, grayish, slatelike, or dark purple discoloration of the skin caused by presence of abnormal amounts of reduced (poorly oxygenated) hemoglobin in the blood; may not appear in patients with severe anemia even though their blood is poorly oxygenated because there is not enough reduced hemoglobin present to cause the blue color to be visible

Defibrillation: Application of direct electric shock to the chest in an effort to return the heart rhythm to normal

Diaphoresis: Profuse sweating

DIC: Disseminated intravascular coagulation

Diplopia: Double vision

Diuresis: Secretion of large amount of urine

Diuretic: Agent that increases the secretion of urine

Ductus Arteriosus: Channel opening between the pulmonary artery and the aorta in the fetus

Dysphonia: Difficulty in speaking, hoarseness

Dyspnea: Air hunger resulting in labored or difficult breathing, normal when caused by vigorous work or athletic activity

Dysuria: Painful or difficult urination

ECG: Electrocardiogram

Ejection Fraction: Portion of the ventricular volume ejected during contraction of the ventricle (systole), normal ejection fraction being approximately 0.70 or 70 percent

Empyema: Collection of pus in the pleural cavity

End-Diastolic Volume: Amount of blood in the ventricle at the end of the diastolic period; represents amount of blood available for ejection during the subsequent contraction of the ventricles

Endogenous: Produced within or caused by factors within the organism

Enuresis: Involuntary urination

Erythema: Redness of the skin caused by congestion of the capillaries

Escharotomy: Surgical removal of burned skin that has formed scabs or dry crusting tissue

Exudates: Accumulations of fluid in a cavity, or matter that penetrates through vessel walls into adjoining tissue, or the production of pus or serum; exudates contain more cells and protein as compared to transudates

Fasciculations: Involuntary contraction or twitching of muscle fibers

Fetus: Infant in utero from the third month of gestation until birth

Fibrosis: Formation of fibrous tissue

Fistula: Abnormal tubelike passage from a normal cavity or tube to another cavity or tube

Flail Chest: Condition of the chest wall caused by two or more fractures on each affected rib that result in a free-floating portion of the rib cage; affected region of the chest wall moves in a paradoxic fashion with breathing

Foramen Ovale: Opening between the two atria of the heart in the fetus, which closes after birth

FRC: Functional residual capacity; amount of gas in the lungs at the end of a normal tidal volume exhalation; represents a combination of the residual volume and the expiratory reserve volume

FVC: Forced vital capacity

Gallop: Abnormal heart rhythm characterized by an extra sound heard during diastole, which, when added to the normal first and second heart sounds, results in a rhythm that resembles the pattern produced by the hooves of a horse during a gallop

Gravida: Pregnant woman, with gravida 1 referring to the woman's first pregnancy, gravida 2 to the second, and so on

Hb: Hemoglobin

HbCO: Hemoglobin bound with carbon monoxide

HCN: Hemoglobin bound with cyanide

Heave: Abnormal pulsation on the chest as the result of ventricular hypertrophy

HEENT: Head, ears, eyes, nose, and throat

Hemolysis: Breakdown of red blood cells, resulting in the release of hemoglobin into the plasma

Hemoptysis: Expectoration of blood arising from hemorrhage of the larynx, trachea, bronchi, or lungs

Hepatomegaly: Enlargement of the liver

Hilum: Depression in an organ in which nerves and blood vessels enter or exit

Hypercapnia: Condition in which the arterial blood contains increased levels of carbon dioxide ($Paco_2$ greater than 45 mm Hg)

Hyperkalemia: Abnormal increase in the serum potassium level

Hypernatremia: Abnormal increase in the serum sodium level

Hyperpnea: Deep breathing

Hypersomnolence: Condition in which the patient is experiencing an abnormal degree of sleepiness

Hypertension: Condition in which the systemic blood pressure is above the normal range

Hypertrophy Enlargement of an organ or part of an organ

Hypoglycemia: Condition of reduced blood glucose levels

Hypokalemia: Abnormal decrease in the level of potassium in the plasma of the circulating blood

Hyponatremia: Abnormal decrease in the level of sodium in the plasma of the circulation blood

Hypoplasia: Underdevelopment of a tissue or organ

Hypopnea: Shallow inadequate breathing

Hypotension: Condition in which the systemic blood pressure is below normal values

Hypoxemia: Insufficient oxygenation of the arterial blood

ICU: Intensive care unit

Idiopathic: Disease occurring without a known cause

Ileus: Obstruction of the intestines

IMV: Intermittent mandatory ventilation

Infarction: Formation of an infarct, an area of tissue in an organ or part, which undergoes necrosis following cessation of blood supply

Inotropes: Medications or compounds that affect the contractility of the heart muscle

Insomnia: Inability to sleep

IPPB: Intermittent positive pressure ventilation

Ischemia: Local decrease in blood flow caused by obstruction of the circulation to a part

Kyphosis: Excessive posterior curvature of the spine, which leads to condition known as humpback or hunchback

Lactic Acidosis: Disturbance in the lactic acid balance of the body; often caused by anerobic metabolism

Leukocyte: White blood cell

Leukocytopenia: Abnormal decrease in the number of circulating white blood cells

Leukocytosis: Transient increase in the number of white cells in the blood

Leukopenia: Abnormal decrease of the circulating white blood cells, usually below 5000/mm^3

Loud P$_2$: Abnormally loud second heart sound that occurs as the result of the pulmonic valve closing more forcefully than normal; often the result of pulmonary hypertension

Lymphadenopathy: Disease of the lymph nodes

Lymphocytosis: Abnormal increase in the number of circulating lymphocytes in the blood

Macrognathia: Abnormal size of jaw

MDI: Metered-dose inhaler

Meconium: Material that collects in the intestines of the fetus and forms the first stool of a newborn

Metaplasia: Change in body cells from normal to abnormal for that type of tissue

Microemboli: Very small blood clots

Micrognathia: Abnormal smallness of jaw, especially the lower jaw

MIP: Maximum inspiratory pressure; a test typically used to determine the strength of the patient's inspiratory muscles and his or her potential ability to wean from mechanical ventilation

Morbidity: Condition of being diseased or unhealthy

Mortality: Condition of being subject to death; often used to refer to death rate for a specific illness

Murmur: Abnormal soft blowing or rasping sound heard on auscultation of the heart

Myocardium: Muscle composing the walls of the heart

Narcolepsy: Chronic ailment consisting of recurrent attacks of drowsiness and sleep

Nasal Flaring: Flaring outward of the external nares with each inspiratory effort; usually indicative of an increase in the work of breathing

Necrotizing: Causing death of areas of tissue or bone surrounded by healthy parts

Neoplasm: Abnormal growth of new tissue, which can be benign or malignant

Nocturnal Dyspnea: Shortness of breath that occurs while the patient attempts to sleep, most often associated with congestive heart failure

Normocephalic: Normal configuration of the head

Nosocomial: Pertaining to or originating in a hospital

Obstructive Sleep Apnea (OSA):　Cessation of breathing for more than 10 seconds owing to obstruction of the upper airway

Obtunded:　Condition of reduced response to stimuli

Oliguria:　Diminished amount of urine formation

Oral Thrush:　Fungal infection of mouth or throat, especially in infants and young children, characterized by formation of white patches and ulcers, frequently fever, and gastrointestinal inflammation

Organomegaly:　Abnormal enlargement of an organ in the body

Orthopnea:　Shortness of breath that occurs in the reclining position

Oxyhemoglobin:　Hemoglobin bound with oxygen

P_2:　Pulmonic component of the second heart sound, with a loud P_2 being suggestive of pulmonary hypertension

Para:　Having produced one or more viable offspring; often used with "gravida" to indicate the number of pregnancies and resulting viable offspring (e.g., gravida 2, para 1 refers to a woman who has been pregnant twice but has produced only one viable child)

Paradoxic Pulse:　Pulse that is abnormally suppressed during each inspiration

Paradoxic Respiration:　Most often used to describe a condition seen with diaphragm fatigue or paralysis in which the diaphragm ascends with inspiration; appears as a sinking inward motion of the abdominal wall with each inspiratory effort by the patient; can also be used to describe a traumatized portion of the chest wall that sinks inward with inspiration in the patient with a flail chest

Parenchyma:　Essential parts of an organ, which are concerned with its function, with lung parenchyma referring to the distal portions of the lung involved with gas exchange

Paresthesia:　Sensation of numbness, prickling, or tingling, often in the extremities

PCWP:　Pulmonary capillary wedge pressure; the pressure used to evaluate left ventricular filling (preload)

PDA:　Patent ductus arteriosus

Pedal Edema:　Abnormal collection of fluid in the soft tissues around the ankles, often caused by heart failure

PEEP:　Positive end-expiratory pressure

Perfusion:　Passing of a fluid through spaces; often used to describe the movement of arterial blood into a certain part of the body

Pericardial Tamponade:　Compression of the heart because of a buildup of blood in the pericardial sac around the heart

Pericarditis:　Inflammation of pericardium (the double membrane sac enclosing the heart and the origins of the great blood vessels)

Perihilar:　Pertaining to the tissues around the hilum of the lung, which is the entrance of the pulmonary artery and veins for each lung

Peristalsis:　Rhythmic, coordinated contraction of smooth muscle that moves a substance through a canal (e.g., peristalsis of the bowel moves food through the intestinal tract)

Peritoneal:　Concerning the peritoneum, the serous membrane lining the abdominal cavity

PERRLA:　*P*upils *e*qual, *r*ound, *r*eactive to *l*ight and *a*ccommodation; part of the neurologic examination during the physical examination of the patient

Pharyngitis:　Inflammation of the pharynx

Plasmapheresis:　Removal of plasma from withdrawn blood and replacement of the formed elements back into the patient

Platypnea: Difficulty breathing in the upright position

PMI: Point of maximum impulse; generated by the contraction of the left ventricle

PND: Paroxysmal nocturnal dyspnea: a sudden onset of difficult breathing that typically occurs during sleep and is associated with congestive heart failure

Pneumoconiosis: Disease of the lung caused by the chronic inhalation of dust—often of occupational origin

Pneumothorax: Presence of air in the pleural space

Polycythemia: Excess of red blood cells, often caused by chronic hypoxemia

Polyphonic: Sound made up of multiple notes

Precordium: Surface of the chest wall overlying the heart

Preload: Volume of blood filling the ventricle just before ventricular contraction

Ptosis: Drooping of an organ, such as the upper eyelid, from paralysis

Pulse Pressure: Difference between the systolic and the diastolic blood pressure

Pulsus Alternans: Pulse characterized by a regular alternation of weak and strong beats

Pulsus Paradoxus: Abnormal decrease in the systolic pressure during inspiration, associated with significant increase in the patient's work of breathing

Purulent: Pus-containing; indicates presence of bacterial infection

Pyrogenic: Producing fever

Radiolucency: Property of being partly or wholly permeable to radiant energy

Radiopaque: Impenetrable to the x-ray beams (e.g., bones, which are usually impenetrable to x-ray beams, leave a white shadow on the radiograph)

Rales: Discontinuous type of adventitious lung sound heard on auscultation of the chest; synonymous with crackles

RDS: Respiratory distress syndrome

Refractory Hypoxemia: Hypoxemia that does not respond adequately to significant increases in the patient's fraction of inspired oxygen (FIO_2)

Respiratory Alternans: Abnormal pattern of breathing in which the patient alternates for short periods of time between breathing with the accessory muscles and breathing with the diaphragm

Respiratory Failure: Failure of the lungs to maintain adequate oxygenation with or without an elevated PCO_2

Retinopathy: Noninflammatory disease of the retina

Retractions: Visible sinking inward of the skin and soft tissues surrounding the bones of the thorax with each inspiratory effort; indicates significantly increased work of breathing

Rhinorrhea: Thin, watery discharge from the nose

Rhonchus: Low-pitched, continuous type of adventitious lung sound heard during auscultation of the chest

S_1:   First heart sound; produced by the closure of the mitral and tricuspid valves

S_2:   Second heart sound; produced by the closure of the aortic and pulmonic valves

S_3:   Third heart sound; may be normal in young people but usually indicates heart disease in adults

S_4:   Fourth heart sound; often heard in adult patients with heart disease

S_3 **Gallop:**   Abnormal third heart sound

Scoliosis: Abnormal lateral curvature of the spine

Segs: Segmented neutrophils; neutrophils that are mature and most able to fight infection

Sensorium: Refers to the patient's level of consciousness or alertness; abnormal when patient is not alert and oriented; abnormal sensorium often indicates inadequate oxygenation of the brain

Sepsis: Pathologic state usually febrile, resulting from the presence of microorganisms or their poisonous products in the bloodstream

Shock: Clinical condition resulting from inadequate blood flow to the vital organs; often characterized by a reduced urine output, diminished level of consciousness, hypotension, peripheral cyanosis, and tachycardia

a. Anaphylactic: Reaction from injection of protein substance to which patient is sensitized

b. Septic: Form of shock that occurs in septicemia when endotoxins are released from certain bacteria in the bloodstream; characterized by hypotension from a significant drop in systemic vascular resistance

c. Toxic: Severe acute form of shock brought on by infection with strains of *Staphylococcus aureus*

Shunt: Blood that passes from the right side of the heart to the left side without coming into contact with gas exchange units of the lung

SpO$_2$: Percent saturation of hemoglobin with oxygen as measured by pulse oximetry

Status Asthmaticus: Persistent and intractable asthma unresponsive to conventional treatment

Stenosis: Abnormal narrowing of a body passage or opening

Stridor: High-pitched continuous adventitious lung sound often heard without the aid of a stethoscope, owing to obstruction of the upper airway

Stroke Volume: Amount of blood ejected by the left ventricle with each beat

Surfactant: Agent that lowers surface tension (e.g., pulmonary surfactant is a phospholipid substance that helps prevent alveolar collapse)

Tachycardia: Abnormal increase in heart rate

Tachyphylaxis: Rapid immunization against the effect of toxic doses of an extract by previous injection of small doses of it

Tachypnea: Abnormal increase in the respiratory rate

Tamponade: Pathologic compression of a body part

Tetany: Nervous system problem that is characterized by spasms of the muscles typically in the extremities

Thyromegaly: Enlargement of the thyroid gland

Vasopressors: Medication given to increase peripheral vascular resistance in an attempt to elevate the blood pressure

VC: Vital capacity

Ventilatory Failure: Inadequate ventilation that causes an increase in the arterial P$_{CO_2}$

Virulent: Very poisonous

Wheeze: High-pitched, continuous type of adventitious lung sound resulting from narrowing of the intrathoracic airways

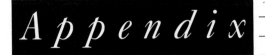

Appendix

Hoai N. Tran

NORMAL LABORATORY VALUES

ADULT

Arterial Blood Gases (ABGs)

pH	7.35–7.45
$Paco_2$	35–45 mm Hg
Pao_2	80–100 mm Hg
HCO_3^-	22–26 mEq/liter
Base excess (BE)	−2 to +2
Arterial saturation with oxygen (Sao_2)	>95 percent

Complete Blood Count (CBC)

Red blood cell (RBC) count	
Men	4.6–6.2 million/mm³
Women	4.2–5.4 million/mm³
Hemoglobin (Hb)	
Men	13.5–16.5 g/dL
Women	12.0–15.0 g/dL
Hematocrit (Hct)	
Men	40–54%
Women	38–47%
Erythrocyte index	
Mean cell volume (MCV)	80–96 μ^3
Mean cell hemoglobin (MCH)	27–31 pg
Mean cell hemoglobin concentration (MCHC)	32–36%
White blood cell (WBC) count	4,500–10,000/mm³
Differential of WBCs	
Neutrophils	40–75%
Bands	0–6%
Eosinophils	0–6%
Basophils	0–1%
Lymphocytes	20–45%
Monocytes	2–10%
Platelet count	150,000–400,000/mm³

Chemistry

Na^+	137–147 mEq/liter
K^+	3.5–4.8 mEq/liter
Cl^-	98–105 mEq/liter
CO_2	25–33 mEq/liter
Blood urea nitrogen (BUN)	7–20 mg/dL
Creatine	0.7–1.3 mg/dL
Total protein	6.3–7.9 g/dL
Albumin	3.5–5.0 g/dL
Cholesterol	150–220 mg/dL
Glucose	70–105 mg/dL

Hemodynamic Values

Variable	Abbreviation	Normal
Cardiac output	$\dot{Q}T$	4–8 liters/minute
Cardiac index	CI	2.5–4.0 liters/minute/m²
Stroke volume	SV	60–130 mL
Ejection fraction	EF	65–75%
Central venous pressure	CVP	0–6 mm Hg
Pulmonary artery pressure	PAP	25/10 mm Hg
Pulmonary capillary wedge pressure	PCWP	6–12 mm Hg
Systemic vascular resistance	SVR	900–1400 dynes/second/cm⁵
Pulmonary vascular resistance	PVR	110–250 dynes/second/cm⁵

Pulmonary Function Tests

Variable	Abbreviation	Normal
Forced vital capacity	FVC	>80% of predicted
Slow vital capacity	SVC	80–120% of predicted
Forced expiratory volume in 1 second	FEV_1	>80% of predicted
Forced expiratory volume in 1 second/Forced vital capacity	FEV_1/FVC	>75%
Forced expiratory flow	$FEF_{25-75\%}$	>80% of predicted
Carbon monoxide diffusing capacity	D_{LCO}	25 mL CO/minute/mm Hg
Total lung capacity	TLC	6000 mL
Functional residual capacity	FRC	2400 mL
Residual volume	RV	1200 mL
Vital capacity	VC	4800 mL

Vital Signs

	Normal Range
Temperature range	36.1–37.5°C
Heart rate	60–100/minute
Respiratory rate	12–20/minute
Blood pressure range	120/80 mm Hg
	Systolic 95–140 mm Hg
	Diastolic 60–90 mm Hg

CHILDREN (AGE 1 to 12 YEARS)

ABGs

Refer to adult values

CBC Tests

RBC count	3.8–5.5 million/mm^3
Hb	11–16 g/dL
Hct	31–43%
Erythrocyte index (refer to adult values)	
WBC count (refer to adult values)	
Differential of WBCs (refer to adult values)	

Chemistry

Na$^+$	135–145 mEq/liter
K$^+$	3.5–5.0 mEq/liter
Cl$^-$	100–106 mEq/liter
Ca^{++}	9.2–10.8 mg/dL
Mg^{++}	1.5–2.0 mEq/liter
Glucose	60–105 mg/dL

Hemodynamic Values

CI	3.5–4.5 liter/minute/m^2
CVP	2–6 mm Hg
PAP	30/8 mm Hg
PCWP	4–8 mm Hg

NEWBORN

ABG

pH	7.25–7.35
$Paco_2$	26–40 mm Hg
Pao_2	50–70 mm Hg
HCO_3^-	17–23 mEq/liter
BE	−10 to −2

CBC Count

RBC count	4.8–7.1 million/mm³
Hb	14–24 g/dL
Hct	44–64%
Erythrocyte index	
MCV	96–108 μ^3
MCH	32–34 pg
MCHC	32–33%
WBC count	
Mean value	18,100/mm³
Range	9,000–30,000/mm³
Lymphocytes	
Mean value	5,500/mm³
Range	2,000–11,000/mm³

Chemistry

Na^+	133–149 mEq/liter
K^+	5.3–6.4 mEq/liter
Cl^-	87–114 mEq/liter
CO_2	19–22 mEq/liter
Total protein	4.8–8.5 g/dL
Albumin	2.9–5.5 g/dL
Glucose	30–110 mg/dL

Hemodynamic Values

Cardiac output	
Newborn	0.8–1.0 liter/minute
6 months old	1.0–1.3 liters/minute
1 year old	1.3–1.5 liters/minute
CI	2.5–4.5 liters/minute/m²
SV	
Newborn	5 mL
6 months old	10 mL
1 year old	13 mL

Vital Signs

Temperature range	36.1–37.5°C
Heart rate	100–160 minute
Respiratory rate	30–60/minute
Blood pressure	75/50 mm Hg

Index

Note: Page numbers followed by f indicate illustrations; those followed by t indicate tables.

A₂, defined, 393

A$_2$, defined, 393
Abdominal paradox, defined, 6, 6f, 393
Acidosis
  lactic, defined, 397
  respiratory, in ARDS, 175
Acquired immunodeficiency syndrome (AIDS),
    pneumonia in, 270
Acrocyanosis, defined, 393
Adenocarcinoma, of the lung, 286–287
Adult respiratory distress syndrome (ARDS),
    173–187
  case study, 179–187, 180f, 183f
  causes, 173–174, 174t
  clinical features, 173, 175
  disorders associated with, 174t
  ECMO in, 177
  exudative phase of, 174
  fibrotic phase of, 174
  mechanical ventilation in, 176–177
    weaning from, 177–178
  monitoring in, 178–179
  multiple organ failure in, 173, 173t
  in near-drowning patients, 154
  pathology of, 174
  pathophysiology, 174–175
  PCWP in, 175
  PEEP in, 176–177
  proliferative phase of, 174
  radiography in, 175, 180f, 183f
  respiratory acidosis in, 175
  synonyms for, 173t
  treatment, 176–179
Afterload, 78, 81
  defined, 393
AIDS. See Acquired immunodeficiency
    syndrome
Airway
  in asthmatics, 16f
  injuries of, pathophysiology, 196–197
  normal, 16f
Airway obstruction
  atelectasis due to, 218
  in COPD, 30f
  following chest trauma, management, 200–
    201
Allergens, asthma due to, 15
Alpha$_1$PI, deficiency of, emphysema due to, 45
Amiodarone, interstitial lung disease due to,
    231
Amniotic fluid, defined, 393
Amyotrophic lateral sclerosis
  case study, 262–267, 266f
  clinical features, 255
  nerve interruption in, 254
  treatment, 257

Anabolic metabolism, defined, 393
Anaerobic, defined, 393
Anemia, defined, 393
Angina, defined, 393
Angiography
  defined, 393
  pulmonary, in pulmonary thromboembolism,
    97
Anion gap, defined, 393
Antibiotics
  in bacterial pneumonia, 275
  in emphysema, 49
  in epiglottitis, 328
  in shock, 85
Anticoagulants, in pulmonary
    thromboembolism, 97
Aorta, rupture of, chest trauma and, 198
Apgar score, defined, 393
Apnea
  defined, 393
  mixed, described, 309
  in respiratory syncytial virus, 341
  sleep. See Sleep apnea
Apnea index, 309
ARDS. See Adult respiratory distress syndrome
Arrhythmia, defined, 393
Asbestos worker, lung cancer in, 286t
Asbestosis, defined, 393
Ascites, 113
  defined, 393
Asphyxia, defined, 393
Aspiration
  defined, 393
  in drowning victims, 151
  in near-drowning patients, 152, 154
Asthma, 15–26
  airway in, 16f
  arterial blood gases in, 18
  bronchial provocation testing in, 18
  bronchospasm in, 15, 16, 16f
  case study, 20–26, 23f
  causes, 15
  chest radiography in, 17
  classification, 15
  clinical features, 16–18, 17f
  decision making in, 19t
  defined, 393
  described, 15
  dyspnea in, 16
  extrinsic, 15
  intrinsic, 15
  laboratory evaluation in, 17
  mechanical ventilation in, 19
  occupational, 15
  pathophysiology, 16, 16f

Asthma—*Continued*
  patient history in, 16
  physical examination in, 16–17, 17f
  schema of, 30f
  stable, 15
  stridor in, 17f
  treatment, 18–19, 19t
  unstable, 15
  wheezing in, 16, 17f
Atelectasis
  case study, 221–227, 224f, 226f
  causes, 217–218, 218t
  defined, 393
  described, 217
  postoperative, 217–227
    airway obstruction and, 218
    arterial blood gas analysis in, 219–220
    auscultation of breath sounds in, 219
    clinical features, 219–220
    CPAP in, 220
    inadequate lung distention and, 217–218
    IPPB in, 220
    mechanical ventilation in, 221
    pathophysiology, 219
    PEEP in, 220
    radiography in, 219, 224f, 226f
    risk factors for, 217
    secretion removal in, 221
    tachypnea in, 219
    treatment, 220–221
  surfactant depletion and, 218
Atopy, defined, 393
Atrophy, defined, 394
Auscultation of breath sounds, in atelectasis, 219

Bands, defined, 394
Beta-adrenergics, in asthma, 18
Bleeding, intrabronchial, pathophysiology, 196
Blood, function of, 77
Blood chemistry, normal values
  in adults, 402
  in children, 403
  in newborns, 404
Blood gas analysis, arterial
  in asthma, 18
  in atelectasis, 219–220
  in bacterial pneumonia, 272
  in chronic bronchitis, 32
  in cystic fibrosis, 62
  in emphysema, 47
  in heart failure, 114
  in infants with respiratory distress syndrome, 355
  normal values
    in adults, 401
    in children, 403
    in newborns, 404
  in persistent pulmonary hypertension of the newborn, 381
  in pulmonary thromboembolism, 96–97
  in respiratory syncytial virus, 341
Blood vessels, function of, 77
Breath, shortness of
  in emphysema, 46
  in lung cancer, 287t, 288

Breath sounds
  auscultation of, in atelectasis, 219
  in respiratory syncytial virus, 341
Breathing
  normal movement of diaphragm and abdominal contents with, 6f
  sleep and, 310–312, 310f-312f
Bronchial provocation testing, in asthma, 18
Bronchiolitis, defined, 394
Bronchitis
  chronic, 29–42
    arterial blood gases in, 32
    case study, 33–42, 36f, 38f, 41f
    causes, 29
    chest radiography in, 32
    cigarette smoking and, 29
    clinical features, 31–32
    complete blood count in, 32
    cough in, 31
    described, 29
    dyspnea in, 31
    hemoptysis in, 31
    laboratory evaluation in, 32
    mucus character in, 30, 31
    oxygen therapy in, 33
    pathology of, 30–31
    pathophysiology, 30–31
    physical examination in, 31–32
    pulmonary function studies in, 32
    schema of, 30f
    sputum production in, 31
    treatment, 32–33
  defined, 394
  patient history in, 31
Bronchoalveolar lavage, in interstitial lung disease, 236–237
Bronchodilators
  in asthma, 18
  in bronchopulmonary dysplasia, 368
  in emphysema, 47
  in respiratory syncytial virus, 342
Bronchopneumonia, 273f
Bronchopulmonary dysplasia, 365–376
  age factors in, 365
  case study, 369–376, 373f
  causes, 365–366
  clinical features, 367
  described, 365
  incidence, 365
  outcome of, 369
  pathophysiology, 366–367
  stages of, 366
  treatment, 368–369
Bronchoscopy, flexible fiberoptic, in lung cancer, 292–293
Bronchospasm
  in asthma, 15, 16, 16f
  defined, 394
Bruit, defined, 394
Burns, 129–148
  case study, 139–148, 143f, 145f
  causes, 130–131, 131t
  clinical features, 135–137, 135t, 136t, 137f
  degrees of, 137
  infections associated with, 139
  mortality due to, 129, 130f
    cyanide and, 131–132

pathophysiology, 131–135, 132t, 133t
pulmonary and systemic changes following
  2–5 days, 131t, 133–134, 133t
  24 hours, 131–133, 132t, 133t
  beyond 5 days, 131t, 133t, 134–135
treatment, 137–139, 138t

Cachexia, defined, 394
Cancer, lung. *See* Lung cancer
Carbon monoxide, poisoning by, clinical
    manifestations, 135, 135t
Carboxyhemoglobin
  defined, 394
  half-life of, 138t
Carcinoma, bronchogenic. *See* Lung cancer
Cardiac index, defined, 78, 394
Cardiac output
  afterload in, 78, 81
  contractility in, 81–82
  defined, 78, 394
  determinants of, 78–82, 79f
  preload in, 78, 79f, 80f
Cardiomegaly, defined, 394
Cardiomyopathy, defined, 394
Carriers, of cystic fibrosis, 59
Catabolic metabolism, defined, 394
Catheter, pulmonary artery, illustration, 80f
Catheterization, pulmonary artery
  in ARDS, 178
  in heart failure, 115, 115t
Central sleep apnea, described, 309
Chemoreceptors, anatomy, 250
Chemotherapy, in lung cancer, 296
Chest
  blunt injuries to, 192t, 193
  flail, 194, 195f, 196
    defined, 395
  penetrating injuries of, 192–193, 192t
Chest pain, in lung cancer, 287t, 288
Chest trauma, 191–213
  airway obstruction following, management,
    200–201
  aortic rupture following, 198
  case study, 202–213, 207f, 210f, 212f
  clinical features, 199
  CPAP in, 201
  ECMO in, 201
  exsanguination following, 198
  injuries following
    causes, 192–193
    distribution of, 191, 192f
    mechanisms of, 192t
    pathophysiology, 193–199, 194f, 195f
    types, 193–199
  myocardial contusion following, 197–198
  PEEP in, 201
  SIMV in, 201
  treatment, 200–202, 200f
  ventilatory support following, 201
Chest wall
  diagram, 36f
  injuries of
    complications, 198–199
    pathophysiology, 193–196, 194f, 195f
Cheyne-Stokes breathing, defined, 394
Children, laboratory values in, 403

Chronic obstructive pulmonary disease
    (COPD)
  airway obstruction in, 30f
  schema of, 30f
Cigarette smoking
  chronic bronchitis due to, 29, 30
  emphysema due to, 45
  and lung cancer, 285–286, 286t
Circulation
  peripheral, in heart failure, 110–111
  pulmonary, 77
    in heart failure, 110–111
  systemic, 77
Circulatory system, described, 77
Clavicle, fractures of, pathophysiology, 193
Clubbing, defined, 394
Complete blood count
  in chronic bronchitis, 32
  normal values
    in adults, 402
    in children, 403
    in newborns, 404
Consolidation, defined, 394
Continuous positive airway pressure (CPAP)
  in atelectasis, 220
  in cardiogenic pulmonary edema, 117–118
  in chest trauma, 201
Continuous positive airway pressure (CPAP)
  system, continuous high-flow mask, 124f
Contractility, 78, 79f, 81–82
  defined, 394
Contusion
  defined, 394
  pulmonary, pathophysiology, 196
COPD. *See* Chronic obstructive pulmonary
    disease
Cor pulmonale, 31
  causes, 107–108
  defined, 4, 394
  described, 107
Corticosteroids
  in asthma, 19
  in croup, 327
Coryza, defined, 394
Cough
  in chronic bronchitis, 31
  in lung cancer, 287t, 288
Coumadin, in pulmonary thromboembolism,
    97–98
CPAP. *See* Continuous positive airway pressure
Crackles
  defined, 394
  in heart failure, 113
Crepitus, defined, 394
Croup, 325–327
  case study, 333–337, 335f
  causes, 325
  clinical features, 326
  epiglottitis and, comparison between, 326t
  pathology of, 325–326
  pathophysiology, 325–326
  treatment, 326–327
Cyanide
  in burn victims, 131–132
  poisoning by, clinical manifestations, 135,
    136t
Cyanosis, defined, 395

Cystic fibrosis, 59–74
  arterial blood gases in, 62
  bronchial hyperactivity in, treatment, 67
  carriers of, 59
  case study, 67–74, 71f
  causes, 59–60
  chest radiography in, 62, 63f-65f
  clinical features, 61–63, 63f-65f
  defect reversal in, 65–66
  described, 59
  gene responsible for, 59–60
  genetic abnormalities in, 63
  history of, 59
  incidence, 59
  laboratory evaluation in, 62–63, 63f-65f
  lung disease in, 60–61
  malnutrition in, 67
  organ systems involved in, 60t
  pancreatic enzyme replacement in, 67
  pancreatic insufficiency in, treatment, 67
  pancreatic involvement in, 61
  pathology of, 60–61
  pathophysiology, 60–61
  patient history in, 61
  physical examination in, 61–62
  problems associated with, 59
  prognosis, 67
  pulmonary function studies in, 62
  respiratory infections in, treatment, 66
  respiratory secretions in, treatment, 66
  sterility in, 61
  sweat electrolyte measurement in, 62
  treatment, 65–67

Defibrillation, defined, 395
Dexamethasone, in croup, 327
Diaphoresis, defined, 395
Diaphragm
  injuries of, pathophysiology, 198
  movements of, breathing and, 6f
Diplpia, defined, 395
Diuresis, defined, 395
Diuretics
  in bronchopulmonary dysplasia, 368
  in emphysema, 49
  in heart failure, 116
Drowning
  aspiration in, 151
  defined, 151
  near. *See* Near drowning
  secondary, 151
Drugs
  inotropic, in heart failure, 116
  interstitial lung disease due to, 230–231, 231t
Ductus arteriosus, defined, 379, 395
Dysphonia, defined, 395
Dyspnea
  in asthma, 16
  in chronic bronchitis, 31
  defined, 395
  in emphysema, 46
  in heart failure, 113
  nocturnal, 113
    defined, 397
Dysuria, defined, 395

ECG. *See* Electrocardiography
ECMO. *See* Extracorporeal membrane oxygenation
Edema
  cardiogenic pulmonary
    CPAP in, 117
    intubation in, 118
    oxygen therapy in, 117
    PEEP in, 118
    respiratory care for, 117–118
    ventilatory support in, 118
  causes, 111–112
  defined, 111
  in heart failure, 111–114
  pedal, defined, 398
  pulmonary. *See* Pulmonary edema
Ejection fraction, defined, 395
Electrocardiography (ECG)
  in emphysema, 47
  in shock, 84f, 85
Electrolytes, serum, evaluation, in shock, 83
Emphysema, 45–57
  age and gender in, 45
  α_1PI deficiency and, 45
  antibiotics in, 49
  arterial blood gases in, 47
  bronchodilators in, 47
  case study, 49–57, 53f, 54f
  causes, 45–46
  centrilobular, 45
  chest radiography in, 47, 48f
  cigarette smoking and, 45
  classification, 45
  clinical features, 46–47
  continuous mechanical ventilation in, 49
  defined, 45
  described, 45
  diuretics in, 49
  ECG in, 47
  laboratory evaluation in, 47, 48f
  methylxanthines in, 47, 49
  oxygen therapy in, 47
  panlobular, 45
  pathophysiology, 46
  patient history in, 46
  physical examination in, 46–47
  pollutants and, 46
  Prolastin in, 49
  pulmonary function studies in, 47
  schema of, 30f
  steroids in, 49
Empyema, defined, 395
End-diastolic volume, defined, 395
Endogenous, defined, 395
Enuresis, defined, 395
Epiglottitis, 327–329, 327f
  case study, 329–333, 332f
  causes, 329
  clinical features, 328
  croup and, comparison between, 326t
  pathology of, 327–328
  pathophysiology, 327–328
  treatment, 328–329
Epinephrine, racemic, in croup, 326–327
Erythema, defined, 395
Escharotomy, defined, 395
Exercise, in respiratory failure, 1

Exhalation, end, diaphragm position in, 4f
Exsanguination, chest trauma and, 198
Extracorporeal membrane oxygenation
(ECMO)
in ARDS, 177
in chest trauma, 201
in persistent pulmonary hypertension of the
newborn, 383
Extubation, in epiglottitis, 328–329
Exudates, defined, 395

Fasciculations, defined, 395
Fetus, defined, 395
Fever, in respiratory failure, 1
Fibrosis, defined, 395
Fires, injuries related to, incidence, 129
Fistula
bronchopleural, pathophysiology, 196
defined, 395
Flail chest, 194, 195f, 196
defined, 395
Flash over, defined, 130
Fluid-electrolyte balance, in heart failure, 111
Foramen ovale, defined, 379, 380f, 395
Fracture(s)
clavicular, pathophysiology, 193
rib, pathophysiology, 193–194, 194f, 195f
sternal, pathophysiology, 194
Frank-Starling response, in heart failure, 109–
110, 110f

Gallium scans, in interstitial lung disease, 234–
235
Gallop, defined, 396
Gas(es), toxic, in house fire smoke, 130, 131t
Glasgow coma scale, 156t
Glycolysis, 152, 153f
Gravida, defined, 396
Great vessels, injuries of, pathophysiology,
197–198
Guillain-Barré syndrome
clinical features, 255
nerve interruption in, 254
treatment, 256

Heart
function of, 77
injuries of, pathophysiology, 197–198
Heart failure, 107–126
arterial blood gas analysis in, 114
case study, 118–126, 121f, 126f
causes, 107–108, 107t
clinical features, 113–115, 115t
congestive, described, 107
crackles in, 113
described, 107
diuretics in, 116
dyspnea in, 113
edema in, 111–114
exercise capacity in, 115
fluid-electrolyte balance in, 111
Frank-Starling response in, 109–110, 110f
hypertension in, 110–111
hypertrophy in, 110

inotropic drugs in, 116
laboratory studies in, 114
liver failure in, 113–114
myocardial performance in, 109–111, 110f
pathophysiology, 109–112, 110f, 112t
peripheral and pulmonary circulation in,
110–111
prevalence, 107
pulmonary artery catheterization in, 115,
115t
pulmonary dysfunction during, 112, 112t
sinus tachycardia in, 114–115
sympathetic nervous response in, 109
tachycardia in, 113
treatment, 115–118, 117f
ventricular hypertrophic response in, 110
wheezes in, 113
Heart rate, regulation of, 109
Heave, defined, 396
Heimlich maneuver, in near-drowning patients,
157
Hemodynamic monitoring, in ARDS, 178
Hemodynamic values, normal
in adults, 402
in children, 403
in newborns, 404
Hemolysis, defined, 396
Hemoptysis
in chronic bronchitis, 31
defined, 396
in lung cancer, 287t, 288
Heparin, in pulmonary thromboembolism, 97
Hepatomegaly, 113
defined, 396
Heroin, interstitial lung disease due to, 231
Hexaxial reference system, 41f
Hilum, defined, 396
"Honeycomb lung," 237f
Hypercapnia, defined, 396
Hypercoagulability, in pulmonary
thromboembolism, 93
Hyperexcitability, in near-drowning patients,
159
Hyperhydration, in near-drowning patients,
158–159
Hyperkalemia, defined, 396
Hypernatremia, defined, 396
Hyperpnea, defined, 396
Hyperpyrexia, in near-drowning patients, 159
Hyperrigidity, in near-drowning patients, 159
Hypersomnolence, defined, 396
Hypertension
defined, 396
in heart failure, 110–111
pulmonary, persistent, of the newborn, 379–
390
Hypertrophy
defined, 396
in heart failure, 110
Hyperventilation, in near-drowning patients,
159
Hyperventilation-submersion syndrome,
defined, 151
Hypoglycemia, defined, 396
Hypokalemia, defined, 396
Hyponatremia, defined, 396
Hypoplasia, defined, 396

Hypopnea
    defined, 396
    described, 309
Hypotension, defined, 396
Hypoxemia
    causes, 2
    classification, 2
    clinical features, 5
    consequences of, 2
    defined, 2, 396
    pathophysiology, 4–5
    refractory, defined, 399
    treatment, 6–7,7t
Hypoxia, described, 152

Idiopathic, defined, 396
Ileus, defined, 396
Immersion syndrome, defined, 151
Infarction, defined, 396
Infection, respiratory, in cystic fibrosis, 66
Inflammation, pulmonary, in interstitial lung
        disease, 232
Inhalation, end, diaphragm position in, 4f
Injury. *See specific type or site*
Inotrope(s), defined, 397
Insomnia, defined, 397
Intermittent positive-pressure breathing (IPPB),
        in atelectasis, 220
Interstitial lung disease, 229–247
    amiodarone and, 231
    asbestos-related calcified pleural plaques in,
        236f
    bronchoalveolar lavage in, 236–237
    case study, 238–247, 242f
    causes, 229–232, 230t, 231t
    chain of events in, 229, 230f
    classification, 230t
    clinical features, 232–237, 234f-237f
    conditions predisposing to, 229
    described, 229
    diffuse reticular nodular pattern in, 234f,
        235f
    drugs and, 230–231, 231t
    gallium scanning in, 234–235
    heroin and, 231
    history, 229
    laboratory data in, 233–237, 234f-237f
    lung biopsy in, 235–236
    lung injury and, 232
    medical history in, 232–233
    narcotics and, 231
    nitrofurantoin and, 231
    oxygen therapy and, 231
    pathology of, 232
    pathophysiology, 232
    physical examination in, 233
    prognosis, 238
    pulmonary inflammation in, 232
    talc and, 231
    treatment, 237–238
Intubation
    in cardiogenic pulmonary edema, 118
    in epiglottitis, 328
IPPB. *See* Intermittent positive-pressure
        breathing
Ischemia, defined, 397

Kidney(s), function of, in near-drowning
        patients, 154
Kyphosis, defined, 397

Laboratory values, normal, in adults, 401–402
Larynx, cross-sectional view, 327f
Left ventricle, ventricular function curves for,
        78, 79f
Leukocyte, defined, 397
Leukocytopenia, defined, 397
Leukocytosis, defined, 397
Leukopenia, defined, 397
Liver failure, in heart failure, 113–114
Lung
    function of, 1
    "honeycomb, 237f
    infections of, in cystic fibrosis, 66
    inflammation of, in interstitial lung disease,
        232
    injury to, interstitial lung disease due to, 232
Lung cancer, 285–306
    adenocarcinoma, 286–287
    in asbestos worker, 286t
    case study, 297–306, 300f-304f, 306f
    causes, 285–286, 286t
    chemotherapy in, 296
    chest pain in, 287t, 288
    cigarette smoking and, 285–286, 286t
    clinical features, 287–288, 287t
    cough in, 287t, 288
    diagnosis, 289–293, 291f, 292f
    distant metastasis in, 294t
    dysfunction associated with, 287
    hemoptysis in, 287t, 288
    incidence, 285
    laboratory studies in, 290–291
    large-cell carcinomas, 287
    metastastic disease, signs, 288–289
    mortality due to, 285
    nodal involvement in, 294t
    pathology of, 286–287
    physical examination in, 288
    preoperative evaluation, 296–297
    primary tumor characteristics in, 294t
    prognosis, 295–297
    radiation therapy in, 296
    radiography in, 290–291, 291f, 292f, 300f-
        304f, 306f
    shortness of breath in, 287t, 288
    small-cell carcinomas, 287
    squamous cell carcinoma, 286
    staging of, 293–295, 294t, 295t
    surgery in, 295–296
    survival rate for, 289
    TNM classification, 293–295, 294t, 295t
    treatment, 295–297
    types, 286–287
Lung diseases
    in cystic fibrosis, 60–61
    obstructive
        airway obstruction in, 30f
        schema of, 30f
Lung distention, inadequate, atelectasis due to,
        217–218
Lung parenchyma, injuries of, pathophysiology,
        196

Lymphadenopathy, defined, 397
Lymphocytosis, defined, 397

Macrognathia, defined, 397
Malnutrition, in cystic fibrosis, 67
Meconium, defined, 397
Mediastinoscopy, in lung cancer, 293
Metabolism, phases of, 152, 153f
Metaplasia, defined, 397
Methylxanthines, in emphysema, 47, 49
Microemboli, defined, 397
Micrognathia, defined, 397
Mixed apnea, described, 309
Morbidity, defined, 397
Mortality, defined, 397
Motor vehicle accidents, injuries from, 191t
Mucus, in chronic bronchitis, 30, 31
Multiple organ failure, in ARDS, 173, 173t
Multiple sleep latency test (MSLT), 310
Murmur, defined, 397
Muscle(s), respiratory, 250, 252f
    innervation of, 253–254, 253t
Myasthenia gravis
    clinical features, 255
    treatment, 256–257
Myocardial contusion, chest trauma and, 197–198
Myocardial fibers, in heart failure, 109
Myocardial performance, in heart failure, 109–111, 110f
Myocardium, defined, 397

Narcolepsy, defined, 397
Narcotics, interstitial lung disease due to, 231
Nasal flaring, defined, 397
Near drowning, 151–170
    ARDS in, 154
    aspiration in, 152, 154
    assessment, 155, 156t, 157
    case studies, 159–170, 162f, 165f, 168f, 169f
    category A (awake), treatment, 157–158
    category B (blunted), treatment, 158
    category C (comatose), treatment, 158–159
    clinical features, 154–155
    defined, 151
    hemodynamic and electrolyte effects in, 154
    hyperexcitability in, 159
    hyperhydration in, 158–159
    hyperpyrexia in, 159
    hyperrigidity in, 159
    hyperventilation in, 159
    incidence, 151
    neurologic insult in, 152, 153f
    pathology of, 152–154, 153f
    pathophysiology, 152–154, 153f
    prognosis, 155, 156t, 157
    pulmonary insult in, 152, 154
    renal function in, 154
    treatment, 157–159
Necrotizing, defined, 397
Neoplasm, defined, 397
Nerve(s). *See also specific types*
    in respiration
        anatomy, 250, 251f
    interruption of, pathophysiology, 253–254, 253t
Neurologic insult, in near-drowning patients, 152, 153f
Neuromuscular disorders, 249–267
    case studies, 257–267, 266f
    clinical features, 254–256
    pathology of, 252–254, 253t
    pathophysiology, 252–254, 253t
    treatment, 256–257
Neuromuscular junction
    anatomy, 250
    pathophysiology, 254
Newborns
    bronchopulmonary dysplasia in, 365–376.
        See also Bronchopulmonary dysplasia
    laboratory values in, 404
    persistent pulmonary hypertension of, 379–390
    respiratory distress syndrome in, 353–362.
        See also under Respiratory distress syndrome
Nitrofurantoin, interstitial lung disease due to, 231
Normocephalic, defined, 397
Nosocomial, defined, 397

Obstructive sleep apnea. *See* Sleep apnea, obstructive
Obtunded, defined, 398
Organ failure, multiple, in ARDS, 173, 173t
Organomegaly, defined, 398
Orlowski score, 156t
Orthopnea, 113
    defined, 398
Oxidative phosphorylation, 152, 153f
Oxygen therapy
    in bacterial pneumonia, 274
    in cardiogenic pulmonary edema, 117
    in chronic bronchitis, 33
    in emphysema, 47
    interstitial lung disease due to, 231
Oxygenation failure
    causes, 2, 2f
    clinical features, 5
    defined, 1
    pathophysiology, 4–5
    treatment, 6–7, 7t
Oxyhemoglobin, defined, 398

Pain, chest, in lung cancer, 287t, 288
Pancreas, involvement of, in cystic fibrosis, 61
Pancreatic enzyme replacement, in cystic fibrosis, 67
Para, defined, 398
Parenchyma, defined, 398
Paresthesia, defined, 398
Patent ductus arteriosus, bronchopulmonary dysplasia due to, 366
PCWP. *See* Pulmonary capillary wedge pressure
PEEP. *See* Positive end-expiratory pressure
Perfusion
    defined, 398
    described, 77
    ventilation to, normal matching of, 2f

Pericarditis, defined, 398
Perihilar, defined, 398
Peristalsis, defined, 398
Peritoneal, defined, 398
Persistent pulmonary hypertension of the
    newborn, 379–390
  case study, 383–390, 387f
  causes, 379, 380f
  clinical features, 381
  diagnosis, 381–383, 382f
  ECMO in, 383
  elevated pulmonary vascular resistance in,
    379
  pathophysiology, 380–381
  treatment, 383
Pharyngitis, defined, 398
Phosphorylation, oxidative, 152, 153f
Phrenic nerve, injury to, 253
Plasmapheresis, defined, 398
Platypnea, defined, 399
Pneumoconiosis, defined, 399
Pneumomediastinum, radiography of, 168f
Pneumonia
  in AIDS, 270
  bacterial, 269–282
    causes, 269–270, 270t
    clinical features, 271–274, 272f-274f
    laboratory data in, 271–274, 272f-274f
    pathology of, 270–271
    pathophysiology, 270–271
    patient history in, 271
    physical examination in, 271
    radiography in, 271–274, 272f-274f, 278f
    treatment, 274–275
  case study, 275–282, 278f
  defined, 269
  incidence, 269
  lobar, 272f
  necrotizing, 270
  nosocomial, 269
  viral, 274f
Pneumothorax, defined, 399
Poisoning
  carbon monoxide, clinical manifestations,
    135, 135t
  cyanide, clinical manifestations, 135, 136t
Pollutants, emphysema due to, 46
Polycythemia, defined, 399
Polyphonic, defined, 399
Polys, nasal, in cystic fibrosis, 61
Polysomnography
  defined, 310
  in sleep apnea, 314–315, 320f, 321f
Positive end-expiratory pressure (PEEP)
  in ARDS, 176–177
  in atelectasis, 220
  auto, defined, 394
  in burn victims, 138
  in cardiogenic pulmonary edema, 118
  in chest trauma, 201
Positive pressure, in hypoxemia, 7
Postimmersion syndrome, defined, 151
Postsubmersion neurologic classification
  system, 156t
Precordium, defined, 399
Prednisone, in croup, 327

Preload, 78, 79f, 80f
  defined, 399
Prolastin, in emphysema, 49
Protriptyline, in sleep apnea, 315
Ptosis, defined, 399
Pulmonary artery catheter, illustration, 80f
Pulmonary capillary wedge pressure (PCWP),
  in ARDS, 175
Pulmonary dysfunction, during heart failure,
  112, 112t
Pulmonary edema
  interstitial, noncardiogenic, radiography of,
    162f
  noncardiogenic, radiography of, 165f
Pulmonary function studies
  in chronic bronchitis, 32
  in cystic fibrosis, 62
  in emphysema, 47
  in infants with respiratory distress syndrome,
    355
  normal values, in adults, 402
Pulmonary injury, in near-drowning patients,
  152, 154
Pulmonary thromboembolic disease, 93–105.
  See also Thromboembolism, pulmonary
Pulmonary vascular resistance, 81, 81t
  elevation of, in persistent pulmonary
    hypertension of the newborn, 379
Pulse, paradoxic, defined, 398
Pulse oximetry, in bronchopulmonary dysplasia,
  369
Pulse pressure, defined, 399
Pulsus alternans, 113
  defined, 399
Pulsus paradoxus, defined, 399
Purulent, defined, 399
Pyrogenic, defined, 399

Radiation therapy, in lung cancer, 296
Radiolucency, defined, 399
Radiopaque, defined, 399
Rales, defined, 399
Respiration
  muscles of, 250, 252f
    innervation of, 253–254, 253t
  paradoxic, defined, 398
Respiratory alternans, defined, 6, 399
Respiratory centers
  anatomy, 249
  pathophysiology, 252–253, 253t
Respiratory distress syndrome
  case study, 356–362, 359f
  in newborns, 353–362
    causes, 353–354, 354f
    clinical features, 353, 355
    cycle produced by, 354f
    maternal history in, 355
    pathophysiology, 354, 354f
    surfactant deficiency and, 353, 354f
    treatment, 355–356
Respiratory failure, 1–13
  case study, 9–13, 12f
  causes, 2–4, 2f, 3t
  clinical features, 5–6, 6f
  defined, 1, 399

exercise and, 1
fever and, 1
pathophysiology, 4–5
treatment, 6–9, 7t, 8t
Respiratory infections, in cystic fibrosis, 66
Respiratory pump
anatomy, 249–250
components of, 249
neural pathways for, 250, 251f
Respiratory syncytial virus, 339–350
arterial blood gas analysis in, 341
case study, 344–350, 347f
causes, 339
clinical features, 340–342
described, 339
diagnosis, 341–342
duration of, 339
history of present illness, 340
laboratory data in, 341
nosocomial, prevention, 343–344
pathology of, 340
pathophysiology, 340
physical examination in, 341
radiography in, 341, 347f
risk factors for, 340t
seasonality of, 339
treatment, 342–344, 343f
Respiratory system, protective mechanisms of, 269t
Retinopathy, defined, 399
Retractions, defined, 399
Revised trauma score, 199t
Rhinorrhea, defined, 399
Rhonchus, defined, 399
Rib, fractures of, pathophysiology, 193–194, 194f, 195f
Ribavirin
administration of, SPAG-2 unit in, 343f
in respiratory syncytial virus, 342–343, 343f
toxic effects, 343

S_3 gallop, defined, 399
Scoliosis, defined, 400
Segs, defined, 400
Sensorium, defined, 400
Sepsis, defined, 400
Shock
anaphylactic, defined, 400
case study, 86–91
causes, 82
clinical features, 83–85, 83t, 84f
defined, 400
described, 77
ECG in, 84f, 85
hemodynamic monitoring and, 77–91
pathophysiology, 82–83
septic, 82
defined, 400
toxic, defined, 400
treatment, 85
types, 82
assessment, 83t
Shunt, defined, 2, 400
SIMV. *See* Synchronized intermittent mandatory ventilation

Sinus tachycardia, in heart failure, 114–115
Sinusitis, recurrent, in cystic fibrosis, 61
Skin, body surface covered by, 137f
Sleep
and breathing, 310–312, 310f-312f
delta, 310, 311f
nonrapid eye movement (NREM), described, 310
normal, types, 310
rapid eye movement (REM), described, 310
slow-wave, 310, 311f
stage I, 310, 310f
stage II, 310, 311f
Sleep apnea, 309–322
case study, 316–322, 320f, 321f
causes, 312–313
central, described, 309
clinical features, 313–315
defined, 309
laboratory data in, 314
obstructive
airway obstruction in, 312f
defined, 398
described, 309
snoring in, 314
pathophysiology, 313
patient history in, 313–314
physical examination in, 314
polysomnography in, 314–315, 320f, 321f
treatment, 315
types, 309
Sleep latency, 310
Smoke inhalation injury, 129–148
case study, 139–148, 143f, 145f
causes, 130–131, 131t
clinical features, 135–137, 135t, 136t, 137f
incidence, 129
infections associated with, 139
mortality due to, 129, 130f
pathophysiology, 131–135, 132t, 133t
pulmonary and systemic changes following
2–5 days, 131t, 133–134, 133t
24 hours, 131–133
beyond 5 days, 131t, 133t, 134–135
treatment, 137–139, 138t
Smoking, cigarette. *See* Cigarette smoking
Snoring, in obstructive sleep apnea, 314
Spinal cord injury
clinical features, 255–256
treatment, 257
Sputum
in chronic bronchitis, 31
evaluation, in bacterial pneumonia, 272–273
Sputum cytology, in lung cancer, 291–292
Squamous cell carcinoma, of the lung, 286
Squamous metaplasia, 61
Static compliance, in ARDS, 178
Status asthmaticus, defined, 15, 400
Stenosis, defined, 400
Sterility, in cystic fibrosis, 61
Steroids
in bronchopulmonary dysplasia, 368
in emphysema, 49
Stridor
in asthma, 17f

Stridor—*Continued*
in croup, 326
defined, 400
Stroke volume, defined, 78, 400
Surfactant(s)
deficiency of, in infants with respiratory
distress syndrome, 353, 354f
defined, 400
depletion of, atelectasis due to, 218
in infants with respiratory distress syndrome,
356
Sweat electrolyte concentration, in cystic
fibrosis, 62
Sympathetic nervous response, in heart failure,
109
Synchronized intermittent mandatory
ventilation (SIMV), in chest trauma, 201
Syncytium, defined, 339
Systemic vascular resistance, 81

Tachycardia
defined, 400
in heart failure, 113
sinus, in heart failure, 114–115
Tachyphylaxis, defined, 400
Tachypnea
in atelectasis, 219
defined, 400
Talc, interstitial lung disease due to, 231
Tamponade
defined, 400
pericardial, defined, 398
Tensilon test, in myasthenia gravis, 255
Tetany, defined, 400
Theophylline, in bronchopulmonary dysplasia,
368
Thoracoscopy, in lung cancer, 293
Thoracotomy, in lung cancer, 293
Thromboembolism, pulmonary, 93–105
angiography in, 97
arterial blood gases in, 96–97
case study, 98–105, 99t, 102f-104f
causes, 93
chest radiography in, 96, 96f, 102f, 103f
clinical features, 94–97, 95t, 96f
differential diagnosis, 99t
hemodynamic and laboratory data in, 96–97,
96f
incidence, 93
pathology of, 93
pathophysiology, 93–94
patient history in, 94, 95t
physical examination in, 95–96, 95t
risk factors for, 93
symptoms, 95t
treatment, 97–98
Thrush, oral, defined, 398
Thyromegaly, defined, 400
Tolazoline, in persistent pulmonary
hypertension of the newborn, 383
Tracheostomy, in epiglottitis, 238

Tracheotomy, in bronchopulmonary dysplasia,
369
Transthoracic needle aspiration biopsy,
percutaneous, in lung cancer, 293
Trauma
deaths due to, 191
causes, 191, 191t
to lung, bronchopulmonary dysplasia due to,
365–366
Tricarboxylic acid (TCA) cycle, 152, 153f

Vasopressors
defined, 400
in shock, 85
Ventilation
mechanical
in ARDS, 176–177
weaning from, 177–178
in asthma, 19
in atelectasis, 221
in bronchopulmonary dysplasia, 368–369
bronchopulmonary dysplasia due to, 365–
366
continuous, in emphysema, 49
in infants with respiratory distress
syndrome, 356
initiation of, 7, 7t
in persistent pulmonary hypertension of
the newborn, 383
in shock, 85
mechanical weaning from, 8, 8t
positive-pressure, in ARDS, 178
Ventilation-perfusion, normal matching of, 2f
Ventilation-perfusion scans, in pulmonary
thromboembolism, 97, 104f
Ventilatory failure
causes, 3–4, 3t, 4f
clinical features, 5–6, 5f
defined, 1, 400
pathophysiology, 5
treatment, 7–9, 8t
Ventilatory support
in burn victims, 138
in cardiogenic pulmonary edema, 118
following chest trauma, 201
Ventricular hypertrophic response, in heart
failure, 110
Virument, defined, 400
Vital signs, normal values
in adults, 402
in newborns, 404
Vitamin(s)
A, in bronchopulmonary dysplasia, 369
E, in bronchopulmonary dysplasia, 369

Wheezes
in asthma, 16, 17f
defined, 400
in heart failure, 113